Mind &Body Health HANDBOOK

David S. Sobel, M.D.
Robert Ornstein, Ph.D.

DR$_X$
Los Altos, California

Editor, Design Director, cover design: Elizabeth Adler
Book design and production: Susan Cronin-Paris
Michael Linkinhoker

Formerly titled "The Healthy Mind, Healthy Body Handbook"

First printing: May 1996 9 8 7 6 5 4 3 2 1

Second Edition: February 1998

Printed in the United States of America

Library of Congress Cataloging-in-Publication Data
Sobel, David S. (David Stuart)
Mind & body health handbook : how to use your mind & body to relieve stress, overcome illness, and enjoy healthy pleasures / David S. Sobel & Robert Ornstein.—2nd ed.
p. cm.
Previous ed. cataloged under title: The healthy mind, healthy body handbook.
Includes bibliographical references and index.
ISBN 0-9651040-1-X (pbk.)
1. Clinical health psychology. 2. Mind and body. 3. Mind and body therapies. I. Ornstein, Robert E. (Robert Evan), 1942- .II. Sobel, David S. (David Stuart). Healthy mind, healthy body handbook. III. Title.
R726.7.S695 1998
613—dc21   98-4698
CIP

DR$_\mathbf{X}$

Box 176
Los Altos, CA 94023
Telephone/Fax: (650) 948-6293

Dedication

*To my son Matt, who teaches me as he learns,
and to the rest of my family, friends, colleagues
and patients, who remind me daily to practice
what I write.*

David

*For René and Jonas, the two mentors who opened
up many new ways to health.*

Bob

Acknowledgements

This book began at HarperCollins where our editor, Carol Cohen, patiently encouraged us. The final book was transformed by the skillful editing and art direction of Elizabeth Adler and design by Susan Cronin-Paris. Their tireless efforts and unflagging enthusiasm made the book much more accessible and attractive.

In addition, we are grateful for the research work and initial drafting provided by Denise Winn, Lynne Levitan, Janet Bailey, Anne Weinberger, Nancy Bruning and Norma Peterson. Mary Ann Cammarota's editorial work on our newsletter also contributed to the final form of many of the chapters. We also wish to thank Sarah Fries, Don Kemper, Michael diCanino and J. Keith Green for their comments, suggestions, and wise counsel on shaping the book as well as Greg Jacobs and Elke Zuercher-White for their review and comments. Shane DeHaven and Patti Schaffer provided much help in coordinating all the little things that need to be done to make a manuscript a book.

Finally, our special thanks to Sally Mallam, our publisher at DRx, who oversees all necessary details to make the book real.

We would also like to thank our colleagues, teachers and friends whose ideas infuse, inform, and inspire this book: Aaron Antonovsky, PhD; Henry L.Bennett, PhD; Herbert Benson, MD; Matthew Budd, MD; David Burns, MD; Margaret Caudill, MD, PhD; Margaret Chesney, PhD; Nicholas Cummings, PhD; Elizabeth Eshelman, MSW; Tom Ferguson, MD; Jerome Frank, MD, PhD; James Fries, MD; Halsted Holman, MD; Jon Kabat-Zinn, PhD; Laura Keranen, MPH; Suzanne Kobasa, PhD; Lowell S. Levin, EdD, MPH; Kate Lorig, RN, DrPH; Robert Most, PhD; Belleruth Naparstek, LCSW; Kenneth Pelletier, PhD; James Pennebaker, PhD; Martin Rossman, MD; Martin Seligman, PhD; David Spiegel, MD; S. Leonard Syme, PhD; Donald Vickery, MD; Redford Williams, MD; and many others.

To Our Readers

This book is not intended to replace common sense or professional medical or psychological help. We strongly encourage you to get appropriate professional evaluation and treatment for problems—especially unusual, unexplained, severe, or persistent symptoms. Many symptoms and diseases require and benefit from specific medical or psychological evaluation and treatment. Don't deny yourself proper professional care.

▶ If your symptoms or problems persist beyond a reasonable period despite using self-care recommendations, you should consult a health professional.

▶ If you receive professional advice in conflict with this book, look first to your health professional. He or she is likely to be able to take your specific history and needs into consideration.

▶ If you are having thoughts of harming yourself in any way, please seek professional care immediately.

This book is as accurate as its publishers and authors can make it, but we cannot guarantee that it will work for you in every case. The authors or publishers disclaim all liability and cannot be held responsible for any problems that may arise from its use. This book is only a guide; your common sense, good judgment, and partnership with health professionals are also needed.

We are continually revising and improving this book. If you have any suggestions or comments that will make the book better, please send it to: DRx, Box 176, Los Altos, CA, 94023. Thank you.

David Sobel, M.D.
and Robert Ornstein, Ph.D.

CONTENTS

HOW TO USE THIS BOOK

Introduction **6**
How to Activate the Most Powerful Healing System in the World—Your Brain

PART 1: STAYING WELL

Ten Essential Skills for Improving and Maintaining Your Health

1. The Power to Change **17**
How to Make and Maintain Healthy Changes

2. Healthy Thinking **35**
How Optimistic Thinking Improves Health and Happiness

3. Humor **49**
How to Use Humor and Laughter to Improve Your Health

4. Enjoy Your Senses **57**
How to Use the Pleasure of Your Senses for Better Health

5. Healthy Sex **71**
How to Enhance Sexual Enjoyment for Better Health

6. Relaxation **81**
How to Focus Your Mind and Relax Your Body

7. Imagery **97**
How to Use Your Imagination to Improve Your Health

8. Enjoy Physical Activity **109**
How to Feel Fit With or Without Exercise

9. Communicate Well **121**
How to Speak and Listen Better to Improve Your Health

10. Healthy Helping **133**
How Helping Others Improves Your Own Health

PART 2: MANAGING COMMON PROBLEMS

How to Use Your Mind to Manage Your Health

11. Anxiety **143**
How to Overcome Excessive Worry, Panic, and Phobias

12. Depression **155**
How to Lighten Depression and Bad Moods

13. Anger **167**
How to Manage Your Anger and Hostility

14. Time Pressure **179**
How to Manage Time and Deal with Procrastination

15. Sleep Better **191**
How to Ease Insomnia and Other Sleep Problems

16. Surviving Trauma **201**
How to Deal with Grief, Loss, and Traumatic Experiences

17. Addiction **209**
How to Control Addiction and Bad Habits

18. Chronic Pain **215**
How to Deal Effectively with Chronic Pain

19. Chronic Illness **225**
How to Live Well with Chronic Disease

PART 3: MANAGING MEDICAL CARE

Becoming an Active Partner in Your Own Health Care

20. Doctor-Patient Partnership **235**
How to Work Effectively with Health Professionals

21. Medical Tests **245**
How to Share in Decisions About Your Medical Tests

22. Medications **251**
Use Your Mind to Manage Your Medicines

23. Surgery **259**
How to Prepare for Surgery and Other Medical Adventures

Resources for More Information **271**

Index **281**

How to Use This Book

We have designed Mind & Body Health Handbook *carefully so that you can find exactly the information you are looking for—quickly and easily. Some chapters are designed to be read through completely, and others to be consulted only if you or a family member has a specific problem. But remember, the techniques described in the book work only if you practice and apply them to your life.*

ORGANIZATION

Mind & Body Health Handbook is organized into three major sections:

PART 1: STAYING WELL

Ten Essential Skills for Maintaining and Improving Your Health

The chapters in this section will give you practical advice and skills on how to prevent disease, recover from illness, and improve your well-being. These ten chapters are like a basic first-aid kit or "medicine chest." If you practice all ten skills, you'll improve your health.

You'll learn about the power of healthy thinking and optimism, humor, using your senses to improve your health, healthy sex, effective relaxation and imagery techniques, physical exercise, effective communication skills, and finally, how helping others can help you.

Chapter 1: *The Power to Change* is an up-to-date summary of steps for successful change. You'll learn how to change bad habits and adopt new healthy ones. You'll also learn problem-solving strategies to help you take full advantage of the advice offered in the rest of the book.

PART 2: MANAGING COMMON PROBLEMS

How to Use Your Mind to Manage Your Health

This section is a guide to helping you understand and manage common problems yourself. Many topics are covered, from pain to insomnia, anxiety to addiction, anger to depression, and time pressure to traumatic experiences. Each chapter in this section:

▶ Describes the problem

▶ Explains the connection between the mind and the body

▶ Discusses the problem in such a way as to lead you to constructive solutions

▶ Offers specific self-help "prescriptions" for improving your ability to cope with the problem

Each of these chapters also refers you to the appropriate basic skills described in

Part 1, which are especially helpful in managing your particular problem. Many of these problems will improve significantly with the self-help advice given in the book. Others will benefit from a combination of self-help and professional help.

PART 3: MANAGING MEDICAL CARE

How to Become an Active Partner in Your Own Health Care

This section reviews the essential skills you need to be a patient these days, including how to work successfully with health professionals. The most effective health care team includes knowledgeable, caring professionals and an active, informed patient—you. In these chapters you'll learn about your rights and responsibilities as a patient, and how to manage your doctor. You'll also find key questions to ask about medical tests, medications, and surgery. You'll discover how to use your mind to enhance the effectiveness of medications, how to prepare for surgery, and how to share in important medical decisions. These chapters encourage true partnerships—between your mind and body, and between you and your doctor and other care providers.

SPECIAL FEATURES

The book includes several features to help you find your way through it.

▶ **Front Cover and Tabs:** All the chapters are listed on the front cover. They line up with the corresponding chapter tabs on right-hand pages throughout the book. By using the cover table of contents and tabs, you can find any chapter you wish easily and quickly. Try it.

▶ **Quick Start Guide:** On the inside of the front and back covers you'll find a guide to the major topics and resources. By answering a few quick questions, you can zero in on what is of most interest to you, and where to go to get started.

▶ **Index:** To locate the specific information you want quickly, there is a complete, easy-to-use index in the back.

▶ **Cross References:** Throughout the book are cross references to other pages that contain related information. Each reference is indicated by a small book icon and specific page numbers (☐ see page xxx). You can use these cross references to find the information you need. You can put together your own program for improving your physical and mental health.

▶ **Key Points:** Key points are highlighted with small "post-it" stickers in the margins. They enable you to skim through the book and pick out essential ideas and advice.

▶ **Rx:** In each chapter specific techniques, suggestions, and self-help advice are highlighted with the symbol "Rx." This symbol is traditionally used for prescriptions. It is derived from the Latin word *recipe*, and means *to take*, as in *remedy* or *cure*. When you see the Rx, think of it as advice that you take as you would a prescription, to better your health and well-being.

▶ **Icons and Boxes:** Icons and boxes highlight key features throughout the book. They enable you to zero in on particularly relevant information as you look through a chapter. For example, if you are interested in the research that supports a certain mind-body technique, look for the box called *What the Research Shows*. This format also allows you to skip sections you are not interested in, and focus on what is most relevant to you. Here are some examples of the icons and boxes:

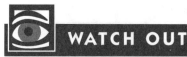

WATCH OUT

PLAY IT SAFE

While the self-help techniques in this book are generally very safe, they should be used with care to avoid side effects. Throughout the book you'll find *Watch Out* boxes that alert you to how to use the self-help advice safely and most effectively. Examples of topics include:

▶ *Healthy Negative Feelings*
   (📖 see page 46)

▶ *Unhealthy Humor*
   (📖 see page 55)

▶ *Changing Bad Moods: What Doesn't Work* (📖 see page 158)

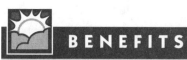

BENEFITS

THE ADVANTAGES

Benefit boxes throughout the book highlight some of the advantages that are associated with specific mind-body techniques. Here are some of the examples:

▶ *Communicating Well Reduces the Risk of Heart Disease*
   (📖 see page 123)

▶ *Imagery Can Boost Your Immune Function* (📖 see page 98)

▶ *Optimistic Thinking Speeds Recovery from Surgery*
   (📖 see page 36)

CHECK YOURSELF

In this book you'll find self-assessment sections that encourage you to check where you stand. Among them are:

▶ *Test Your Hostility*
   (📖 see page 170)

▶ *Are You an Optimist?*
   (📖 see page 37)

▶ *Are You Addicted?*
   (📖 see page 211)

▶ *How Assertive are You?*
   (📖 see page 126)

▶ *Eliminating and Solving Problems*
   (📖 see page 31)

WHAT THE RESEARCH SHOWS

SCIENTIFIC EVIDENCE

In each of the chapters you'll find what the latest research shows on the importance of the mind-body connection. Here are some examples:

▶ *Mood Influences Immunity to Cold Viruses* (📖 see page 14)

▶ *Volunteering is Associated with Lower Death Rates*
   (📖 see page 136)

▶ *Laughter Can Raise Pain Thresholds* (📖 see page 50)

▶ *Looking at Nature Reduces Time in the Hospital* (📖 see page 62)

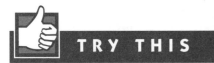

TRY THIS

SELF-HELP EXERCISES

These boxes include practical, step-by-step exercises that will show you how to take action and develop specific, relevant skills. For example, you'll learn how to:

▶ *Be More Assertive*
 (📖 see page 128)

▶ *Deflect Others' Anger*
 (📖 see page 176)

▶ *Wake Up Your Senses*
 (📖 see page 68)

▶ *Communicate Directly About Sex*
 (📖 see page 76)

▶ *Practice Self-Hypnosis*
 (📖 see page 100)

▶ *Use Writing to Deal with Traumatic Experience* (📖 see page 207)

▶ *Counter Anxious Self-Talk*
 (📖 see page 149)

▶ *Rehearse Success*
 (📖 see page 47)

▶ *Let Music Change Your Mood*
 (📖 see page 65)

▶ *Relax Your Muscles*
 (📖 see page 92)

▶ *Practice Mindfulness*
 (📖 see page 94)

▶ *Use Guided Imagery*
 (📖 see page 104)

▶ *Distract Yourself*
 (📖 see page 162)

SPECIAL INTEREST

This book includes many boxes on topics that may be of special interest to you. Here are some examples:

▶ *Four Keys to Listening Well*
 (📖 see page 122)

▶ *Procrastination*
 (📖 see page 188)

▶ *Try to Cry* (📖 see page 56)

▶ *Somatization: Dealing with Unexplained Physical Symptoms*
 (📖 see page 232)

▶ *The Faith That Heals*
 (📖 see page 39)

▶ *The Grieving Process*
 (📖 see page 204)

▶ *Getting A Second Opinion*
 (📖 see page 268)

We hope you enjoy, use, and benefit from the advice and special features in *Mind & Body Health Handbook*.

Dear Reader,

Sometimes after a busy day as a physician in a general medical clinic, I discuss the patients I've seen with my colleague, Robert Ornstein, a psychologist.

▶ A 42-year-old warehouse worker with back pain

▶ An 18-year-old first year college student with headaches

▶ A 24-year-old new mother with fatigue and dizziness

▶ A 72-year old retired machinist with chest pain

These patients seem so different: in age, background, and symptoms, but we are struck by how much they have in common. They are all suffering and in distress; they all are whole human beings with feelings, thoughts, frustrations, and talents. They are not mindless machines or collections of flesh and bones. Their symptoms are the common language through which they express their distress and illness.

For most of these patients, no physician, including me, can identify a clear physical problem, and we can't simply fix them with medications or surgery. More than 80% of them have emotional distress. They aren't mentally ill—they just have difficulty coping with the demands in their daily lives. Their symptoms, if not directly caused by stress, are certainly made worse by it. The majority would benefit greatly from learning how to better use the most powerful healing system in the world—their brain.

Based on our clinical experience as well as the latest scientific evidence, we are convinced that what goes on in people's minds influences every part of their body. *No bodily system is immune to the effects of our thoughts, emotions, and behaviors.* And the brain's chemical messengers transform our thoughts and feelings. Our minds and bodies are truly united. We can't ignore the power of our minds to harm or to heal.

This book is a true collaboration of a physician and a psychologist. Each brings our knowledge and discipline to the book to bridge the gap between mind and body. We firmly believe that the best, most effective health care addresses the needs of both. The emerging mind-body medicine combines age-old practices, common sense, and the latest science. We have written *Mind & Body Health Handbook* to help you use your mind to improve both your physical and emotional health, and have carefully selected the most effective mind-body techniques for you to try. This book contains the "prescriptions" we like most to recommend to patients and would like to share with you. We invite you to enjoy the benefits of a healthy mind and healthy body.

David Sobel

David S. Sobel, M.D. and Robert Ornstein, Ph.D.

Introduction

How to Activate the Most Powerful Healing System in the World: Your Brain

magine a new drug or medical treatment that can:

▶ Lower blood pressure

▶ Decrease heart disease and cancer risk

▶ Boost the immune system

▶ Block pain

What if the treatment could also:

▶ Extend the life of those with cancer

▶ Improve the lives of those with arthritis, diabetes, and other chronic conditions

And say this new medical treatment could:

▶ Heighten mood

▶ Lighten depression

▶ Calm anxiety

▶ Defuse hostility

▶ Ease insomnia

As well as:

▶ Shorten the duration of labor in pregnant women

▶ Speed discharge from the hospital following surgery

▶ Decrease visits to the doctor

This treatment is now readily available, inexpensive, safe and makes you feel good.

It isn't a new miracle drug, and it can't be obtained in any pharmacy. In fact, this prescription can be filled only by you in the "internal pharmacy" of your own brain.

The benefits described here—and many others—come from mind-body medicine. The power of the techniques in this book result not from the magic in any medication, but from taking advantage of the natural healing capacities of your mind.

Your body is not a mindless machine. Your thoughts, feelings, moods and actions have a significant effect on your health. They determine the onset of some diseases, the course of many, and the management of nearly all. What goes on in your mind also shapes your overall happiness, and sense of well-being.

> Key Point

At this moment you have in your hands a practical guide to the science and practice of mind-body medicine. This handbook shows you how to use your mind to:

▶ Relieve stress

▶ Improve your mood

▶ Stay well

▶ Boost your immunity

▶ Manage illness

▶ Reduce your medical costs

MEDICINE FROM YOUR MIND

Mind & Body Health Handbook contains strong medicine. The "mind-body prescriptions" are based on well-proven behavioral techniques drawn from scores of studies and clinical programs (see box page 14). For each technique, we provide a summary of the potential benefits, the research on effectiveness, what to watch out for, and practical instructions on when and how to use the technique. The information and advice in this book will enable you to prescribe wisely for yourself and take advantage of your internal pharmacy.

We urge you to take these prescriptions seriously, just as you would take prescriptions for medications seriously. Like medications, mind-body medicine techniques are:

▶ Able to change powerfully body chemistry and function

▶ Useful in preventing or treating a variety of symptoms and diseases

▶ Most effective when used regularly

While there are many similarities between drugs and "mind-body prescriptions," the mind-body approach offers some major advantages:

▶ Mind-body techniques are generally safer than medications (fewer negative side effects, adverse reactions, and less risk of overdosing). The most common "side effects" are a positive sense of well-being, increased self-confidence, and better mood.

▶ Mind-body techniques generally cost less than long-term drug treatment for chronic medical conditions, and they often lower overall medical costs.

▶ Since the mind-body approach often involves learning and practicing certain new skills, the benefits may be longer lasting than with medications. With many medications, the improvement may stop as soon as you stop the medicine.

▶ Unlike most medications, mind-body medicine invites you to take a more active role in maintaining and improving your own health. The techniques described in this book allow you to be more in control.

▶ While most medications are used to treat disease *after* it appears, mind-body medicine techniques are most effective in *preventing* symptoms and disease.

Fortunately, you don't always have to choose between medications or mind-body medicine. You can use either or both. The mind-body techniques described in *Mind & Body Health Handbook* can enhance the effectiveness of appropriate medications and other medical treatment.

Limitations

Neither drugs nor the mind-body prescriptions are cure-alls or panaceas—both have their usefulness and their limits (see box page 13). Mental imagery, relaxation, or other mind-body techniques alone are not effective treatments for infections, cancers, heart disease, and other serious conditions. But treatment with drugs and surgery alone is not complete for most medical problems either. Mind-body medicine techniques can work side-by-side with your usual medical care.

"Knowing It" and "Doing It"

For a prescription to be effective, you must take it. Just knowing a technique is not enough. If you want to learn, grow, and become healthier, you need to take some risks. You must actually do something different. Learning requires new actions, not just new information.

Key Point

WATCH OUT

GET PROFESSIONAL HELP

Don't ignore symptoms that might require medical attention. Many symptoms and diseases require specific medical or psychological help. This book is designed to *supplement* medical care, not to be a substitute for it. Be sure to get appropriate medical evaluation and treatment, especially if you have any unusual, unexplained, or severe symptoms. If they persist beyond a reasonable period despite self-care treatment, consult a health professional. Don't deny yourself professional care when you need it.

If you receive professional advice that is in conflict with the information in this book, follow the advice of your health professional. He or she can base your treatment on your personal history and specific needs.

As you read this book, if the thought "I already know that" or "that's too simple to work" crosses your mind, reconsider it. Knowing something and putting it into daily practice are two different things.

Don't be frustrated if you don't have time or energy to try out all the suggestions and advice in this book. Even the authors can't practice all they preach.

But can a book alone make a difference? Yes. Studies show that just reading and practicing these self-help strategies can improve symptoms and prevent problems by themselves. Bibliotherapy (therapy based on what you read) can also be supplemented by classes, programs, groups, and individual counseling.

Millions of years of evolution have shaped your remarkable brain to mind your health. It is at your command. Many of the most powerful prescriptions are ready for you to use now in the pharmacy of your own brain.

EMERGING NEW RESEARCH

Mind-Body Medicine Can:

Change Body Chemistry

▶ Imagery, hypnosis, and relaxation techniques have helped diabetics stabilize blood sugar levels and hemophiliacs control bleeding.

▶ Positive expectations about treatments can alter cholesterol levels, blood counts, stomach acid, immune function, and levels of endorphins—the body's own pain relieving chemicals.

▶ Massage and pleasurable touch can reduce stress hormones. In one study, a group of older children hospitalized for anxiety and depression got a 30-minute back massage each day for five days. A similar group saw relaxing videos instead. The group that got the massages were less depressed and slept better. Many of them also had lower levels of stress hormones.

Boost Immune Function

▶ Antibodies in the saliva that protect against colds are higher on days when people are in a positive mood.

▶ Imagery techniques can enable healthy people voluntarily to increase antibodies and change the activity of disease-fighting white blood cells.

Prevent Disease

▶ Church-goers have nearly half the risk of a heart attack than nonchurch-goers, and their blood pressure is lower.

▶ A long-term study of college graduates found that optimistic men were healthier, and had less chronic illness in later life.

▶ Depressed coronary heart disease patients are more likely to have heart attacks, undergo bypass surgery, and suffer other heart-related problems. In those patients who had had a heart attack, depression predicted future heart problems better than the severity of artery damage, high cholesterol levels, or cigarette smoking. In heart attack survivors, depression triples the risk of dying within six months.

▶ Deaths due to lack of regular physical activity are comparable to those from smoking, high blood pressure, and an elevated cholesterol level.

▶ Inadequate social support is as dangerous to your health as lack of exercise, smoking, and elevated cholesterol.

▶ Reducing anger and hostility may prevent heart disease and reduce risk of recurrent heart attack.

Treat Illness

▶ Positive expectations and beliefs can help headaches, arthritis, hay fever, colds, warts, constipation, angina, insomnia, and pain after surgery.

▶ Patients who take an active role in their health care and ask more questions report better overall health. For example, diabetic and hypertensive patients who regularly interact with their doctors have more control of blood sugar and blood pressure levels.

▶ An education program in skills for arthritis patients led by other patients reduced pain levels by 20%,

Continued on next page

decreased doctor visits by 43%, and saved an average of $400 per patient over four years.

▶ Patients with chronic pain who had ten sessions of mind-body techniques saw the doctor 36% less in the following two years. They felt more in control, and less depressed and anxious.

Speed Recovery from Surgery

▶ Mentally prepared surgery patients have fewer complications, less discomfort, recover more quickly, and leave the hospital sooner.

▶ Patients undergoing open-heart surgery who received strength and comfort from religion were three times more likely to survive than those without religious support.

Extend Lives

▶ Nursing home residents who were given more control over things such as what to have for lunch or what night to see a movie were happier and more active. After 18 months, they had half the death rate as those who were not offered as much control.

▶ Confidence in your health appears to predict future health better than lab tests or doctor's exams. In one study, senior citizens who believed they were in "poor" health were nearly three times more likely to die over a seven-year period than those who rated their health as "excellent." These self-ratings more accurately predicted who would die than their doctors' objective reports.

▶ One group of patients with a deadly skin cancer (malignant melanoma) received a group support and education program for six weeks in addition to standard surgical treatment. They learned about their condition, stress management, relaxation, and coping skills. The group receiving this training had a 60% reduction in death rate six years later.

Save Money

▶ Patients with psychosomatic complaints who attended a group to learn and practice mind-body skills reduced their medical expenses by over $85 each in just six months.

▶ Patients with unexplained physical symptoms were helped with a mind-body approach that decreased their annual medical charges by an average of $289 (a 33% reduction). They also reported greatly improved physical functioning.

▶ Patients receiving focused mental health treatment reduced their overall medical costs by 22% over a year and a half. Costs for those not offered any mental health treatment rose by 22%.

▶ Providing continuous emotional support during labor and delivery can result in shorter labor, 56% fewer caesarean sections, and decreases the need to keep the baby in the hospital longer than two days.

▶ Treating premature infants with music therapy (Brahms' Lullaby) resulted in greater weight gain, and earlier discharge from the hospital by one week, producing a savings of $4,800 per infant.

Have You Ever Wondered:

▶ Why do some people cope better with illness and stress in their lives than other people?

▶ Why are some patients with minor physical problems disastrously disabled, while others with serious diseases not only survive, but maintain an active, fulfilling life?

▶ Why is it that some people exposed to germs develop infections while others remain healthy?

Part of the answer lies in inheriting good genes and a strong constitution. Another part comes from the good fortune of living in a clean, healthy environment with adequate nutrition. *But a good portion of the explanation of who stays healthy and who gets sick lies in our own minds, and within our control. Your thoughts, moods, attitudes and behaviors strongly influence the quality of your health and vitality.* You are not a defenseless victim of microbes, toxins, or stressors. You can learn to use your mind to prevent illness and improve your health.

Key Point

Life Skills Worth Mastering

Evidence suggests that the healthiest, hardiest people are able to:

▶ Transform pessimistic, negative thoughts into health-affirming, optimistic ways of thinking

▶ Refocus their minds and relax their bodies to counteract stress

▶ Master skills that can boost immunity and resistance to disease

▶ Communicate in a satisfying way that connects them with others

▶ Enjoy a laugh that dispels tensions and brings a happier perspective

▶ Enjoy the relaxing and revitalizing pleasure of their senses

▶ Extend beyond themselves by helping others, and thereby nourishing themselves

▶ Cope effectively with bad moods, anger, time pressure, trauma, and chronic illness

▶ Become active, involved partners in their own health care

Mind & Body Health Handbook will help you strengthen these vital health-promoting skills.

📖 *For more information, see page 271*

1 The Power to Change

How to Make and Maintain Healthy Changes

▶ *"I'd like to exercise more, but I just can't seem to get started."*

▶ *"Every year I make some great New Year's resolutions, but within a week or two I'm back to the same old habits."*

▶ *"I started doing a 15 minute relaxation exercise everyday, and felt great. I just couldn't keep it going."*

▶ *"When I get in a bad mood, I know there are things I can do, but I just never seem to do them."*

▶ *"I'd like to quit smoking and drinking, but I just don't have the will power."*

This book describes many ways to make your life healthier and more pleasurable. You may have already adopted some of these ideas; others may strike you as new, and things you'd like to try. Still others may be changes you've attempted in the past, but they haven't yet become a part of your life.

Even when we're aware of the benefits of change, there's often a gap between thinking about it and doing it. Understanding the nature of change helps bridge that gap, increasing the odds that your new efforts will be successful and lasting.

Change isn't always hard. Most of the time it comes easily and naturally. Take a look at a photo of yourself 15 years ago. Your hair and clothing have probably changed a great deal without much deliberate effort on your part. We adopt new behaviors, learn new information, and acquire skills continuously, often without even thinking about them. Our environments shape our behaviors all the time, for better or worse.

When change is difficult, it's important not to wallow in self-criticism, telling yourself you're "lazy," "stupid," or "worthless." You may genuinely be trying to manage your time at work efficiently, but the company is always making unexpected, last-minute demands on you. Instead of blaming yourself for poor time management, figure out what's really getting in the way. Then see what you can and cannot do about it.

Pathways to Change

Different people have different styles of change. For example, some people make elaborate written plans and follow them; others don't bother to plan at all. *It's* *important to discover the style of change that works for you, and in what situation.*

Many big changes—such as stopping smoking or getting into better physical shape—happen as the result of a series of small steps (getting rid of ashtrays and buying fewer cigarettes, for instance, or using the stairs instead of the elevator). Other changes come from a more radical conversion; they often involve a major shift in our hearts and minds. The change may result from a conviction that the old way of behaving is no longer compatible with who you are.

We have identified three of the basic pathways to change: *Pleasurable Change,* *Breakthrough Change,* and *Step-By-Step Change.* They are described below.

1. Pleasurable Change

We make some changes just because they are so enjoyable—things like getting a massage, drinking a glass of wine, taking a nap, or watching a funny movie, for instance. And all of this fun pays off in immediate gratification as well as better health. Part 1 of this book, *Staying Well,* suggests many healthy pleasures you can easily add to your daily life.

So try changing the easiest and most fun things first! Playing with a pet, taking a siesta, or listening to your favorite music all can make you feel good. And they may fit easily into your life, so you're likely to keep doing them.

Changing some unhealthy habits can even be a healthy pleasure. An immediate reward for successfully giving up a bad habit or addiction is the increased sense of mastery and control you feel. The pleasure from the increased self-confidence can sometimes more than make up for the lost enjoyment of smoking, excessive drinking, or other bad habits.

2. Breakthrough Change

Some changes, even controlling addiction and other bad habits, occur without much planning. People "Just Do It." Sometimes these changes involve a major crisis or trauma, and they are not always comfortable.

Many people who face life-threatening illness, family crises, or natural disaster make sweeping changes in their lives. A person suffers a heart attack and suddenly his life priorities undergo a radical shift. These changes often occur as dramatic breakthroughs, shattering old beliefs and habits. They give rise to new ways of thinking and acting. For some, the change results from a profound spiritual experience, a religious conversion, or deep insight.

The Chinese ideogram for "crisis" contains two symbols—one means "danger," the other "opportunity." It is difficult to engineer a crisis, but when such an opportunity occurs, you may take advantage of it to make some rapid progress and health improvements.

Sometimes radical changes are easier than successive, step-by-step changes. Some people find it easier to go "cold turkey" and make the change in one giant step. Others prefer "warm turkey." For them, gradual change is the ticket to success.

Susan adopted a low-fat diet by degrees. First she eliminated margarine and butter from her cooking, then she switched to skim milk, and then prepared fish instead of meat.

For Diane, this incremental approach would be too difficult. It would mean that every time she sat down at the table, she'd have to choose between her old and new ways to eat. Instead, Diane decided that she would no longer eat high-fat food. Fatty foods are gone from her diet, and that's that. No more decisions. This path to change, although it can be difficult at first, is sometimes less stressful in the long run because there's no continuous struggle with choices and decisions.

3. Step-By-Step Change

For some people, small incremental stages of change work best. Here's where deliberate planning is most helpful.

Recent research has uncovered some valuable information about the stages of change (📖 see box page 20). If you know the stage of change you're in, you can select the tips and strategies that are most likely to help you succeed. The stages are:

Stage 1. Not Interested in Changing

Stage 2. Considering Change

Stage 3. Ready to Make Plans

Stage 4. Ready to Take Action

Stage 5. Maintaining the Change

Here are two examples of people at a different stage of readiness to change. Perhaps you can identify with one of them.

Joe has been a smoker for 40 years. "So what?" he says. "It doesn't harm anyone but me. And I don't think it does me any harm. My uncle smoked 80 cigarettes a day and lived to be 90."

Angela has smoked for 20 years. After months of carefully considering all her reasons to change, she finally enrolls in a local stop-smoking class. At last, Angela manages to quit. Three weeks after quitting, her teenage daughter runs away from home, and Angela reaches for a cigarette.

Readiness to Change

Joe and Angela have the same habit, but they are very different in their thoughts, feelings, and stage of readiness to change. They are more likely to be successful if the strategies they try are closely matched to their stage. Whether you want to break a bad habit or start a new healthy one, you can learn how to increase your chances of success. Start by understanding your own readiness to change. Then choose the strategies that are likely to be most effective for you. *Don't worry about the ultimate goal. Just focus on moving to the next stage. Your success will boost your confidence.*

Key Point

HOW PEOPLE CHANGE

Thousands of studies have been done to learn how people change—or why they don't change. Here's what we have learned:

▶ Most people change by themselves, when they are ready. While physicians, counselors, spouses, and self-help groups coax, persuade, nag, and otherwise try to assist people to change their lifestyle and habits, most do so without all that much help from others.

▶ Change is not an all-or-nothing process. It occurs in specific stages. Most of us think of change as a regular sequence: each step is an improvement over the one before it. Although a few people do make changes this way, it is rare. More than 95% of people who successfully quit smoking do so only after a series of setbacks and relapses.

▶ In most cases, change resembles a spiral more than a straight line, with people reverting to previous stages before proceeding further ("two steps forward, one step back"). So relapses aren't failures but setbacks, which are an integral part of change. And dealing with relapse is frequently a helpful way for people to learn how to maintain change. Relapsing provides feedback about what doesn't work.

▶ Efficient self-change depends on doing the right things at the right time. There's evidence that people who are given strategies inappropriate to their particular stage are less successful in changing than people who receive no assistance at all. Making an elaborate written plan of action, for example, when you really haven't decided you want to change, is a prescription for failure. You're likely to get bored, discouraged or frustrated before you even decide to start!

▶ *Confidence in your ability to change is the key ingredient for success.* Your belief in your own ability to succeed predicts whether you will:

Key Point

▶ Attempt change in the first place

▶ Persist if you relapse

▶ Be ultimately successful in making the change

Success Improves Health

The benefits of change go beyond the payoffs of adopting new, healthier habits. *Obviously you will feel better when you exercise, eat well, keep regular sleeping hours, stop smoking, and take time to relax. But regardless of the behavior that's altered, there's evidence that the feelings of self-confidence and control over your life that come from making any successful change improves your health.*

Key Point

As we age or develop a chronic illness, physical abilities and self-image may decline. For many it is discouraging to find that they can't do what they used to or want to do. By changing and improving one area of your life, whether it is improving your physical fitness or learning a new skill, you regain a sense of optimism and vitality. By focusing on what you *can do,* rather than what you *can't do,* you're more likely to lead a more positive and happier life.

How to Make and Maintain Healthy Changes

When you have trouble putting your good intentions into practice, the strategies described below can help you. They are tailored to your particular stage of change. These self-help strategies are effective whether you are making a positive change such as adding more physical activity to your life, or ridding yourself of a bad habit like addiction. For more information on addiction see Chapter 17: Addiction *(📖 page 209).*

℞ Just Do It

Russell Baker said: "To give up smoking, you quit smoking." *The first way to try beating a destructive habit is to simply stop—stop without a lot of planning, techniques, or group support. This advice may seem too simple, but this is the way most people quit or control bad habits.* They decide that it is unacceptable to continue the habit. After a firm decision, the rest is often surprisingly easy. You can just quit.

Key Point

℞ Are You Ready For Change?

If you are not prepared to "just do it," then start by determining how ready you are to make a particular change. Which of the stages described on page 19 best fits how you feel right now? In some areas you may be ready for action; in others, you just need some help maintaining the positive change. In still others you may need more information before deciding to take action. Decide which stage you're in, then skip ahead to the specific techniques below matched to your stage.

Start by asking yourself these four key questions:

1. **What's the problem?**
2. **Do I really want to change?**
3. **How ready am I to make that change?**
4. **What are the best strategies for me to use to be successful?**

STAGE 1: NOT INTERESTED

Perhaps someone is nagging you to fix something about your life you don't think needs fixing. If you change only to please other people, you won't be motivated to keep it up, no matter how great the rewards might be.

People in this stage, like Joe, typically have no intention of changing in the foreseeable future. That's not because they don't see a solution; it's because they don't even see a problem. People in this stage need more awareness, information, and reasons to change. If you are in this stage, it is unlikely you are even reading this chapter.

℞ Examine Your Excuses

You may have good reasons for not wanting to change, or they may be excuses for not changing. Take a critical look at your reasons. For example, you may have been putting off taking a couples communication class because you think you "communicate just fine." This may be true, or it may be an excuse blocking you from making some changes that could improve your health and enrich your life.

Or say you smoke. You may have many "good reasons" for continuing to smoke: you're crabby when you can't smoke; you take pleasure in the rituals associated with smoking; you assume that lung cancer won't strike you.

What's the evidence for and against these claims? If someone else used these excuses would you agree or dispute them? Is it possible that once you go through the discomfort of change and break the habit, you will feel even stronger, calmer, and more satisfied?

If you don't want to change and others are urging you to, try complaining. Ranting and whining about the problem helps you begin to examine your reasons for not wanting to change. Just talking about them at least gets you thinking about change. This gets the wheels turning, and can open up the possibilities for future change. Remember, thinking is the first step to doing.

℞ Recognize When You Hit Bottom

When dealing with addictive behaviors, hitting bottom is sometimes necessary. This may seem cynical, but for some people, it takes a life-threatening medical problem, bankruptcy, divorce, job loss, or other serious crisis to get themselves to change. A crisis often leads people to realize that life with the addictive behavior is no longer tolerable.

Surprisingly, those with either the mildest or most severe addictions seem to be the ones most likely to recover. Those caught in the middle with problems too difficult to solve easily and no disaster to shock them into action have the most difficulty changing.

Key Point

STAGE 2: CONSIDERING CHANGE

At this stage, you're aware of the benefits of change, but not sure you're ready to do it. What you need now is more information, motivation, inspiration and encouragement.

℞ Get Informed

Reading this book is a good start in gathering new information. As you go though each chapter you can review the benefits of change (improvements in your health, mood, and sense of well-being), as well as some easy first steps you can take. But don't limit yourself. Also:

▶ Talk to friends

▶ Discuss it with your doctor

▶ Call a community service hotline

▶ Read a community college course catalog

▶ Check out a computer bulletin board

▶ Find a discussion group

▶ Explore the resources in your own community

℞ List the Pros and Cons

Write down all the pros and cons of changing the particular behavior you can think of. Even if it doesn't convince you to move forward, this "cost-benefit analysis" at least helps you see the situation more clearly, and prepares you to take action.

So if smoking is your problem, for example, list your reasons for quitting, and the benefits you see for yourself in doing so. Write down both the immediate and longer-term gains. You may have such reasons as "to please my spouse or daughter or boss." Your motivation to stop (and stay stopped) must be stronger than just the wish to please someone else. Once you stop, you may resent the person who urged you to do it. This can lead to a quick relapse.

Consider how you hurt yourself and others by continuing the bad habit, and list the consequences of the habit. They might include getting lung cancer, or, with other unhealthy behaviors, injuring or killing someone while driving drunk, or causing financial ruin due to compulsive gambling. Linking these disasters with the bad habit removes some of its pleasure, and paves the way to change.

On a separate piece of paper, list the benefits of *not* making the change. What do you give up by changing? What is the cost, in terms of time, energy, pleasure, stress, image, or status? Some people see cigarettes as friends, for instance, and drinkers may be unable to imagine a life without bars and fellow drinkers. *Being honest about the benefits or pleasures of bad habits helps prepare you for possible feelings of deprivation and self-pity. These can undermine your efforts to change. Plan ways that your life can be full and enjoyable without keeping your bad habit.*

Key Point

Keep the lists you wrote. After you've quit, you may need a boost to help keep you on track. Look back at your reasons for wanting to change.

℞ Brainstorm Your Options

There are many ways of changing. You don't have to get locked into a single strategy. You may need to experiment until you find the method (or combination of methods) that works for you.

Hold a personal brainstorming session. Write down anything that occurs to you. Don't reject any ideas. If you want to enjoy your job more, for instance, your options might include trading duties with a colleague, asking for more challenging assignments, enrolling in a class that would qualify you for promotion, investigating opportunities at other companies, or visiting a career counselor to explore the possibility of a career change. Then add the input of people whose ideas you respect. When asking others for advice, don't ask what you should do. Instead, just brainstorm. Generate some options, choices, and possibilities together.

Once you've come up with a list of options, write out the possible consequences of each action. Then decide which alternatives seem most promising (they're probably the ones that most closely match the stage you're in). Get more information on the ones you're not sure about. Pick one or two you might be willing to try as an experiment.

STAGE 3: READY TO MAKE PLANS

At this point, you're pretty sure you want to make a change, but you need specific plans to help you do so.

℞ Write Down a Specific Plan

A written action plan makes your intentions clear and real. Think of it as a kind of contract with yourself. It's a way to help

MONITOR YOURSELF

It may help to keep a diary on the habit you want to change. Record:

- ▶ When you engage in the behavior
- ▶ Where
- ▶ With whom
- ▶ Events preceding it
- ▶ Feelings preceding it

This self-monitoring alone may reduce the behavior and help you become aware of what triggers it.

Identifying your triggers enables you to develop strategies—the ones you need to break the automatic link between the situations, feelings, thoughts, and the behavior you want to change. For example, smokers who record each cigarette may find they are most likely to smoke when they drink coffee. Or a problem drinker may find that attending business lunches or feeling lonely leads to drinking.

If you're thinking about working on your excessive anger, start noticing what situations and thoughts trigger your angry feelings. Look for a pattern. Do you get angry when you have to wait in line? When someone doesn't seem to understand you? When you feel out of control?

Monitor what you tell yourself about change. For example, you might ask yourself:

- ▶ *If I _____ (stop smoking, start exercising, etc.), what am I afraid might happen?*
- ▶ *When I think of making a change, what thoughts come to mind?*
- ▶ *Am I making statements like, "That's just the way I am" or "I can't do it"? Counter those beliefs (see page 42).*

Remind yourself that many people have successfully done what you're setting out to do. Recall some examples of successful changes you have made in the past. If you are wondering, "Is this worth it?" think of all the reasons that led you to consider the change in the first place.

you keep your goals in mind, monitor your progress, and evaluate what is and isn't working. Here are keys to an effective plan:

1. Be specific. First, spell out exactly what you'll do, how often, when, and how you will know you have successfully achieved your goal. If your plan is to get more exercise, specify how often you'll exercise, the type of workout, where you'll do it, and for how long. For example, you might write something like, "Beginning next Monday, I'll take fast walks around the neighborhood for 20 minutes twice a week, and on Saturdays I'll swim 15 laps at the city pool." Limit the contract to a week or two, then renegotiate the goals for the next week.

2. Break your goal into small, do-able steps. Let's say you want to conquer chronic anxiety. That's a terrific goal, but you'll be disappointed if your goal is to be a completely calm person by the end of the first week. Instead, come up with concrete actions that will decrease your anxiety. Resolve to learn a relaxation technique, cut your coffee intake to one cup a day, or spend more time on an engaging hobby like gardening.

Don't demand of yourself more than you can handle. If you want to expand your circle of friends, committing yourself to a class or club seven nights a week doesn't leave much room for the rest of life. *You're more likely to be successful—and less inclined to abandon the whole effort—if you build in some flexibility.* If your plan includes walking five days a week for the next week, and you miss a day or two, you haven't automatically failed. Allow room for "lapses."

3. Make sure your plan is realistic. Picture a scale from one to ten, with ten representing your final goal or achievement (quitting smoking, riding 10 miles on your bicycle, or practicing a relaxation exercise for 20 minutes a day). Decide which number on that scale represents your *current* level toward that final goal. What would it take to move just one notch higher on that scale? Too often we want to move from a "three" to a "ten" in one step. Planning to move up only one number at a time sets you up for success. There's time to take the steps one at a time.

4. Apply the confidence test. Ask yourself if you are at least 70% certain that you can accomplish your proposed goal within your planned time frame. If you're not that confident, lower your goal until you are. Plans that fall short of this confidence test usually fall short in practice. If you are 100% confident, then you might want to revise the goal upward to make it a bit more challenging.

5. Write it down. Once you have made a contract you're satisfied with, write it down, and post it where you'll see it every day. Each day you can check your progress (📖 see box page 26).

Remember, a successful plan or contract includes:

▶ Something *you* want to do

▶ Reasonable changes that you can accomplish within the next week or so

▶ Specific actions (what? how much? when? how often?)

▶ Confidence of 70% or more that you can achieve your short-term goal

℞ Working Around Barriers

You can defuse potential problems by identifying the situations that are likely to throw you off your agreement with yourself. (The self-monitoring described in the box on page 24 can help you with this step.) Once identified, can you avoid any of these situations? If not, how can you prepare for them? Or cope with them differently than you did in the past?

If, for example, you're trying to learn to handle anger better, and you know that a visit to your in-laws always prompts an outburst, think about alternatives to blowing up. How can you assert yourself without losing your temper? When your usual trigger topic comes up in conversation—politics or sports—can you change the subject, take a walk, or head for home before the after-dinner argument begins?

Learn from past successes. Think of a time when you were able to make a change and stick with it. Ask yourself:

▶ *What did I do?*

▶ *How did I overcome obstacles?*

▶ *How did I get back on track?*

CHECK YOURSELF

MAKING A CONTRACT WITH YOURSELF

For this week:

▶ What activity or action are you going to do? _____

▶ How much are you going to do? _____

▶ When are you going to do it? _____

▶ How often are you going to do it? _____

▶ How will you reward yourself (optional)? _____

▶ Who is your support person (optional)? _____

▶ How confident are you that you will successfully complete your contract and goal *(adjust contract until you are at least 70% confident)?*

Not at all 0% 10 20 30 40 50 60 70 80 90 100% **Totally Confident**

Your Signature _____ Date _____

Perhaps, after many tries, you finally got into the habit of jogging regularly. After thinking about what made it work, you realize that it wasn't the new cross-training shoes, the pedometer, or the stopwatch; it was finding a friend to run with. Consider working a social component into future plans for change.

℞ Imagine You've Already Changed

You may be so used to thinking of yourself in a certain role such as a workaholic or lazy person that you can't really picture yourself any other way. Use your imagination to help you feel more comfortable with a new, healthier identity.

Key Point *Create a vivid mental picture of yourself having already made the desired*

change, easily and confidently. Imagine yourself enjoying the benefits: having more energy, sleeping more soundly, being in a better mood. Get in the habit of calling up this happy scenario whenever you begin to doubt your ability to change. Use imagery, self-hypnosis, and affirmations to create a clear, strong, positive image of yourself succeeding at change (📖 see page 97).

℞ Get Committed

Sometimes people get so caught up in techniques for doing actual things differently that they neglect their decision to change. But without that commitment change isn't likely to last.

Keep in mind that actions, thoughts, and feelings influence each other. Even if

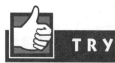

TRY THIS

ONE DAY TO LIVE

Here's an exercise that can be useful in nudging yourself toward commitment. Ask yourself, "If I had only one day to live, (or three months, or a year) how would I live it?" When faced with a life-threatening illness or other crisis, people often make dramatic changes in their lives—changes they never thought possible before. And they often wish they'd gotten around to them earlier.

Why Wait for a Crisis?

▶ What would you do differently if you really understood how precious time was?

▶ Can you make some of those changes now?

you don't always feel like it, act as if you believe in your ability to achieve your goal successfully. Take an action step. Seeing the positive results may bring your thoughts and feelings back into line.

Since thoughts influence actions as well, pay attention to the language you use in thinking about change. Expressions like "I'll try" suggest that failure looms. Say "I do," "I am," or "I will" instead.

Reframe your problems by stating them in the past tense. Transform "I *have* a hard time communicating" into "I *had* a hard time communicating." This allows you to be different in the future.

Think positively. You may hear yourself saying, "I can't do it." "I'm addicted. It's hopeless." "I don't have enough will power." "Just one more cigarette or drink won't

hurt." If you do, challenge those incorrect negative thoughts.

℞ Set Up a Support System

Changing is much easier if friends or family support your effort. Be sure to state explicitly what kind of help you'll need. It may be cheering your progress, refraining from nagging, or storing alcohol out of your sight. Or you may prefer that the people close to you treat you normally, and don't tiptoe around, hiding their cigarettes or drinks when you come in. Be clear about your needs. Be aware that needs may change as time goes on, as different issues arise.

Unfortunately, you can't always count on other people's support. If you get a new job, stop smoking, or start exercising, some of those around you may think it is great. But others may feel threatened because they still have your bad habit or because they're uncomfortable with a "different" you.

Sometimes it helps to "go public" and announce to the world your intention to change. Share your plans with the people closest to you. Come up with ways to make the change a "win" for everyone. Hiring a skywriter or airplane to fly your banner may be overdoing it a bit, but letting others know your intentions may help channel peer pressure into support.

If you decide not to tell anyone that you are quitting a bad habit, examine your reasons. For some people it's important to deal with the problem on their own. Others don't want anyone watching how they handle it. If no one knows, failure will be less humiliating. But you could also be setting yourself up for failure. You may also be depriving yourself of very much needed vital support and encouragement.

STAGE 4: READY TO ACT

Now you're ready to put your plans into practice. Here are ways to help keep yourself on track:

℞ Manage Your Environment

New habits take time to become familiar, and we often forget to do what we want to do. So rearrange your environment to remind you. Sometimes a small sign is all you need. A Post-it® note on your telephone reminds you to take a deep breath and relax. A cartoon strategically placed invites you to smile. Placing your pills by your toothbrush prompts you to take them.

Sometimes we have to change our environment in order to change ourselves. The alcoholic who's giving up drinking, for example, avoids bars. Start by removing anything associated with your habit. If you smoke, remove ashtrays and throw away your lighter. If you drink, clear out the alcohol cupboard, give away your favorite beer mug, and press the mute button during beer commercials. If you eat too much, remove tempting foods.

Some things may be difficult to do if you share your home. You may have to negotiate with your family, partners, or roommates, or come up with some new arrangements.

℞ Celebrate Your Quit Day

Make a big deal of the day you quit your habit. Set this date in advance so that you can prepare for it. Celebrate the day in a way that seems appropriate. Have a last drink or cigarette the night before; then do something that makes you feel good about your new life the next day. Plan fun things for your quit day.

℞ Substitute Healthy Pleasures

It can be difficult to just stop without replacing an addiction with another activity. But don't exchange one bad habit for another! Don't eat too much to avoid cravings for cigarettes, for example, or don't get drunk instead of high on cocaine.

Replace your bad habit with something healthy. For instance, chew carrot sticks when you give up smoking; go to the movies instead of the pub; take a walk; do an enjoyable hobby; and eat your favorite fruit at lunch time instead of chowing down a high-cal dessert. "Positive addictions" or "healthy pleasures" can balance the loss when you give up an unhealthy habit (📖 see page 57).

℞ Revise Your Plan

When your initial short-term plan is complete, evaluate the results:

▶ Were you able to stick to the plan? If not, what got in the way?

▶ How can you revise the plan to be more successful for the next step?

Successful plans are often just revisions of unsuccessful ones. Review the recommendations for making a plan on page 23. Remember, to achieve your overall goal, you will require a series of successful (or revised unsuccessful) short-term plans.

Key Point

STAGE 5: MAINTAIN PROGRESS

By this stage, you probably have a good sense of which of the previous strategies worked best for you. And you may have added a few techniques of your own. You're starting to get used to this new behavior. Or you have changed your habit, but you're not quite confident that the change is permanent. To maintain your progress, continue to use the techniques that have already worked for you, and learn how to deal with relapse.

℞ Don't Be Surprised If You Lapse

"Quitting smoking is easy. I've done it a hundred times."

—*Mark Twain*

Relapse is a common occurrence on the road to change. Don't blame yourself when you fall short of a goal. Remember that setbacks are not a sign of failure. They are part of the very process of change, and they provide an opportunity to learn. Many times you'll find yourself cycling through the stages of change several times before succeeding. The key to successful, long-term change is managing and preventing the inevitable lapses.

Total abstinence is a near impossibility for many people. To expect perfection is unrealistic. Nearly everybody lapses; slips in behavior happen all the time. Yes, it's okay to lapse—if you turn a lapse into a renewed commitment to stop again.

Rebecca began eating a healthy diet and exercising regularly. She always skipped dessert. As she had hoped, her weight gradually dropped about 10 pounds. One fine summer night she went out to dinner with good friends, and they persuaded her to taste the delicious double chocolate cake. She not only tasted it, she finished the entire plate.

Okay, so she lapsed. But what occurred next was her undoing. Rebecca misinterpreted what happened. Instead of enjoying the cake and then resuming her healthy diet the next day, she thought that having eaten the cake, her diet was "broken"; that

it no longer existed. She went back to her old pattern of unhealthy eating, and her weight went right back to where it had been.

℞ Anticipate Cravings

Some people do not understand a craving. They mistakenly imagine that it is a physiological withdrawal symptom that can't be controlled. But in fact, cravings are urges for immediate gratification. They are usually brought on by such things as:

▶ Seeing others indulge in your former habit

▶ Associating the habit with certain events (like smoking while talking on the phone)

▶ Feeling miserable, bored, lonely, angry, or deprived

Cravings to return to your bad habit are natural. Expect them and plan for them. Most urges are temporary and short-lived. A good way to deal with a strong urge is to detach yourself from it. Instead of thinking, "I'm dying for a smoke," think, "I am now experiencing an urge to smoke," or, "Oops, here comes the urge. It won't last."

By watching an urge as though you were outside it, you can let it pass. Urges and cravings are like waves in the ocean: they rise, crest, and fall. Wait out the urge; look forward to it passing, and it will. Or distract yourself by doing something different and fun.

℞ Manage Relapses

Lapses enable you to revise your plan. The revision will improve your chances of success. Analyze what happened when you slipped off track.

- What can you do about the situation that triggered it?
- How could you have prepared for (or responded to) this situation differently to have avoided the relapse?
- Do you need to make changes smaller?
- Can you modify your timetable for achieving your goal?
- Can you remove barriers or temptation from your environment?
- What new rewards can you add to reinforce the change?
- Who can you ask for help or advice?
- What can you learn from this experience to decrease chances of future lapses? (see box this page)

℞ Stay in Control

The most common triggers for relapses are negative emotional states. You can learn to deal better with anger (see page 167), depression (page 155), and negative thoughts (page 35). This will help you stay in control. And remember, in order to have a lapse, you need to have made some progress first. Congratulate yourself for getting this far.

What counts is how you think about the lapse. If you can sort out why it happened and take responsibility for it ("I was feeling nervous and I took that one drink"), then you can remain in control ("So feeling nervous is a danger point for me and I need to work on a different way to handle it"). Choose not to let your one-time lapse become a relapse.

If you quit smoking and light up a cigarette, you do not have to smoke it. If you start it you don't have to finish it. And if you finish it, you don't have to smoke another one. You stopped once, and you can stop again. Abstinence is not undone

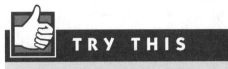

TRY THIS

WHAT TO DO IF YOU RELAPSE

Here are some suggestions for what to do if you relapse:

- Keep calm
- Remove yourself from the danger zone (go out of the room, or leave the casino, bar, or shopping center)
- Review what has just happened as objectively as you can, without self-criticism
- Renew your commitment
- Remind yourself of your goal

It can be helpful to rehearse what to do if you lapse. For example, you might imagine that you have smoked one cigarette after having quit successfully for a month. What would you do next? Imagine yourself successfully coping with this challenging situation. Each time you successfully handle such a situation—even an imaginary one—you reduce the chances of relapse.

with the first throw of the dice for a compulsive gambler or the flick of a cigarette lighter for an ex-smoker. At every moment you have choices that can put you back in control.

The most important thing to remember about stopping a bad habit or starting a good one is that you have to keep at it. You need to repeat it over and over, just like learning any new skill. The side-effect of successful, healthy change is an increased sense of control and confidence.

Key Point

℞ What You Can't Change, Accept

The Serenity Prayer

"God, grant me serenity to accept the things I cannot change, courage to change the things I can, and wisdom to know the difference."

—*F. Oetinger and R. Niebuhr*

Whether they're due to genetics, social forces, or powerful psychological barriers, some problems are difficult to change. Although many people adopt healthier eating habits and feel much better as a result, dieting to achieve permanent weight loss is rarely successful. Also, trying to change someone else's behavior is notoriously ineffective. That doesn't mean that change in resistant areas is impossible, but it does suggest that it makes sense for you to be realistic about the limits of change.

Sometimes, you find yourself repeatedly blocked even in areas that "should" be within your control. Don't reinforce a negative self-image by dwelling on repeated efforts that fall short of goals. Instead, it may make more sense to accept the situation and choose a new target, at least for a while.

By refocusing energy on easier goals, you can regain a sense of competence and enjoy the fruits of success. When change is elusive, remember that a full life embraces not only action, but also acceptance of the things that can't be changed.

CHECK YOURSELF

ELIMINATING AND SOLVING PROBLEMS

1 Identify Your Problems and Stresses by Making a List

Consider every area of your life. It probably includes:

- ▶ Family
- ▶ Love
- ▶ Relationships
- ▶ Health
- ▶ Money and financial security
- ▶ Work or school
- ▶ Social life
- ▶ Living environment

2 Sort Your Problems

Evaluate each problem as:

- ▶ Important or Unimportant
- ▶ Changeable or Unchangeable

Make four boxes on a piece of paper, and label each box like the sample on the next page. Now write each of your problems in the appropriate box. Needing to quit smoking is changeable, and for most people, important. The bad record of your very favorite sports team is unchangeable, and may or may not be important. What really counts is your perception of how important or changeable each problem is.

SORTING YOUR LIFE PROBLEMS

IMPORTANT & CHANGEABLE	UNIMPORTANT & CHANGEABLE
▶ Arguments with partner	▶ Irritating phone calls
▶ Problems with boss	▶ Errands
▶ Meeting job deadlines	▶ Chores
▶ Quitting smoking	▶ Unnecessary meetings
IMPORTANT & UNCHANGEABLE	**UNIMPORTANT & UNCHANGEABLE**
▶ Death of a loved one	▶ Bad weather
▶ Loss of job	▶ Spilled food on clothes
▶ Serious illness	▶ Traffic jams
▶ Natural disaster	▶ Neighbor's opinion

You can use this space to jot down your problems.

IMPORTANT & CHANGEABLE	UNIMPORTANT & CHANGEABLE
▶ _____	▶ _____
▶ _____	▶ _____
▶ _____	▶ _____
▶ _____	▶ _____
IMPORTANT & UNCHANGEABLE	**UNIMPORTANT & UNCHANGEABLE**
▶ _____	▶ _____
▶ _____	▶ _____
▶ _____	▶ _____
▶ _____	▶ _____

3 Match Your Coping Strategy to the Problem

For each type of problem and situation a different coping skill might work better. Below are some strategies to help you be more effective in managing each type of problem.

Important and Changeable

These types of problems are best managed by taking action to change the situation and to reduce the stress associated with them. Useful problem-solving skills include:

- ❏ Planning and goal setting (📖 see page 23)
- ❏ Self-monitoring (📖 see page 24)
- ❏ Dealing with relapse (📖 see page 29 and 209)
- ❏ Imagery (📖 see page 99)
- ❏ Time management (📖 see page 183)
- ❏ Assertive communication (📖 see page 127)
- ❏ Seeking social support (📖 see page 142)

Important & Unchangeable

These stressors are often the most difficult to manage. They can make you feel helpless and hopeless. No matter what you do, you cannot make another person change, bring someone back from the dead, or delete traumatic experiences from your life. Even though you may not be able to change the situation, you may be able to:

- ❏ Change the way you think about the problem
- ❏ Find some part of the problem that you can reclassify as changeable (you can't stop the hurricane, but you can take steps to rebuild)
- ❏ Reassess how important the problem is in light of your overall life and priorities (maybe your neighbor's criticism isn't so important after all)
- ❏ Change your emotional reactions to the situation, and thereby reduce the stress (you can't change what happened, but you can help yourself feel less distressed about it)

Here are some useful coping skills that can help you deal with what you cannot change, and feel better about it:

- ❏ Challenge negative thoughts (📖 see page 42)
- ❏ Think how much worse it could be (📖 see page 47)
- ❏ Focus on the positive (📖 see page 48)
- ❏ Deny or ignore the problem (📖 see page 204)
- ❏ Deal with traumatic experiences (📖 see page 205)
- ❏ Write and confide your deepest thoughts and feelings (📖 see page 207)
- ❏ Distract yourself (📖 see page 148)
- ❏ Desensitize your fears and anxiety (📖 see page 151)
- ❏ Help others (📖 see page 134)

☐ Seek social support and help
(📖 see page 142)

☐ Enjoy your senses
(📖 see page 57)

☐ Relax (📖 see page 88)

☐ Use imagery (📖 see page 99)

☐ Enjoy humor (📖 see page 51)

☐ Exercise (📖 see page 114)

☐ Accept what you can't change
(📖 see page 31)

Unimportant & Changeable

If the problem is unimportant, first try just letting it go. But if you can control it with relatively little effort, go ahead and deal with it. Solving small problems helps build your skills and confidence to tackle bigger ones. Use the same strategies described above for important, changeable problems.

Unimportant & Unchangeable

The best solution for these problems is to ignore them. *Starting now, you are given permission to let go of unimportant concerns.* These are common hassles, and everybody has their share of them. Don't let them bother you.

Key Point

If you can't let go of one of these problems, consider reclassifying it as an "important" problem, or try:

☐ Distractions and thought stopping
(📖 see page 175)

☐ Challenging negative thoughts
(📖 see page 42)

☐ Relaxation (📖 see page 88)

☐ Imagery (📖 see page 99)

☐ Humor (📖 see page 51)

📖 *For more information, see page 271*

2 Healthy Thinking

How Optimistic Thinking Improves Health and Happiness

▶ *Doug, Lydia, and John make a sales presentation after weeks of preparation. The response from their new manager: "Lousy. You've completely missed the boat."*

▶ *Doug gets angry, and rages about his boss. "He doesn't know anything about the client or this product. He hates everything I do. I could do his job better than he does. It's not fair." Doug becomes more and more difficult to work with and develops frequent stomach pain.*

▶ *Lydia worries. "I knew he wouldn't understand what I was trying to do," she thinks. "I don't fit here anymore. I'll probably be fired soon. I'll never get anything right. I'm a failure." Lydia finds it harder to go to the office in the morning, can't concentrate on her work, and has trouble sleeping.*

▶ *John feels disappointed at first; then challenged. "He certainly sees things differently," he reflects. "I'd better find out what he was expecting." John sets up a meeting with his boss to discuss revisions of the presentation.*

Here's the same situation, and three different ways of responding to it. Each interpretation has a different result. Before reading on, take a moment to reflect honestly on how you would have responded to this situation. How would you "explain" it to yourself? What would you feel? What do you think the consequences of your response would be?

The Attitude That Works

Doug, Lydia, and John each interpreted the same event in different ways, and each one led to very different feelings, actions, and consequences. Doug's and Lydia's responses illustrate two different forms of negative thinking. Doug blamed unfair circumstances, and Lydia blamed herself. Both of these attitudes are most likely to result in more negative feedback and more bad feelings.

John's response was much more optimistic and allowed him to take constructive action. Though he didn't like being criticized, he didn't let it keep him down. He saw himself as having some control over the situation, and that strengthened his competence.

Key Point

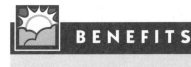

You Feel What You Think

"There is nothing either good or bad, but thinking makes it so."

Hamlet—*Shakespeare*

We often assume that outside events are the cause of our moods and symptoms. But it's remarkable how different people's reaction can be when faced with the same event. Even when we experience the exact same situation at different times or in different moods, it's surprising how differently we can feel and respond to it.

We are constantly talking to ourselves. This "self-talk" is how we explain the events of our lives to ourselves. And it is the way we interpret these external events in our minds that determines how we feel, and determines what actions we decide to take. Some explanations we give ourselves are positive and empowering. Others arouse anger, feed our frustration, or lead us to depression and despair.

Key Point

We are usually not aware of the continuous, automatic chatter in our heads. We may feel anger, depression, or anxiety, but we don't connect these feelings with the negative thoughts that are going on in our minds and bodies. We don't notice how these thoughts shape our mood.

Learn to recognize these patterns. Specific negative thoughts lead to different types of bad moods. For example:

▶ *Thoughts of loss* like, "I've lost everything—my job, my home, and my spouse," are often followed by *sadness or depression*

▶ *Thoughts of unfulfilled expectations* such as, "Why is my spouse always late?" give rise to *frustration and anger*

▶ *Thoughts of possible danger or threat* like, "What if I can't find my way back?" lead to *anxiety and worry*

Negative self-talk greatly limits us. If you are constantly saying to yourself, "I'm not very smart," or "I won't ever amount to much," you probably won't try to learn a new skill. That's because learning a new skill doesn't fit with what you are telling yourself. You become a prisoner of your own beliefs.

But the walls of our prison are made of thoughts, and thoughts can be changed. Self-talk is not something fixed in our biology, and our feelings are not completely out of our control. New, healthier thoughts can be cultivated.

Try Rose Colored Glasses

"Sometimes you just need to look reality in the eye and deny it."

—*Garrison Keillor*

Healthy thinkers see the world through rose-colored lenses. They distort their reality in a positive direction, and most of

CHECK YOURSELF

ARE YOU AN OPTIMIST?

Do you agree or disagree with the following statements? Don't respond with what you think you *should* say, but how you typically view your life.

- ❏ In uncertain times, I expect the best

- ❏ I always look on the bright side

- ❏ I'm optimistic about my future

- ❏ Every cloud has a silver lining

- ❏ If something can go wrong, it will

- ❏ Things never work out the way I want them to

- ❏ I rarely count on good things happening to me

If you *agree* with the first four statements and *disagree* with the last three, you are an *optimist*.

If you *disagree* with the first four statements and *agree* with the last three, you are more *pessimistic*.

Adapted from The Life Orientation Test by Michael Scheier and Charles Carver

the time their rosy illusions benefit them. Healthy thinking *is not* necessarily more realistic; it's just healthier.

Optimists believe that their ability to influence events is much greater than it actually is. If they are playing dice, they believe they have greater control if they are the ones who are throwing the dice, even though the outcome is random. If they are working on a project, optimists believe that the positive aspects of the project stem from them, and the negative ones from their collaborators.

Most of our self-talk—either positive or negative—is simply just not true. That's because no one perceives the outside world with complete accuracy. *Data from our senses is always filtered through and interpreted by our brains. We tell ourselves inaccurate stories, and then believe these stories as though they were true.* Our negative self-talk may appear reasonable, but when challenged, it often falls apart. So if you're going to distort reality anyway, you may as well distort it positively. It's healthier.

Key Point

What Makes an Optimist?

Optimists seek out, remember, and expect positive experiences. With an optimistic frame of mind, they reshape the stories they tell themselves about their past, present and future. Optimists learn to:

- ▶ Be selective, remember mainly the positive events in the past

- ▶ Focus on the present

- ▶ See the future in terms of what can be done instead of what can't happen

- ▶ See threats as challenges—problems to be solved

- ▶ Believe the world is coherent, and their actions make a significant difference

Optimistic thinking doesn't mean you're not touched by life's misfortunes, or never have a negative thought. Even optimists don't feel great all the time. *No one enjoys losses and setbacks, but you don't have to be demolished by them either. How you feel about negative events is usually based on what you tell yourself about them.* Similarly, how good

Key Point

Continued on page 42

OPTIMIST'S AND PESSIMIST'S SELF-TALK

Optimists and pessimists explain their fortunes to themselves in completely different ways. Optimists thoroughly enjoy good events, while pessimists minimize them.

EXPLAINING BAD EVENTS

Optimists

Optimists see setbacks as temporary:

▶ *My daughter and I fought because she was in a bad mood*

▶ *I was exhausted at the time*

Optimists see failure or adversity as specific to the immediate problem:

▶ *I was nervous about giving the speech because the audience was so large*

▶ *I'm not a very good skier*

Optimists explain bad events in terms of external causes:

▶ *I caused a fender bender because all the traffic distracted me*

▶ *I never got a good education*

Pessimists

Pessimists see setbacks as permanent:

▶ *My daughter and I never get along no matter what I do*

▶ *Things never work out for me*

Pessimists generalize the problem to their whole life:

▶ *I was nervous about giving the speech because I always screw up*

▶ *I'm not at all athletic*

Pessimists explain bad events by blaming themselves:

▶ *I caused a fender bender because I'm a lousy driver*

▶ *I'm stupid*

EXPLAINING GOOD EVENTS

Optimists see good events as permanent:

▶ *I'm always lucky*

▶ *I'm really skilled; things go easy for me*

Optimists generalize good outcomes to their whole life:

▶ *I got the job promotion—my whole life is working well*

▶ *I'm smart*

Optimists attribute good events to themselves:

▶ *I know how to take advantage of luck*

▶ *My ability made a big difference*

Pessimists dismiss good events as temporary:

▶ *I'm just lucky today—it won't last*

▶ *Things take lots of extra effort*

Pessimists limit good outcomes to a specific area:

▶ *It went well at the office, but it's still a mess at home*

▶ *I'm good at math*

Pessimists attribute good events to external causes:

▶ *I just got lucky*

▶ *Other people made it work*

THE VALUE OF FAITH

For the majority of people, religious and spiritual beliefs are a vital part of how they think about their lives, and cope with it. These beliefs can provide:

▶ A sense of meaning and purpose
▶ A framework for setting priorities
▶ A way to place stresses in perspective
▶ Comfort during illness or crisis
▶ Support for a healthy lifestyle
▶ Opportunities for social contact
▶ A means of developing supportive relationships
▶ Reasons to help others
▶ A sense of being part of something larger than oneself

Recent research suggests that maintaining religious and spiritual beliefs may improve health. In a study of hospitalized male patients, one in five reported that religion is "the most important thing that keeps me going." Nearly half rated religion as very helpful in coping with their illness. And those that found comfort in religion were significantly less depressed.

A seven-year study of seniors showed the more their religious involvement, the less their physical disability and depression. One interesting finding was that death rates were lower than expected before important religious holidays. This suggests that faith may even postpone death.

Church-attendees have lower blood pressure and half the risk of heart attack than non-attendees, even after making adjustments for smoking and income.

The patients undergoing open-heart surgery who received strength and comfort from religion were three times more likely to survive than those who had no comfort from religion.

A variety of studies find that religious belief and practice is associated with:

▶ Less stress
▶ Less risk of self-destructive behaviors (suicide, smoking and drug abuse)
▶ Greater overall satisfaction with life

Keep the Faith

Many people turn to religion for solace when they're in situations over which they have little control. Religious involvement may counteract feelings of helplessness. It may also give meaning to challenging life situations, and restore a sense of control.

Religion cannot be "prescribed" for you. Such beliefs and values often come from one's family, and are an intensely personal matter. As one way to improve your mental and physical health, we invite you to explore your own beliefs.

▶ If you are religious, tell your doctor. Most won't ask. Help him or her understand the value of your beliefs in managing your health and life.

▶ Consider consulting a religious or spiritual counselor. Choose someone you feel comfortable with. Their advice and counsel can supplement your medical and psychological care.

▶ Find beliefs and practices that suit you. Remember, the comfort and support that faith offers appears to be more important to your health than believing in any particular faith.

Confidence Counts

Changing the way you think is one of the best things you can do to enhance health. Research suggests that positive thinking—optimism, confidence, and a sense of control—has very positive health benefits. It can affect your immune system, your susceptibility to disease, and perhaps even your life span. Here are some studies that demonstrate the power of optimistic thinking:

Optimism and Immunity

▶ In one study, researchers measured chemical substances in saliva that protect us from infections like colds. Immunity was higher on days when people felt positive about their lives than on days when they felt down.

▶ Blood samples were taken from both optimistic and pessimistic people. The optimists had a higher ratio of disease-fighting "helper" immune cells to "suppressor" immune cells than the pessimists.

Optimism and Cancer

▶ Mice and rats were implanted with tumors in several studies, and given electric shocks. The ones who fought the tumors more successfully were those who could turn off the shock by pressing a bar. This gave them some control over a stressful situation.

▶ Confidence and optimism also appear to help those facing life-threatening diseases. Women who had a second occurrence of breast cancer survived longer if they felt joy in living, and talked to themselves optimistically.

▶ There is evidence that people can learn to think more positively, and so improve their physical health. For example, one group of patients with cancer were taught more constructive thinking habits. They also received relaxation training. These patients' natural killer cells showed much higher activity than patients who received similar medical treatment, but no counseling.

Attitude Affects Longevity

▶ In one study, seniors who believed they were in "poor" health were nearly three times more likely to die within seven years than those who rated their health as "excellent." The self-ratings more accurately predicted who would die than the doctors' objective reports.

▶ People who thought they were in poor health (despite the fact that their doctors had given them a clean bill of health) had a slightly greater risk of dying sooner than health optimists. Those who saw themselves as well (even though doctor's reports suggested that they had poor health) lived slightly longer.

▶ Even a sense of control over minor daily events can improve health. Nursing home residents who were given a choice of what to have for breakfast or what night to see a movie were happier and more active. After 18 months, they had half the death rate of those not offered as much control.

Continued on next page

Attitude Affects Illness

▶ In a company undergoing major reorganization, executives who felt a sense of control over their situations felt challenged rather than threatened by the change. They were less likely to get sick than the executives who saw the change as a threat, and felt powerless.

▶ A long-term study of college graduates found that men with optimistic self-talk were physically healthier later in life, and had less chronic illness than more pessimistic alumni. Optimistic students at another college reported fewer sick days, doctor visits, and symptoms (such as fatigue, sore muscles, and coughs) than the students with negative self-talk.

▶ In another study, elderly people were asked to list all the good and bad things they expected to happen in the future. Two years later, those with a more positive outlook had better health (including fewer physical symptoms, less tension, greater energy, and fewer colds) than people who were more negative about the future.

Attitude and Surgery

▶ Optimistic patients facing open-heart surgery develop fewer complications, including heart attacks during surgery. They recover more quickly, and return to work, hobbies, and exercise sooner than their pessimistic counterparts.

▶ Patients undergoing surgery who were given the suggestion that they could control blood flow during the procedure cut their blood loss by half.

Believing Beats Reality

Surprisingly, just believing that you have control—even when you really don't—can affect your physiological response to stress, and your health.

Key Point

In one experiment, people were asked to solve math problems while being distracted by irritating noise. They showed less stress if they were told they could stop the noise by pressing a button. Even though no one pressed the button, and the button didn't really shut off the noise, they still experienced fewer stress symptoms (sweaty hands, racing hearts, ringing ears, and headaches).

Beliefs Become Biology

Because optimists are more active than pessimists, they are more likely to do something for their health (go to the doctor, change their diet, or exercise). Optimists may also be more active than other people in seeking out support—another factor that's been shown to promote health.

We don't yet understand exactly how optimistic thinking translates into better health. But we do know that thoughts determine moods, and moods reflect changes in both hormonal activity and immune function. However it works, the evidence clearly shows that it's worthwhile to learn to think as optimistically as possible.

events benefit you is largely shaped by how you explain them to yourself. Optimistic, healthy thinking helps you cope better with whatever life throws at you.

You may think that optimism and pessimism are traits you're stuck with, but they're not. To a large extent, optimism and pessimism are just *learned habits*. Changing the way that you think and talk to yourself can improve your physical and emotional well-being. Remember, your body speaks its mind (📖 see page 232).

℞ How to Think in a Healthier Way

Inaccurate thoughts can be challenged and changed. On the following pages you will find the best techniques for changing your negative thought patterns to positive ones. It will improve your mood, your happiness, and your health.

℞ Track Your Thoughts

Recognizing unhelpful negative thoughts is the first step to stopping them. The best way to change your thinking is to write it down.

▶ At the top of a piece of paper, briefly describe what is bothering you. Just record the facts of the situation without judgment or interpretation.

▶ Next, draw three columns. On the left side, write down "Feelings/Body Response," and what you feel (angry, depressed, anxious, guilty, headache, weak, etc.).

▶ In the middle column, write "Negative Thoughts," and list the thoughts that went through your mind just before and during the situation. If there are many, pick the stronger ones.

▶ On the right put down "Alternative Responses," and list the arguments against each of your major negative thoughts. Write down a more rational response to it (📖 see box page 43).

Think of your thoughts as hypotheses or guesses. Then critically examine them. Take a good look at the evidence, and compare your thoughts to alternative ways of seeing the situation.

Just reading this exercise won't help straighten out your thinking. *You need to practice it. At first, be sure to do this exercise in writing, not just in your head.* Later you will be better able to recognize some of your negative patterns and correct them as they go through your mind.

℞ Question Pessimistic Self-Talk

Here are ten questions to ask yourself when you challenge your automatic negative thoughts. Each time you discover a pessimistic thought, rethink it to reflect a more positive, optimistic story.

1. Have I really identified what's bothering me?

When you are feeling badly, it's sometimes difficult to put your finger on the real

TRACK YOUR THOUGHTS

__Situation:__ I didn't get the promotion I expected.

Feelings/Body Responses	Negative Thoughts	Alternate Responses
I'm upset, headache	I'm not good enough	I'm successful in many ways
I feel depressed, fatigue	I'll never be successful	I earn a good living
I'm discouraged	Nothing works	My co-workers respect me
		I'll get more training
		I'm a loving husband and father
		I'll keep my eyes open for other opportunities

__Situation:__ I am preparing dinner for guests.

Feelings/Body Responses	Negative Thoughts	Alternate Responses
I'm nervous, sweaty	I'll never get dinner finished on time	There is actually time to finish making the dinner
I'm worried, heart racing	They won't like the meal	If not, I'll ask for some help
I'm angry, tight jaw muscles	They may not even show up	The guests are coming to spend time with me, not to be restaurant critics

__Situation:__ _____

Feelings/Body Responses	Negative Thoughts	Alternate Responses
_____	_____	_____
_____	_____	_____
_____	_____	_____
_____	_____	_____

cause. Review your activities for the past day or two:

▶ What have you been doing recently?

▶ With whom have you been talking?

Try to identify a specific event, situation, or encounter that might have triggered the negative thoughts that led to feeling bad.

2. Am I exaggerating the situation?

Automatic thoughts often exaggerate the importance of situations and events. Put an exaggerated response into a healthier perspective. Ask yourself, "What difference will this make next week, in a year, or in ten years?" Will anyone remember (let alone care) that you made a stupid remark or had dandruff on your sweater a few years from now? Our mistakes are rarely fixed permanently in others' minds.

Or imagine yourself in a hot air balloon looking back down at Earth. How important do your worries appear from that perspective?

3. Am I over-generalizing?

A common mistake is to assume that because something happened once, it will happen again. The truth is, no two situations are exactly the same. You usually have a choice and can respond differently. By generalizing, you lock yourself into a future that's the same as the past. Words like "always" and "never" are tip-offs:

▶ *I'm always late*

▶ *I'll never find another job*

▶ *I'll never find the right person for me*

Watch out for "all-or-nothing" or "either-or" thinking. Other common mistakes are:

▶ Thinking in black or white; most situations are shades of gray

▶ Trapping yourself between two unrealistic viewpoints (*I didn't exercise*

yesterday, and I've blown my regimen completely; I'm pretty stupid and everyone else is brilliant)

▶ Allow for partial successes (*This was not my best moment; even Einstein failed math in high school*)

The tip-off for this type of over-generalization are words like "all," "completely," "nothing," "totally," and "always." And be aware of the labeling trap: "I'm a loser." "He's a jerk." Labels don't accurately reflect the true complexity of real people.

4. Am I overworrying?

We all worry. For example, we think things like:

▶ *I won't get the report done on time*

▶ *David will catch cold in that rain*

▶ *My stomach ache means I have cancer*

Ask yourself what the odds are of each of your worries coming to pass: 50%? 90%?

Most worries are just automatic thoughts with little basis in fact. We often worry about things that are very unlikely to happen. If you worry, make sure you've got a good reason. If you do, then do what you can to fix the situation.

Make a list of your worries and check it periodically. Notice how the vast majority of your anticipated calamities never occur.

5. Am I assuming the worst?

If something does go wrong, would it be a catastrophe? When you consider the *worst* thing that could happen, would it truly be a disaster? Are you underestimating your ability to cope with the situation? Do you think such thoughts as:

▶ *This turbulence means the plane will probably crash*

▶ *I can't stand this anymore*

- *This is the worst thing that ever happened to me*

- *I'll lose my job if I make a mistake*

With catastrophic thinking, small events become disasters. Even big problems or crises become exaggerated. Counter your thoughts of calamity with facts and a more reasonable perspective:

- *Turbulence is very common; it rarely brings a plane down*

- *I'm still here, so I obviously can stand this; I just need a better way of coping*

- *Worse things have happened to me*

- *Everyone makes mistakes; my overall work is actually quite good*

6. Am I making an unrealistic or unfair comparison?

Key Point

Remember, we face the reality our mind makes up, not reality itself. And our minds judge by comparison: experience vs. expectation, this year vs. last, them vs. me, and so on. Our feelings about events are shaped by how much better or worse it was compared to what we expected. Once we understand how our mind works by using comparisons, we can begin to evaluate them with greater insight.

If you find yourself thinking, "I'm not a very good basketball player," for example, ask yourself: "Compared to whom?" Michael Jordan? Your next-door neighbor who played four years of basketball in college? Your 8-year-old son?

If your expectation and comparison level is unrealistic, change it. Try to get a better perspective. Tell yourself, "I play basketball as well as I can." Only one person can be President. Does that mean everybody else has to feel bad?

7. Do I have the evidence for my conclusion?

You may jump to conclusions as though you know what the future holds and think, for example, "I'll never find another job." Or you may assume you're a mindreader: "Sally thinks I'm irresponsible." That may be true, but unless you check it out with Sally, you'll never know. Or you may think: "Keith didn't smile at me. He's mad at me."

Challenge these assumptions, and use alternative responses: "I really don't know why Keith didn't smile. Maybe he didn't see me, or he was in a grumpy mood. I'll call him soon and check it out." Believing that you know what other people are thinking and feeling leads to mistakes more often than not. Don't confuse your feelings with facts.

8. Am I taking it too personally?

"It's all my fault." "I'm responsible that everyone didn't have a good time at the party." "If only I would have treated her better, she wouldn't have left me." Are you blaming yourself for something that is not entirely under your control?

Accepting personal responsibility makes sense only when you're dealing with something you can really influence. To blame yourself because it rained on the date you chose for the party doesn't make sense. Weather, the financial markets, and the actions of others are things that you can't realistically expect to control.

9. Am I discounting the positive?

Are you focusing only on the negative aspects of the situation, and ignoring the positive? Do you think things like, "She only said those nice things about me to make me feel better," or "I was just lucky"? When you filter out the positive, that leaves only the negative to determine your mood.

HEALTHY NEGATIVE FEELINGS

Life is not only about thinking positive, happy thoughts. Emotions, both positive and negative, give texture and meaning to life. There are times when negative feelings are healthy and appropriate. For example:

▶ When a loved one dies, it's okay to feel sad (📖 see page 204).

▶ When someone offends you, anger may be the appropriate response. It may change the offender's behavior (📖 see page 171).

▶ When you feel threatened, anxiety may prepare you to take effective action. It's obviously better to have a suspicious lump checked out than to ignore it; it's better to make lifestyle changes after a heart attack than to hope you'll regain health without doing anything differently (📖 see page 144).

The Limits of Optimism

Optimistic attitudes are certainly not always the major factor in determining who gets sick and who stays well. Your genetic inheritance, environmental conditions, nutrition, exercise, smoking, and other factors all play a role.

Sometimes biological factors dominate, and no amount of positive thinking will reverse them. Still, optimistic thinking can help you to prevent some illnesses, and cope better with others. | Key Point |

Healthy thinking may not prolong your survival, but it can help you maximize your health and functioning in the meantime.

10. Am I expecting perfection?

Do you really think that people should never make mistakes? If you do, you're going to be disappointed frequently. Give everyone (including yourself) a break. Making mistakes is part of being human. Why hold yourself to an impossible standard? Put your energy to better advantage rather than feeling bad. Mistakes can be opportunities to learn and grow if you don't paralyze yourself with self-blame.

℞ Uncover Your Core Beliefs

You can learn a lot by identifying the deeper beliefs that give rise to your negative self-talk. One way to get at them is to take each negative statement and ask yourself, "If that were true, what would it mean and why would that be bad?" For instance, if you're worried that the report you're about to turn in isn't absolutely accurate, you might ask yourself, "If there are errors in this report, why would that be bad?" Your reply might be, "It would mean I haven't done a perfect job."

That leads to the question, "If I didn't do a perfect job, why would that bother me?" *You might find yourself up against an entirely unreasonable belief that nothing short of perfection is acceptable.* | Key Point | Here are some examples of other common (but irrational—and often deep-seated) beliefs:

▶ *Fear and anxiety are the only reasonable responses to anything that is unknown and uncertain*

TRY THIS

REHEARSE SUCCESS

When you aren't happy with the way you handled a particular situation, try this exercise:

▶ Write down three ways that it could have gone better

▶ Write down three ways it could have gone worse

▶ If you can't think of alternatives to the way you handled it, imagine what someone whom you greatly respect would have done

▶ Or think what advice you would give to someone else facing a similar situation

Remember that mistakes aren't failures. They're good opportunities to learn. Mistakes give you the chance to rehearse other ways of handling things. This is great practice for future crises.

▶ *When people disapprove of me, it means I am wrong or bad*

▶ *There is a perfect love and a perfect relationship*

▶ *My worth as a person depends on how much I produce and achieve*

▶ *It's easier to avoid life's difficulties than to face them*

▶ *I'm very fragile and vulnerable*

▶ *If I feel something, then it must be true*

▶ *Unusual physical symptoms always mean that something is seriously wrong with me*

℞ Challenge Your "Shoulds"

Underlying beliefs often involve the word "should":

▶ *I should be thin*

▶ *I should be at the top of my profession*

▶ *I should be a more devoted daughter*

Also watch for the words "must," "have to" and "ought to." They often substitute for "should." Many of us are stuck with "shoulds" that are no longer relevant to us. We may have adopted them many years ago in order to earn someone's approval— perhaps our parents or peers.

When you become aware of a "should," write it down and trace it back to where it came from. Does it represent something you really care about? Does it empower you or drain you? Do you still need it?

If a "should" statement does represent a genuine value which you aren't living up to, try substituting "want" or "could" for "should." So instead of thinking, "I should go visit my mother," say, "I want to go visit my mother." It's a much more positive statement. And it becomes a desire or intention upon which you choose to act, without the added burden of guilt.

℞ Use an Affirmation

To break the cycle of automatic, negative thoughts, many people find it helpful to repeat positive statements called affirmations. *Over time, these affirmations become just as powerful as the negative statements used to be.* Think of a few strong, positive statements about yourself. Put them in the present tense, as though they were already true, such as: "I take care of my body" or "I'm good at my job."

Key Point

Set aside a few minutes each day to repeat the statement to yourself (see page 103).

℞ Get a Sense of Control

A sense of control is important to having an optimistic outlook. "Control" in this context doesn't mean a false sense of power, or freedom from unexpected events. It refers to the belief that you can always have some impact on your situation, and some degree of choice.

One way to build up a feeling of control is to achieve success in small ways. Often we try to change too much at once, and fall flat on our faces. Then we feel like failures.

It's important to find at least one small area in which you can cultivate a sense of competence and confidence. Take time to work on a favorite hobby, cook a special meal, or deal with an annoying home maintenance problem. Get your taxes organized early, or discuss a difficult situation with a co-worker. Your success puts an end to negative generalizations such as, "I can't do anything," and it encourages you to take more steps toward success (📖 see page 149).

Humor can also lighten your thoughts and increase your sense of control. Remember, when faced with a stressful situation you can fight, flee, or laugh (📖 see page 51).

℞ Focus on What You've Got

Key Point *Use your thoughts to increase your happiness. Make it a goal to think about positive events and experiences in your daily life as much as possible.* Focus on what you have, not what you lack. Rather than mulling over your shortcomings or difficulties, think about the good things in your life. It might be your family, your friends, your work, or something you are looking forward to. Every one of us can find something to be grateful for.

Make a personal inventory of your talents, skills, achievements, and qualities—big and small. Celebrate your accomplish-ments. When something goes wrong, consult your list of positives, and put the problem in perspective. It then becomes just one specific experience, not something that defines your whole life.

℞ Act As If...

By acting *as if* something good were true, you can generate positive feelings and thoughts. So you can act yourself into a new way of feeling as easily as you can think yourself into a new way of acting. By changing your facial expression alone you change your physiology as well as your mood.

Even when you don't feel like doing something differently, *just pushing yourself to try* can sometimes shift your mood in a positive direction. Don't worry that you don't feel like doing it. Fake it. Pretend self-esteem. Assume optimism. Be outgoing. Act as if you were confident. Just going through the motions can cause a powerful change. Soon you'll be enjoying the feelings that go along with your new behavior. Give it a try.

℞ Be Mindful

Set aside some time to simply observe your thoughts, *without trying to change them.* With practice, you can learn to sit quietly and watch the endless flow of thoughts as they move in and out of your mind. Don't judge them as positive or negative, just watch them come and go. Over time, this practice removes the emotional dominance of your thoughts. And it opens up more space for a deeper awareness of your present experience (📖 see page 94).

📖 *For more information, see page 272*

3 Humor

How to Use Humor and Laughter to Improve Your Health

"A cheerful heart is a good medicine." — *Proverbs 17:22*

"The arrival of a good clown exercises more beneficial influence upon the health of a town than twenty asses laden with drugs."
— *Thomas Sydenham, 17th century physician*

"Caution: Humor may be hazardous to your illness." — *Anonymous*

When was the last time you laughed really hard? You know, a hearty, sidesplitting belly laugh—the kind that suddenly grabs you and sends you reeling out of control? Or when was the last time you laughed so hard that you forgot what triggered it, leaving you laughing without reason? This kind of laughter is not only enjoyable, it's also health-promoting. And modern science is beginning to confirm that laughter can indeed be good medicine.

Laughter is an invigorating tonic that heightens and brightens mood, gently releasing us from tensions and social constraints. What strikes us as funny is usually triggered by a mismatch between what we expect and what we see.

Humor offers a valuable perspective on ourselves and our world. Psychologist Gordon Allport says, "No person is in good health unless he can laugh at himself...noticing where he has over-reached, where his pretensions have been overblown...where he is too sure of himself, too short-sighted, and above all, too conceited." Laughter is an affirmation of our humanness.

Laughter can be a face-saving way to express our anxieties, fears, and other hidden emotions to others. It breaks the ice, builds trust, and draws people together into a common state of well-being. Entertainer Victor Borge once quipped, "Humor is the shortest distance between two people." Nothing like a rolling tide of laughter to sweep away inhibitions and express warmth and friendliness.

Our culture often inhibits humor, even though it is a most natural, pleasurable response. We are made to associate growing up with "getting serious." We are told we won't get anywhere if we aren't serious about our work. And being "serious" is somehow equated with being solemn—and perhaps humorless.

We are ordered to "wipe that smile off your face." We are told that things are "no laughing matter," as if it's impossible for laughter to coexist with a responsible attitude. Sometimes we repress our good humor, because we're afraid that others will think we're frivolous or foolish. Our

49

What Happens When You Laugh?

A robust laugh gives the muscles of your face, shoulders, diaphragm, and abdomen a good workout, and sometimes even your arms and legs. Heart rate and blood pressure temporarily rise, breathing becomes faster and deeper, and oxygen surges throughout your bloodstream.

Your muscles go limp and your blood pressure may fall after a good laugh. You're in a mellow euphoria. Laughter is called "inner jogging." The total workout of a good laugh can burn up as many calories per hour as brisk walking. And you don't need fancy shoes or even have to get off the couch.

During a good hearty laugh your brain orchestrates hormonal rushes that rouse you to a high-level alertness and numb pain. Researchers speculate that laughter triggers the release of endorphins, the brain's opiates. This may account for the pain relief that accompanies laughter.

Laughter Raises Pain Thresholds

Norman Cousins claimed to nurse himself back to health from a crippling arthritic condition, in part with old tapes of *Candid Camera* television program and Marx Brothers movies. He claimed that ten minutes of belly laughter had an anesthetic effect and would give him at least two hours of pain-free sleep.

Controlled studies suggest that laughter can indeed raise pain thresholds. People listening to twenty minutes of Lily Tomlin joking about the telephone company were far less sensitive to pain than those who listened to an academic lecture. The Tomlin tape also blocked pain as effectively as a standard relaxation tape—and you know which one was more fun.

In a second experiment, a non-humorous but attention-grabbing tape was shown. It had no effect on pain. This proved that it is humor itself which is important—not just any distracting material. So it may be more correct to say, "It only hurts when I don't laugh."

Laughter Reduces Stress

People who use humor a lot are less likely to get upset when faced with negative events. In one study, students had to solve increasingly tricky math problems, becoming highly stressed in the process. Afterwards, they could listen to relaxation tapes, watch an exploration film on Icelandic River, or see a funny *Candid Camera* scene. The relaxation and funny tapes both reduced stress. But humor only worked for people used to laughing a lot. Laughter needs to be a regular part of your life to get its full benefit.

Laughter Enhances Immunity

There's even a hint that laughter may put your immune system in a better humor. Researchers found that watching a funny tape of *Richard Pryor Live* temporarily boosted levels of antibodies in saliva (they help defend us against infections like colds). Those who reported using humor frequently as a way of coping with stress had consistently higher baseline levels of these protective antibodies. And finally, people with a strong sense of humor don't have the expected drop in immune function following exposure to stress.

DEFINITION

THE SCIENTIFIC DEFINITION OF A LAUGH

"A psychophysiological reflex, a successive, rhythmic, spasmodic expiration with open glottis and vibration of the vocal cords, often accompanied by a baring of teeth and facial grimaces." Sounds more like a disease than a cure!

BENEFITS

THE BENEFITS OF LAUGHTER

Humor and laughter can:

▶ Brighten your mood and improve your sense of well-being

▶ Facilitate positive social interaction

▶ Reduce anxiety, tension, depression, anger, and hostility

▶ Lower stress levels

▶ Exercise your heart and cardiovascular system

▶ Reduce pain

funny bone has been broken. We have to repair our sense of humor and relearn how to use laughter because, for many, it doesn't come naturally anymore. But fortunately, laughter is not a bitter pill to swallow.

Humor may be one of our best antidotes to stressful situations. When confronted with a threatening situation, animals have two choices: they can flee, or they can fight. We humans have a third alternative: to

laugh. By seeing the humor in a stressful situation, we may be able to change our response to the threat. Humor allows us to distance ourselves and replace paralyzing feelings of anxiety with mirth. When we laugh, we simply cannot be worrying deeply at the same time.

How to Use Humor to Stay Healthy

"Humor isn't for everyone. It's just for those who want to have fun, enjoy life, and feel alive."

—*Anne Wilson Schaef*

℞ Expose Yourself to Humor

There is a lot of funny material around. Actively seek out things that make you laugh:

▶ Take in regular doses of funny films, joke books, and comedians.

▶ Browse through the humor section of a book store or library.

▶ Make a point of looking at the cartoons in the newspapers and magazines. Cut out the ones that appeal to you, and keep them posted in places where you can see them: on the refrigerator, bulletin board, or in your wallet, and change them regularly.

▶ Laugh at other people's jokes: you'll feel better, they'll feel better, and they'll like you more.

▶ Expose yourself to different styles of humor. If you hate the Marx Brothers it doesn't mean you don't have a sense of humor. Perhaps you prefer political cartoons or dry British humor. The more you tune in to how much that's funny in this world, the more you will enjoy yourself.

℞ Keep a Humor Journal

Get into the habit of listening for the unintentionally amusing remark and note it down in a diary.

Watch for the wonderfully funny things young children spontaneously say or write. One child was lying between his parents enjoying being in the middle. One parent got up and the somewhat dismayed child asked, "What happened to the *middle*?" Another child wrote:

Dear God,

Thank you for the baby brother but what I prayed for was a puppy.

Emily

Listen for the amusing slips of the tongue, or the amusing error or the clever pun ("Seven days without laughter makes one weak").

Watch the newspapers. Sometimes a grammatical error or inappropriate choice of words in a particular context can make a sentence funny: "The sale has fallen through so we now have 100 pairs of surgical boots on our hands."

Other entries you might include in your journal: humorous newspaper headlines, clever bumper stickers, license plates, witticisms, funny events that happen to you or a friend, or stories:

Two space scientists were struggling for months with how to protect a rocket being sent into the intense heat of the sun's surface. Finally, one said, "I've got

a great idea. We'll launch the rocket at night!"

Find (or make up) some funny saying to repeat to yourself whenever the going gets rough, or you start feeling stressed or disappointed. For instance, "When life hands me lemons, I make lemonade," or "When you get to the top of the ladder, you find it is leaning against the wrong wall," or as Charlie Brown said, "I have a new philosophy. I'm only going to dread one day at a time." The saying will give you a wry smile and serve as a pick-me-up. The saying can become an old friend reminding you to see the humorous side, even when things don't feel very funny.

℞ Tell a Joke

Having a good sense of humor doesn't mean you have to have a store of jokes or tell them perfectly. Lots of people who know a good joke say they can't tell them properly, so they keep them to themselves. Or they forget them the moment after they hear them.

Nurture your jokes. If you hear a good one, write it in your journal and tell five other people as soon as possible, so it imprints on your mind. Don't worry about how well you are telling it. Sometimes screwing up the delivery can create something that's even funnier than the original joke.

If you *can't* remember a joke, tune in to everyday situations. Become aware of the sitcom of your own life. Sooner or later we all have experiences that strike us as funny—notice them, collect them, and tell them.

℞ Laugh at Yourself

Focus the humor on yourself rather than others. If you expect to do everything right all of the time, then you can't afford to have a sense of humor. But if you can allow yourself the inevitable mistakes and stupidities that we all make, then you can

MAKE UP A COMEDY ROUTINE

Imagine sitting at a table on which an old tennis shoe, a drinking glass, and an aspirin bottle have been placed. Now make up a comedy routine for three minutes describing the objects on the table in as humorous a manner as you can.

Research shows that the funnier monologue you are able to produce, the less likely you are to become tense, depressed, angered, fatigued, or confused when confronted with stress in your life. And it can be freeing, enabling us to get detached from our problems. After watching funny movies, people solve problems with more ingenuity and innovation.

laugh at yourself. Being able to laugh at yourself helps you to accept that your shortcomings don't really matter that much. The people who are able to laugh at themselves have a much stronger sense of self-worth and higher self-esteem than those who can't.

If you think you are taking yourself too seriously, try to back up and give yourself a sense of perspective. Keep a pair of Groucho glasses to put on at such moments, then twirl in front of the mirror and ask, "just how serious is this?"

When you have a private moment, look at yourself in the mirror and try to compose 10 different funny faces, e.g., sucked-in cheeks, pressed-in nose, crossed eyes, tongue as far above or below your mouth as possible. Work all your face muscles—it will reduce tension. When you have perfected your faces, dare to use one of them on some

appropriate occasion: having fun with the kids, fooling around at work, or to strangers on vacation.

Or do a *Candid Camera* on yourself. Take a step back from your office or your kitchen and see what is going on there with outsiders' eyes. How would they react to the scenario that just now seems of such vital importance to you—your clash with the boss or ambitious colleague or disgruntled salesperson, or your broken dishwasher that's spilled water all over the kitchen floor?

The real test of seeing whether or not you can laugh at yourself is if you can take a bit of teasing. We all need a few things that we are willing to be teased about by our nearest and dearest—things like our clumsiness, forgetfulness, or getting our words twisted, or perhaps a few physical ones such as flat feet or balding. But they really do have to be things you can see the funny side of too. If you don't feel okay about it, gently let the joker know the subject is off limits.

℞ Look for the Funny Side

A stressful situation can sometimes be transformed into a bit of fun if you can see the humor in it. One traveler tells of an airport "horror story":

After a long flight, the group of weary travelers finally arrived, but their baggage didn't. After a long wait one suitcase finally appeared. But it was obviously damaged, and clothing and personal items spilled all over the conveyor belt.

Everyone was becoming quite upset when one group member commented: "Relax, this is really funny. In a few weeks we'll be telling stories about tonight, and we'll be laughing about it. Why wait? If it'll be funny then, it's funny now!"

That comment broke the tension and drew the travelers together. When the other bags didn't arrive, they smiled. When the car rental agency ran out of

HOW MUCH SHOULD YOU LAUGH?

Babies start to laugh when they are 10 weeks old: six weeks later they are laughing about once every hour. Four-year-olds laugh once every four minutes. The average American grown-up is said to laugh only about 15 times per day. Very happy people laugh several hundred times a day, so most of us have a way to go.

cars, they laughed. And when they heard there was a taxi strike, they howled.

Ŗ Exaggerate

Try using humorous exaggeration to help put things into perspective. Expand situations into mock life and death proportions. Woody Allen once remarked:

"More than any other time in history, humankind faces a crossroads. One path leads to despair and utter hopelessness. The other to total extinction. Let us pray we have the wisdom to choose correctly."

Here's another example of how humor puts things in perspective. A daughter at college writes to her parents:

Dear Mom and Dad,

I am sorry that I have not written, but all my stationery was destroyed when the dorm burned down. The car crash that followed when we drove away wasn't as bad as it seemed at the time, for we were all alive. I am now out of the hospital and the doctor said that I will be fully recovered within a few years, and I may well be able to walk one day. I have also moved in with

the boy who rescued me, since most of my things were destroyed in the fire.

Love,
Hilary

PS. There was no fire, no accident and my health is perfectly fine. In fact, I do not even have a boyfriend. However, I did get a D in French and a C in Math and Chemistry, and I just wanted to make sure that you keep it all in perspective.

Ŗ Try a Retake

Ever been stuck in the supermarket line that doesn't move an inch while the lines you rejected are flying past you? You might find yourself thinking, "Oh no, why me, why now, I'm late!"

Try taking another attitude. Reframe the situation. Make your moans into a comic routine for yourself. Exaggerate, add funny extras, explore the humorous possibilities:

"Just my luck. The man at the head of the line knows the checker and they want to chat. So they pretend they don't know the price of canned tuna. In fact, the shopper probably looked everywhere for a can with no price so that he could bring it to his friend the checker. Maybe he has lots of items with no prices. It probably takes him hours to do his shopping, looking for those items. He's just lucky that by the time he's finished collecting all his unpriced items, his friend hadn't gone on break."

Ŗ Try Humor Instead of Anger

Next time you are really livid about an inconvenience—like poor service, try making your point with humor instead of anger:

David went with his family to a fancy

When Laughter is Dangerous

While laughter is generally safe and effective, vigorous laughter should probably be limited if you have a rib fracture, uncontrolled hypertension (high blood pressure), or acute respiratory distress such as an asthma attack. It's probably also not a good idea to make people laugh immediately following abdominal, thoracic, or pelvic surgery.

Unhealthy Humor

Not all humor is positive and healthful. Following are kinds of negative "humor" to watch out for:

▶ **Scorn, sarcasm, ridicule, and contempt.** These can be used to discharge hostile, cynical, and resentful feelings, and are harmful.

▶ *Inappropriate humor.* When people are deeply distressed by the death of a loved one, a joke designed to "cheer them up" is unlikely to be appreciated. Similarly, people who are severely depressed are unable to respond to humor. It may make them feel worse because they realize that once they would have laughed, and now cannot. Someone seeking advice for a troubling personal problem may or may not be helped by a humorous approach. And don't joke about people's names. They have to live with them. Whatever clever comment you think you come up with is probably a very old remark to them. It is important to be sensitive to each occasion and know when humor really helps.

restaurant. Everyone ordered clam chowder. David noticed a gritty texture in the soup, scowled and began to complain angrily. His nine-year-old son, Matt, also noted the grit but replied with a grin, "The clams are so fresh, you can still taste the sand in them!"

℞ Use Humor to Handle Anxiety

Think of something humorous to say when you need someone to know that you are frightened, anxious, or in some way unhappy. It can lighten a tense moment and break the ice.

Nick was lying on a hospital gurney after he mysteriously collapsed in the street. His wife was beside him, anxiously wringing her hands. The atmosphere was extremely tense as a young doctor took down his medical details and asked, "Do you get breathless at night?" "Only when I get lucky," he replied. Everyone suddenly exploded into laughter and the unhelpful tension was broken.

Humor can help reduce anxiety in many different ways. If you are terrified of speaking in public or fear making a presentation at work, for example, imagine your audience wearing funny hats or sitting there without their clothes on. Suddenly they won't seem so threatening. Practice by imagining a stressful situation. Then invent a humorous response, and rehearse it.

℞ Hang Out with Happy People

Make sure there are people in your life whom you find it fun to be around—ones

A GOOD CRY

Have you ever felt better after a good cry? If so, there could be a reason for it. It has been discovered that emotional tears have a different composition than those we shed when something gets in our eye or we chop onions. It's likely that research will reveal that emotional tears contain more of the chemicals released during stress. Even without hard scientific evidence, crying does seem to help release tension and sadness.

If you often prevent yourself from crying, make sure you find times when you do let yourself go, either alone or with someone supportive. If you find it difficult to cry, it is worth getting into practice. Listen to moving music. It can start you off. Or watch a sad film, and then allow the sadness to focus on yourself. But be cautious: as with anger, crying has its limits. *Excessive* tearfulness sometimes offers little relief, and only reinforces sad feelings.

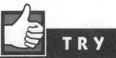

TRY THIS

PUT ON A HAPPY FACE

Try a brief experiment. First, raise your eyebrows and show your teeth. Hold this posture for 30 seconds. What kind of thoughts go though your mind? How do you feel (besides silly)? Now try bringing your eyebrows together and clench your jaw. What are you thinking and feeling now?

℞ Put On a Happy Face

Research has shown that just changing your facial muscles can set off different physiological changes. It can also trigger different thoughts that affect moods of sadness, happiness, and anger. So when we "put on a happy face" in times of adversity, or say "have a nice day" or "smile at a camera and say cheese," we are actually changing our neurohormone levels, and they change our moods. A smile-like pose produces pleasant feelings, whereas a pout produces feelings of unhappiness. So even when you don't feel particularly cheerful and you smile, blood flow to the brain increases, and the production of positive neurotransmitters are stimulated. In other words, if you *look* happier, you might actually start to *feel* happier. So if you can't laugh, smile. And if you can't smile, fake it.

Humor can be a powerful medicine, and laughter can be contagious. It's reassuring in these days of deadly epidemics and sometimes painful, expensive medical treatments that laughter is cheap and effective. And the only side effects are pleasurable.

📖 *For more information, see page 272*

who lighten the atmosphere and make you feel good about yourself.

Often people who aren't especially witty as a rule can be razor-sharp when they get together with someone who inspires them, amuses them, or just loosens them up. Certain people make you feel relaxed and happy. Others are too full of gloom and doom, or are just relentlessly serious. Try to avoid getting brought down by those who are negative. Spend more time with people whose presence gives your mood a boost. If you don't know such people, seek them out.

4 Enjoy Your Senses

How to Use the Pleasure of Your Senses for Better Health

Today many of us aren't getting our minimum daily requirement of sensory pleasures—pleasures that are vital to our health and well-being.

Human beings evolved to find pleasure in natural sensory experiences: the sweetness of ripe fruit, the satisfactions of sex, the chorus of a flock of birds, the peaceful view stretching from a mountain top all the way to the horizon.

But many sensual pleasures we're designed to experience are thwarted in the modern world. We miss the glory of the sunrise and sunset as we hustle in our commute; we miss the stars in our city-lit nights. The synthetic foods in our markets often bear little resemblance to the natural foods we were built to eat. Our ancestors heard the pleasant sound of a stream and the wind rustling in the trees, but for us it's the din of traffic, jackhammers, and deafening leaf blowers.

Source of Survival and Pleasure

Our senses provide information about the world that is critical for our survival. They warn us of danger. Without sight, avoiding traffic, a cliff edge, or a raging river becomes dangerous. The sound of a snapping twig warns us of an approaching predator. The stench of spoiled food stops us from eating poison. A flash of pain prevents a serious burn. The chill of freezing weather inspires us to dress warmly, preventing frostbite.

But our senses do more than alert us to danger. Through pleasure, they guide us to experiences that enhance health. The pleasures of touch and sex make procreation more likely. Our taste for variety helps us to eat many different kinds of foods, thus insuring a wide range of nutrients. Sensory pleasure and positive mood is nature's way of letting us know that we are doing things that are contributing not only to our survival, but to our health as well.

Certainly there are unhealthy pleasures: cigarette smoking, excessive drug and alcohol use, prolonged sunbathing, and eating junk food, to name a few. *But for the most part, pursuing things that make us feel good is one of the simplest routes to better health.*

Key Point

We are not recommending senseless pleasures at the sacrifice of the rest of life. But the modern world has deprived us of too many of our natural sensory requirements for comforting touch, stimulating taste, aromatic fragrances, soothing sounds, and relaxing nature scenes. Happily, it turns out that one of the best ways we can help extend and enrich our lives is to spend more time enjoying life. We are designed for pleasure, and we need doses of it daily.

BENEFITS

Take Your Senses Seriously

Enjoying your senses can:

▶ Improve your mood

▶ Enhance relaxation

▶ Help you focus on the present

▶ Lower your blood pressure

▶ Reduce stress, anxiety and depression

▶ Possibly enhance immune function

▶ Decrease pain

WATCH OUT

Don't Tune Out

Brad sits down to enjoy a delicious meal. He eats the first bite and smiles, enjoying the flavor. Then it's "off to the races" in his mind. He thinks about the day's events, his plans for tomorrow, his worries, his fears, and his hopes—everything but the food. Then he discovers he is finished with his meal.

The same thing happens with sound, touch, smell, and even sex. We are often only vaguely aware of what's going on. *To fully enjoy your senses, you have to pay attention. Since we often go on automatic pilot, focus on the pleasures your senses can bring.* Mindlessness is the enemy of sensual pleasure. Stay tuned in to the moment.

Key Point

Avoid the habit of substituting words and thoughts for direct sensory experience. As you listen to the sounds around you, your mind often jumps to label them: there's a car, a bird, a child's voice. But once it's labeled you stop hearing it. So when you listen, *really listen.* When you eat, *really taste.* Also:

Avoid Repetition and Sameness

Try grasping your hands together. Hold them still. When they first join, there is immediate tactile stimulation. You rapidly adapt to it, and lose awareness of it. *Things that are constant and repetitious no longer bring sensory pleasure.*

Key Point

Watch for Undermining Thoughts

You can undermine your pleasure with thoughts. You might tell yourself, "I don't have time to listen to music." This thought tells you that sensory pleasures are not important—certainly not as important as work or making money. Or you might hear yourself say, "I don't deserve this," or "if it feels this good, it's got to be bad for me." Guilt undoes the pleasure. Monitor your thoughts about pleasure (📖 see page 42).

Treat Yourself to Therapeutic Touch

Touch is essential to survival. Without it you wouldn't know to pull your hand away from a hot fire, or keep your tongue out of harm's way while chewing. Touch helps you eat, mate, and procreate. And you need the sense of touch to control everyday tools from steering wheels to keyboards. Touch is a form of communication: it often expresses what words cannot. Touching, hugging, and cuddling make us feel closer to other people, and to our pets. It can also be a supremely pleasurable experience. So satisfy your skin hunger!

YOUR SENSE OF TOUCH

Our skin is our body's largest organ, with millions of nerve receptors. No wonder touch is so important. Yet in the United States it is often the most neglected sense.

Our society distances us from others. Today's parents use strollers and don't carry their children as often as their parents did. American caregivers touch their children primarily to control and discipline, whereas those in Mediterranean countries touch mainly to soothe and comfort.

We don't give each other massages, baths, or hugs very often. Couples in cafes in the U.S. and England are rarely seen touching each other, whereas in other countries such as France and Puerto Rico couples touch and caress frequently: as much as 180 times an hour!

℞ Get More in Touch

▶ Get or give a hug or massage.

▶ Take a massage break instead of a coffee break. Exchange a quick head, neck, or shoulder rub with a colleague.

▶ Practice self-massage: gently rub the muscles of your face, neck, and shoulders.

▶ Try rubbing your hands together rapidly and then place your warm palms like cups over your eyes. Feel them relax in the darkness and warmth.

▶ Explore the roughness of tree bark, the smoothness of a flower petal, the coolness of a stone.

▶ Take up an art or craft and enjoy the tactile sensation—savor cool, wet clay, or soft warm yarn.

▶ Take off your shoes and socks and walk on soft grass; wiggle your toes in mud or wet sand; stroll through the surf.

▶ Ride a bike and feel the wind blowing through your hair.

▶ Pet an animal.

▶ Enjoy the weather: the sensation of cool mist on a foggy day, or the warm soothing heat of the sun.

▶ Treat yourself occasionally to a long soak in a bath, hot tub, or sauna. For added pleasure and relaxation, add fragrant, healing oils or herbs.

TOUCH: AN ESSENTIAL NUTRIENT

In the early part of this century most healthy institutionalized orphans died before the age of two. When researchers realized that babies who were doing poorly responded to tender loving touch, they changed the way the babies were handled. By incorporating touch regularly into their care, the death rate plummeted to less than 10 percent.

Healthy animals—including humans—know instinctively that their young need to be touched in order to thrive. Both animal and human offspring deprived of touch grow more slowly than normal.

All infants require touch. One group of premature infants were treated to 15-minute massages three times a day for ten days. They gained nearly 50% more weight, and were discharged from the hospital six days earlier than untreated infants who received no massage.

Massage Works

In one study, a group of older children who were hospitalized for depression and adjustment problems received a 30-minute back massage every day for five days. Another similar group saw relaxing videos instead. The group that got the massages were less depressed and anxious. They slept better, and had lower levels of stress hormones. An interesting sidelight to this study is that the hospital staff also requested massages!

Massage can also help adults with chronic anxiety. Patients with chronic muscle tension, body aches, and pain who failed to improve after anti-anxiety medications, antidepressants, muscle relaxants, and relaxation exercises were given 10 sessions of massage. Afterwards, most reported less tension, pain, and need for medications.

Massage may even have a positive effect on the immune system. In a study of HIV-positive patients, regular massage appeared to increase natural killer cells. These cells are one of the immune system's first lines of defense.

Touch Helps Both Sick and Well

Touch speaks to our hearts, and our hearts respond. If a nurse quietly holds the hand of an unconscious patient, rapid, irregular heartbeats decease.

Touch may also be helpful for the healthy. Office workers who received brief massages twice a week for a month were more alert, finished math problems quicker, and made fewer mistakes.

Heat Can Also Help

Our skin also has sensors for temperature. We tend to seek out warm, sunny climates, saunas, steam baths, and hot tubs.

Saunas can decrease muscle and joint pain, and may help sleep. One study found that sitting in a sauna for 30 minutes increased beta-endorphins, the internally-produced chemicals that relieve pain and produce a sense of well-being. It may not be far-fetched to speak of a "sauna bathers' high."

Regular saunas may also help boost the immune system and prevent colds. In a study of German children, those who took weekly saunas lost only half as many school days due to colds and ear infections as those who took no saunas.

℞ Treat Yourself to Visual Medicine

Watch birds nest in a tree. Observe brilliant white clouds in a clear blue sky. Notice blossoms about to bloom. Gaze deeply into a wood fire. Watch fish wander slowly, hypnotically, back and forth.

YOUR SENSE OF SIGHT

We have a deep-seated hunger for natural beauty. When given a choice between looking at a scene from nature with lots of foliage or a city landscape without vegetation, we choose the natural scene.

This may come as no surprise, but such choices may mean more than personal preference. Looking at natural beauty helps us recover from surgery, tolerate pain, and manage stress.

Sight is our most dominant sense. For millions of years we have evolved to be comfortable in a natural environment. In evolutionary terms, it hasn't been very long since we began spending most of our time indoors, trading books for fields, televisions for forests, and mirrors for mountain vistas. Even when many of us are surrounded by nature, we ignore it. We drive to and from work without noticing the clouds, the trees, or the stars. But our connection to nature is still strong, even if we aren't always aware of it.

℞ Get More from What You See

You may not need a meditation technique, a long course in biofeedback training, or weeks of instruction in stress management to relax. Just watch a bird out the window or waves at the seashore, or look at a bouquet of flowers. Spend some time each day noticing nature. If you have access to a window with a view, look out often, if only for a moment. Wherever you go, notice the beauty of nature around you.

You may not have the Grand Canyon or a view of majestic mountains at your doorstep, but no matter where you live, you can find some small part of nature to contemplate. *Any natural view can get your attention outside yourself, and stop the internal monologue of thoughts and worry. This sight reconnects you with the larger natural world around you.*

Key Point

℞ Bring the Outdoors In

Small things can help keep you in touch with nature. Bring some of these things into your home or work environment:

▶ Plants: a bonsai plant (it can make a small pot seem like a forest), a potted bulb, or an herb garden

▶ Photographs or paintings of outdoor scenes

▶ A pet (fish, bird, cat, or dog)

▶ A collection of beautiful stones

▶ Autumn leaves

▶ A basket of pine cones

▶ Blossoming spring branches

VISUAL TREATS

When people are shown slides of natural scenes, they say they have more positive feelings such as friendliness and elation. They also have fewer feelings of sadness and fear than when they look at man-made urban scenes. And our bodies respond to nature:

▶ Compared to cityscapes, images of natural habitats such as lakes, trees, and vegetation produce lower blood pressure, less tension, and more relaxation.

▶ Patients recovering from surgery develop fewer complications, need less strong painkillers, and leave the hospital sooner if their bedside window looks out on trees rather than a brick wall.

▶ Office workers with a view of nature said they had fewer ailments, better health, more job satisfaction, less frustration, more enthusiasm, and were generally happier with their lives than those who had no view, or a view of buildings.

▶ And the more satisfied these workers were with the natural environment surrounding their homes, the better their health was.

Faster Stress Recovery

What we see also influences how quickly we recover from stress. After watching a graphic film of bloody accidents, viewers had an increase in anxiety, muscle tension, blood pressure, and skin conductance—all measures of a stress reaction. But when the stress-provoking film was followed by ten minutes of nature scenes of trees and water, their recovery from stress was faster than if they watched urban scenes.

Gazing at Fish Helps

A group of volunteers were stressed in order to raise their blood pressure. Then they stared at a blank wall for twenty minutes, and after that, they looked at an aquarium containing colorful tropical fish for twenty minutes. Aquarium-gazing reduced blood pressure and relaxed the volunteers more than looking at the blank wall did. In some people with hyper-tension, their blood pressure fell to normal after gazing at the fish.

But the relaxation effect was lost if people were asked to stare into an *empty* fish tank. They quickly became bored, and their blood pressure rose.

In another study, aquarium gazing before dental surgery decreased patients' anxiety and discomfort as much as hyp-nosis during the surgery.

Pleasant Views Restore

Mental fatigue makes you less able to concentrate, more likely to make mis-takes, more irritable, and even more hostile. Encounters with nature appear to be an excellent remedy for mental fatigue.

Looking at a natural environment is restorative because it gives you a feeling of "being away"—like a tiny vacation for the mind and soul—a brief respite in a moment's glance at a tree or bird in flight. Yet many people regard access to natural environments as a luxury rather than a necessity for health and well-being.

Treat Yourself to Musical Medicine

Would you believe that some people find music more thrilling than sex? That's what one survey found. Music and other sounds are a powerful part of our lives.

YOUR SENSE OF SOUND

We live in a "sound soup." From the first moment we first hear our mother's heartbeat in the womb to the strains of the funeral march, our ears are always active. In between we hear a continuous array of sounds, from endless hours of shopping mall Musak, jackhammers, rock concerts and classical recitals to happy sounds of children's laughter, cats purring, clocks ticking, and rain falling. *Whether it's Bach, jazz, rock, or gospel, music can powerfully alter your moods, your emotions, and even your physiology.*

Key Point

You may have noticed that certain music puts you in a romantic mood or makes you feel like dancing. Although we all have our unique preferences, most of us agree that high-pitched music is "happy" and "playful," fast beats make us "alert" and "aroused," and low-pitched music is "sad" or "serious." Slow, quiet music calms and relaxes us. Several experiments show that music has a greater positive effect on mood and anxiety when people can *choose* what they like. Many classical and New Age pieces may be intended to soothe, but if you dislike them, they can make you more anxious. Experiment, and find what kind of music you really like.

Perhaps music's allure stems from its ability to absorb your attention and distract you from unpleasant thoughts, feelings, and memories. The right music at the right time brings you joy or serenity, soothes your frazzled nerves, or lifts you up when you're feeling down.

℞ Listen to Nature

Sounds of nature can be refreshing, renewing, and soothing. Take time out to experience natural sounds: the chatter of squirrels, songs of birds, or wind through the trees. Take walks in the woods, by a lake, or by the ocean. Listen to audio tapes of nature sounds—the sound of a soft summer rain, the twitter of birds, or waves gently breaking on the shore.

℞ Make Your Own Music

Over 2,500 years ago, Pythagoras, the Greek philosopher, advocated singing and playing an instrument every day to purge the body of worry, sorrow, fear, and anger. That advice is still good today. Learning to play a musical instrument enhances the pleasure you get from music. It also increases appreciation, sense of mastery and pride of accomplishment.

Take up a musical instrument—perhaps a drum, a recorder, a guitar or a harmonica. Find the best learning situation for you: private lessons, classes, how-to books, or tapes. You might prefer playing with others, or by yourself.

MUSICAL MEDICINE

Since ancient times, healing with sound and chanting has been practiced all over the world. Today modern medicine is using music for a number of conditions.

Physiological Effects

Music influences respiratory rate, blood pressure, stomach contractions, and hormone levels. Heart rates slow down or speed up to synchronize with a musical beat, and music can alter our brain's electrical rhythms.

Immunity

Music may help healthy people stay well, possibly through its influence on the immune system. In one study, night shift nurses with stress-related problems listened to tapes of music, relaxation exercises, and guided imagery. Afterwards, their biological rhythms were more in sync, and their stress hormone levels—the ones that can suppress immune function—didn't rise as fast.

Surgery

Patients who listen to music before, during, or after surgery feel less pain and anxiety, require less medication, and recover faster. Music blocks distressing sounds that provoke anxiety. In one study, music in the operating room throughout surgery cut the amount of sedative required in half. In another study, music was estimated to be as effective as 2.5 milligrams of Valium.

Pain Relief

When patients listen to the music of their choice, they report less anxiety and discomfort while undergoing uncomfortable medical examinations. "Dentist music" enhances the effect of anesthesia. Music can reduce the pain and duration of labor by as much as two hours.

Intensive Care

Premature infants who listened to Brahms' Lullaby gained weight faster and left the hospital sooner than babies not treated to music. In intensive coronary care units music reduces rapid, irregular heart rates, lowers blood pressure, increases pain tolerance, and lessens anxiety. In one study of patients after a heart attack, music was more relaxing than meditation.

Easing Sleep

In a geriatric nursing home, light, sedative music was introduced before bedtime. After three months, the number of residents who needed sleeping pills was reduced by more than two-thirds. Lullabies work for all ages.

Chronic Disease

Music reduces depression, and anxiety in burn, kidney dialysis, organ transplant patients, and those isolated with contagious diseases. Music also eases the pain, calms the anxiety, and lifts the spirits of the chronically or terminally ill.

Mental Health

When music accompanies guided imagery, it facilitates psychotherapy. It is also useful in treating conditions that have a strong emotional component such as headaches and digestive problems.

LET MUSIC CHANGE YOUR MOOD

See how music affects your mood by listening to a variety of musical styles. Note whether the music makes you sad, happy, relaxed, or energized so that you can create that feeling again whenever you wish.

Try listening to music to change an anxious mood, or relieve chronic pain. You can begin with "tense" music that matches your mood. As you get in sync with it, make a gradual transition to pieces that are more calming.

Or take singing lessons. Join a singing group, or just sing along with recorded music. Singing is a natural "breathing exercise" that can relax and invigorate you.

℞ Move with Music

Try exercising to music for more gain and less pain. Music gets you in tune with your body, increases endurance, regulates breathing, and gets you in the mood to exercise. In one study, moving to an even rhythm made muscles flex and extend more smoothly. Upbeat, fast tempo music tends to make you feel less tired, but light rock seems to improve endurance and lower heart rate more effectively than the booming, bone-jarring variety.

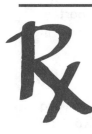

Treat Yourself to a Pleasure Diet

Eating involves more than taste. When you eat, use all your senses. Eat slowly, savor the food, and pay attention to the different tastes, textures, and aromas.

YOUR SENSE OF TASTE

We eat to celebrate, to commemorate, and to nourish our bodies, but most of all, we eat for pleasure. A German survey rated "a fine meal at home" as one of the major pleasures in life. It ranked above parties, hobbies, sleeping, TV, and movies.

But our enjoyment of food is diminishing in modern times. On the one hand, we often short-circuit the enjoyment by gulping down our meal without really tasting it (how often have you finished some delicious treat only to realize that you hardly tasted it?). On the other hand, we sacrifice the pleasures of the palate in the name of low-fat, high fiber fare and weight-loss diets. Can you still eat a piece of chocolate, banana cream pie, or a high-fat ice cream cone without guilt undermining your enjoyment? When you decide to indulge, at least enjoy it!

FOOD FOR THOUGHT

Through the release of certain brain chemicals called neurotransmitters, some foods act like weak drugs. For example, protein foods release chemicals that tend to keep us awake, alert, and mentally energetic. Carbohydrates and fatty foods often make us calm, relaxed, and drowsy. You can take advantage of this knowledge.

Enjoying Food Aids Absorption

The enjoyment of food may influence its nutritional value. A Swedish study showed that people absorbed more iron when they ate attractively presented food than when they ate the same food blended into an ugly gloppy goo. In another study, people from Thailand were given Swedish food and Swedes were given Thai food. Neither group was happy with their meal and members of both groups absorbed less iron than when they ate their favorite food.

A Flavorful Diet Helps

One researcher increased the weight loss and satisfaction of a group of dieters by boosting food flavor, but not calories. One group of the dieters ate standard, low-calorie foods. A second group ate similar meals but with the taste boosted with noncaloric flavoring and spices. A third group treated themselves to a burst of chocolate or vanilla spray on their tongues before meals, and any other time they had a craving for food. Enhancing the flavor boosted weight loss and made for happier, more satisfied dieters.

Spicy Food is Good for You

Chili peppers, which many people enjoy because of their fiery hot sensation, also pack a healthful wallop. Spices and herbs boost flavor without boosting calories or fats. The active ingredient in chili peppers—capsaicin—has beneficial effects. It may loosen congestion due to colds, burn up excess calories, thin the blood to help prevent heart attacks, lower cholesterol, prevent certain cancers, and trigger mood-elevating endorphins.

Garlic is Good for You Too

Garlic lovers can rejoice: the "stinking rose" may do a lot more than flavor food and show us who our true friends are. Several studies suggest garlic may reduce "bad" (LDL) cholesterol, increase "good" (HDL) cholesterol, prevent blood clots and avert heart attacks, lower blood pressure, protect against cancer, and boost the immune system.

THE EVOLUTION OF GOOD TASTE

It is possible to recapture the pleasures of taste and enjoy better health, but it requires some understanding of how our tastes evolved. Taste and smell help us avoid poisons and seek out nutritious foods. We are evolutionarily programmed with a "sweet tooth"—one that guided our ancestors to ripe fruits, a ready source of energy and vitamins.

A taste for fatty foods also served our ancestors well. Since fats are a rich source of calories and fat-soluble vitamins, they could tide them over during difficult times of famine.

We also evolved to seek out foods with different tastes. We get bored eating the same things day after day. Our craving for variety helps insure our intake of a full range of nutrients.

But unfortunately, our inborn appetites can no longer guide us through an overabundance of delectable foods available in the modern world. Evolution's safety mechanisms are fooled by synthetic foods that taste, smell, and look like what they're not. We consume liters of sweet liquids that don't contain a single nutrient. In just one trip to the supermarket we have access to more fatty foods than our ancestors had in a year.

How can we turn nature around in our favor? Paradoxically, by paying more attention to the flavor of what we eat. If we really savor every bite, we're likely to eat less, but enjoy it more. Thorough chewing breaks food down, and this releases more taste-filled molecules. Longer chewing also creates more air currents. These carry odor molecules up the back of the throat to the nose, and they increase the flavor. And eating at a leisurely pace also allows time for your body to realize it is full.

℞ Use All Your Senses

The many different qualities of food are amazing: the crisp sweetness or tartness of an apple, the startling visual beauty of a kiwi, the sensual ruby-like seeds of a pomegranate, the crunch of a carrot, the flavor explosion of a single sac in a section of an orange. So make the effort to prepare foods that are flavorful, aromatic, and colorful. Baking bread smells wonderful. Fresh fruits and vegetables such as bright red peppers, blueberries, orange cantaloupes, and brilliant green vegetables—are not only good looking, they're good for you because they are particularly high in healthful nutrients. Enjoy selecting, chopping, and serving food. Arranging food attractively also enhances the taste.

℞ Taste With Your Nose

Remember, most flavor comes from your nose. If you bite into an apple or an onion with your nose pinched, or when you have a stuffy nose, you can't tell the apple from the onion. So be aware of the aromas of foods, and enjoy them. Sometimes smelling the food alone can satisfy your hunger for sensation, providing more pleasure and fewer calories.

℞ Cultivate Your Palate

We often get stuck in a routine of consuming the same old foods week after week. Arrange a special evening (or several) with friends or family and seek out a new cuisine that you haven't tried before. Try new recipes, and don't rule out anything until you have tasted it.

One little American boy's favorite food is a Japanese sushi dish of grilled eel. How would he ever have discovered that unless he was willing to taste it in the first place?

And since our taste changes, be willing to try foods you rejected in the past.

℞ Eat What You Are Hungry For

Since eating is such an easily available pleasure, we often reach for food. Many people can't even recognize true hunger because they eat so often and so much. But it's a good idea to find out what you're hungry for before you start automatically eating. Perhaps you really want ice cream, but you distract yourself with pounds of other foods first. Tune in to what you are really hankering for, and go for that.

℞ Don't Use Food as a Substitute

You don't always have to eat when you feel hungry. Try a day of fasting: it will allow you to experience real hunger. And the next time you automatically reach for something in the refrigerator, consider if it's food you really want. Perhaps you're feeling emotional hunger and need companionship, nourishing talk, or comfort. Or perhaps another type of sensual pleasure would satisfy you more. Try going for a walk or to a movie, listening to music, getting a massage, or, if available, try some comforting cuddling instead of food.

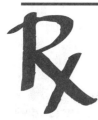

TRY THIS

WAKE UP YOUR SENSES

Take a single piece of chocolate and pretend it is the last chocolate on earth. Imagine that you will never again have a chance to experience this food again. To fully enjoy it:

▶ Concentrate on the beautiful, rich brown color before you put it in your mouth

▶ Feel the weight and texture of the chocolate as you gently toss it from hand to hand

▶ Slowly inhale the rich chocolate aroma—that complex, earthy smell

▶ Now take the smallest bite you can, and extract as much taste as possible from that speck

▶ Take a larger bite; see how it melts from solid to liquid in your mouth

▶ Savor the creamy feel of the chocolate as it melts at exactly body temperature

▶ Then swallow and enjoy the lingering after-taste

℞ Treat Yourself to Aromatherapy

The sense of smell can make our lives delightful. The crisp fragrance of a pine forest invigorates, the smell of a certain flower triggers memories, the scent of a lover arouses. Our noses can also save our lives by warning us of gas or smoke or spoiled food.

AROMATHERAPY

The ancients used the power of smell for healing. They worked with fragrant oils, herbs, flowers, and other natural substances. Modern science is discovering the value of some of these practices. For example, modern aromatherapy is being tried in patients with insomnia, anxiety, phobias, panic attacks, depression, nausea, back pain, migraine, and food cravings. And one company now offers a strawberry scented surgical mask to help calm patients under anesthesia.

In Japan, a fragrance company claims that a lemon scent boosts office workers' energy, jasmine calms hotel guests, and lavender reduces mental fatigue during prolonged business meetings.

Fragrances may also improve concentration and learning. In one study on aromatherapy, subjects did connect-the-dot puzzles. When asked to repeat them, the test-takers who sniffed scented oil finished about 30% faster than those breathing unscented air.

Some smells invoke positive memories or emotions that have beneficial physiological effects. Others focus our awareness, distracting us from less pleasant thoughts. When we savor a pleasant aroma we take slow, deep, breaths, and become more relaxed.

One study measured physiological responses to stress-provoking questions. If people were treated to a whiff of spiced apple before the mental stress, the stress response was blunted. Blood pressure declined, breathing and heart rate slowed, and muscles relaxed. The scent also increased their alpha brain waves, which are associated with a relaxed but alert state. With exposure to the scent people also felt happier, less anxious, and more relaxed.

YOUR SENSE OF SMELL

Ever since our ancestors stood upright and left the trees, our "distance senses"—sight and sound—became our main source of information about threats and opportunities in our environment. So we don't appreciate smell as much. But smell has a great (though often subconscious) influence on our moods and memories. That's because of its connection with the brain's emotion-generating areas.

Smell is the only sense that leads from the world directly to the brain. Odors are registered in the "oldest" part of the brain, responsible for our most basic emotional reactions: pleasure, fear, and the "fight-or-flight" response. This "nose-brain" also governs memory, sexual behavior, hunger, and basic body processes such as heart rate, respiration, and temperature. Smell is deeply linked with each of these functions, making it powerful and immediate.

While particular scents may have an inborn effect on our mood and physiology, most of our reactions to them are colored by our previous experiences. As people have very different associations with smells, they

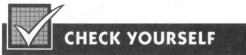

CHECK YOURSELF

Take turns with a friend holding familiar things under each other's noses, and guess what they are (the sniffer keeps her or his eyes closed). Try coffee, toothpaste, soap, wine, food, vanilla, garlic, and other spices and herbs. With each odor, see how many components you can identify.
Is the aroma:

❑ Earthy?

❑ Flowery?

❑ Spicy?

❑ Citrus-like?

❑ Cedar-like?

❑ Fresh-smelling?

❑ Musty?

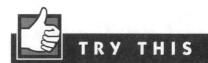

TRY THIS

PROGRAM YOUR NOSE

Take advantage of the power of scents to trigger intense, vivid recall of a particular mood or memory. Or you can program your mind and body to respond to certain scents. For example, try practicing a relaxation exercise (📖 see page 88). Once deeply relaxed, take some sniffs of a pleasant scent, such as lavender.

Gradually you will learn to associate relaxation with that specific scent. Once your mind has got it, you can quickly evoke the sense of relaxation or well-being just by taking a whiff of the scent alone. You can then use fragrance-enhanced relaxation to calm yourself before or after entering stressful situations.

have different responses to them. A whiff of cinnamon may remind some of a kitchen in childhood; other smells bring to mind vivid memories of a terrible tasting medicine.

℞ Know Your Nose

You may want to test various odors in perfumes, colognes, spices, and foods to find out what their effect is on your mood and memory. When you know your responses, you can use the scents at a particular time to create a desired mood.

℞ Expand Your Sense of Smell

There are more than 10,000 known scents. When asked to identify an odor such as toothpaste, bubble gum, lemon, or coffee by smell alone, the average person can

usually get it right 70% of the time.

Many people such as Helen Keller, great perfumers, and wine connoisseurs, have developed highly acute and sensitive olfactory talents. With practice nearly everyone can increase his or her odor vocabulary (📖 see box this page). Developing your olfactory vocabulary can enhance your awareness and enjoyment of the scentual world around you.

Enjoying your senses can be a powerful natural medicine. Remember to use them well to manage your moods and improve your health.

📖 *For more information, see page 272*

5 Healthy Sex

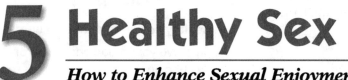

How to Enhance Sexual Enjoyment for Better Health

"Sex can deplete the body of precious elements."
— *An Ancient Greek Text*

"Masturbation can cause blindness, hairy palms, warts, and madness."
— *Folk Tale*

Although the above quotes are myths which are no longer widely held, the simple act of sex is still shrouded in a cloud of misunderstanding, dissatisfaction, and guilt. To make matters worse, today we have to contend with a growing risk of sexually transmitted diseases. **AIDS**, gonorrhea, syphilis, and herpes are on the rise. So it may seem strange to recommend sex as a valuable antidote for disease, but it can be a valuable pathway to better health.

How to Enhance Sexual Enjoyment

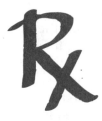

Many of us think that good sex should just come naturally—we should instinctively know how to be good lovers without instruction or practice. We are blessed with a primary biological drive for sex and procreation, but satisfying lovemaking is more often than not a learned skill. Lack of knowledge of the body and sexual techniques is common, and it limits our potential for satisfying sex. While we're not offering a sex manual, we can highlight the types of thoughts, feelings, and actions that lead to a healthy and satisfying sex life.

℞ What is Good Sex?

Enlighten yourself about what lovemaking really is all about: the sharing of an emotional closeness through physical interaction. Healthy sex is:

▶ Freely chosen

▶ Conscious of consequences

▶ Respectful

▶ Erotic

▶ Playful

▶ A way to be closer

▶ An expression of love

▶ Caring

Good sex doesn't always have to mean intercourse, orgasm, ejaculation, or even sexual arousal. Make love sometimes just by holding your partner, and concentrate solely on the physical and emotional closeness you feel.

Try to get a clearer picture of what *you* really want and value about sex. Is it:

▶ The setting?

▶ What you do before and afterward?

▶ The degree of emotional commitment?

Think about the qualities that make a sexual experience satisfying to you, and communicate them to your partner.

℞ Time for Sex

Sex takes time. Work and other interests compete for our time and energy. Sex is often the first thing to go during times of mental stress, illness, parenting, pregnancy, or aging.

You may take it for granted that you can return to it later on. Don't. *If your sex life isn't working, give it the same attention you'd give to other problems in your life.*

Key Point

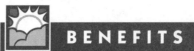

BENEFITS

HEALTHY SEX

A healthy sexual relationship can:

▶ Improve your mood and sense of well-being

▶ Reduce a sense of isolation

▶ Improve your satisfaction with your relationship

▶ Reduce pain, menstrual, and reproductive problems

▶ Possibly lessen your risk of heart disease, depression, anxiety, and hostility

Make touching, cuddling, loving, and sex a real priority. Don't let other events interfere. Sure it may cost you points at work to take a long weekend off with your lover, but what are you working for?

Many lawyers now say that sexual incompatibility is a primary but often hidden issue in divorce. The complaints usually focus on cruelty, lack of commitment, or broken promises, but the real problem often boils down to difficulties with the couple's sex life.

People have very different sexual appetites. If your sexual relationship is a problem—even a small one—heed it. Give this essential pleasure the attention it needs to make it nourishing.

℞ Misconceptions about Sex

Many of our sexual attitudes and beliefs are learned—they are not automatic or instinctual. Indoctrination begins at a very early age. It comes from friends, older children, parents, and other adults. We also learn it through jokes, magazines, TV, and movies. Much of what we learn about sex is interwoven with inhibitions, "shoulds," "musts," "should nots," "must nots," and misconceptions.

To maximize your sexual enjoyment, you often have to break down your misconceptions so that you are free to discover and explore your own sexuality. For example, many people believe that:

▶ Older people can't enjoy sex

▶ Sex is for people with beautiful bodies

▶ A "real man" is always ready for sex

▶ A "real woman" should be sexually available whenever her partner is interested

▶ Lovemaking has to involve sexual intercourse

▶ Sex must lead to orgasm

▶ Orgasm should occur simultaneously in both partners

▶ Kissing and touching should only be done when they lead to sexual intercourse

Challenge your beliefs. What do you gain or lose by believing such things? Replace fiction with fact. Learn more about the anatomy and physiology of the human sexual response.

℞ Change What You Think

Have you ever thought:

▶ *I can't really satisfy my partner*

▶ *All my partner really wants is sex*

▶ *I can't tell my partner what I really feel*

▶ *I won't be able to maintain an erection*

Such thoughts produce and sustain feelings of frustration, hopelessness, and fear, and can dampen the flame of arousal.

Learn to control these automatic and negative thoughts (📖 see page 149). Many of them can be changed into positive, rational, and helpful statements. For example, if you think that lovemaking means intercourse and orgasm, turn that thought around. Tell yourself, "Lovemaking means physical and emotional closeness with someone I care about." Or if you notice yourself thinking during lovemaking, "I'm not enjoying this," say to yourself, "I often enjoy sex, but I can't expect to enjoy it as much or as intensely every time."

Tackle one negative thought at a time. This will help you cultivate more positive attitudes towards yourself, your partner, and sex.

℞ Eliminate the Negative

The ability to feel sexual desire and pleasure can take a nose dive when you are tired or under a lot of stress. You often don't realize the amount of stress you are feeling, or how it saps your energy. And sometimes you don't connect it with a sputtering sex life.

Take care of any physical factors that could be contributing to a lowered sexual desire or diminished pleasure. These include certain blood pressure medications, tranquilizers, alcohol and antidepressants as well as physical discomfort or pain. Techniques for relaxation (📖 see page 88) or time management (page 183) may also help you to feel more in the mood for this sensual pleasure.

℞ Sexual Communication

A woman yawns and says to her husband, "I think I'm going to bed. Are you coming?" He replies, "Yeah, you look really tired."

THE VALUE OF SEX

While much is known about sexual problems and dysfunction, surprisingly little is known about how a satisfying sex life contributes to better health and well-being. The most obvious benefit of sex is survival of our species—no sex, no babies. But humans have sex far more often than is required for procreation. We have sex because we find it intensely pleasurable. But lovemaking also gives us much more. It can bring us closer to others, and strengthen our vital sense of connectedness.

Most personal experience attests that people feel better after good sex. It puts a spring in your step, a sparkle in your eye, a glow in your skin, and the world seems like a more wonderful place. Some people report that sex helps them relax and sleep better; others say it helps ease menstrual cramps or other aches and pains. And there is some research that it may also bring you better health:

▶ **Sex may be important for the health of your heart.** One study found that two-thirds of heart attack victims reported sexual problems preceding their heart attacks. Sex may provide a heart healthy workout. During vigorous sexual intercourse you can burn four to five calories a minute, which is roughly equivalent to dancing, hiking, or doubles tennis, and is certainly more fun than equally vigorous lawn mowing, wall scrubbing, or floor mopping. When it comes to physical activity, every minute counts.

▶ **Sex eases pain.** Climaxing appears to raise pain thresholds, making arthritis and similar complaints less annoying. One quarter of migraine sufferers report that orgasms relieve their headaches. So even though sex may be the last thing on your mind when you have a splitting headache, you might consider sexual medicine as an alternative to two aspirins.

▶ **Regular sex can help reproductive function.** Women who have sex regularly with men tend to have more regular menstrual cycles. Researchers found that healthy doses of sex during the year before becoming pregnant reduces the risk of pre-

Continued on next page

What just happened? She might have been extending a sexual invitation. He might have been thinking she's always tired, with no time for sex. They'll never know.

Bill comes up behind Claire and puts his hands around her waist. She's startled and pushes his hands away. She thinks he is making a sexual advance, and she's just not in the mood. He was just fooling around with no sexual intent, but now he feels angry and rejected.

Good sex depends upon good communication. But you may assume (along with many other *people) that your partner knows intuitively what will sexually satisfy you without your saying what that is.* Many couples spend more time talking about what furniture to buy than they do discussing what they

eclampsia, a life-threatening rise in blood pressure that complicates nearly 10% of pregnancies.

To improve the chances of fertilization, the new prescription for men with low sperm counts is to have intercourse every day (or even twice a day) in the days just before his partner's ovulation.

Frequent sexual intercourse may also help prevent one distressing change associated with menopause: vaginal atrophy. As hormone levels drop, the tissue lining the vagina becomes thinner, less elastic, and less able to produce lubrication, causing discomfort during intercourse. But women who maintain an active sex life by having intercourse three or more times a month have much less vaginal atrophy than those who have intercourse less than ten times a year. This confirms the adage, "use it or lose it."

▶ **Sex contributes to mental health.** A survey showed that people who were satisfied with their sex life were less likely to report depression, anxiety, hostility, and a variety of complaints such as fatigue and lightheadedness. Sexual satisfaction may also give you an increased sense of control and feeling of positive well-being.

▶ **A good sexual relationship predicts a happy marriage.** Sex is important to marital satisfaction, happiness, and bonding. It is often assumed that a poor sex life is the result of a troubled relationship, but the reverse can also be true. Many relationships are undermined or severely strained by the lack of satisfying sex.

Sometimes the most direct way to improve a relationship is by focusing on enhancing sexual satisfaction. One study revealed that the best predictor of marital happiness could be based on the following formula: the frequency of sexual intercourse minus the frequency of fights. More intercourse or less fighting equals happier couples. So while you improve your communication and decrease your fights, increasing sex may be another helpful way to improve your relationship.

want, need, and feel about sex (📖 see box page 76).

We are also often hesitant to ask our partners directly:

▶ What turns you on?

▶ Does this feel good?

▶ Do you want to make love now?

It's all supposed to happen magically, without words. But unless you or your partner are very good mind readers, neither one of you will have a very clear picture of the others' sexual likes and dislikes.

℞ Overcome Sexual Monotony

Even when sex starts out fantastically intense, it's easy to slip into routine, automatic sex during a long-term relationship—even when you still love each other very much. As Erica Jong puts it, there

COMMUNICATE DIRECTLY

People vary tremendously in their degree of comfort in talking about sex. You must learn to communicate your likes and dislikes with your partner, even if it's difficult. Asking for what you want is the only way to insure healthy sexual communication. Here are some concrete things for you to try:

▶ Ask: "Where do you like to be touched?" "How?"

▶ Make a list of your 10 favorite turn-ons (such as candlelight, talking dirty, surprise, slow undressing).

▶ Then make a list of turn-offs (such as talking about household matters in bed, not brushing teeth, no kissing, no foreplay).

▶ Share your lists with your partner.

▶ Be specific and positive. Instead of saying, "I wish you would be more affectionate to me," try something like, "I really like it when you kiss me when you come home." Instead of saying, "I hate it when you're so passive and just lie there," try, "I really liked it when you climbed on top of me."

▶ Listen carefully to your partner's feelings.

▶ After you have both had the opportunity to state your preferences, come up with a tentative solution that is acceptable to both of you.

▶ Agree to try it out for a specified period of time before you decide how well it is working. If it wasn't satisfactory, negotiate a new tentative agreement and test it out.

▶ After a sexual experience, talk about it. Tell your partner what you liked about it, and what you would have preferred to have been done differently. Immediate feedback can be helpful in improving sexual communication.

A word of caution: Not feeling turned on one night or losing an erection is really no big deal. It happens sooner or later to everyone. And you can talk too much about a sexual problem, especially if it is an isolated incident, or one due to a temporary external stress. Dwelling on the difficulty can stir up performance anxiety and make the problem more likely to occur.

---

comes a time when sex "turned as bland as Velveeta cheese: filling, fattening even, but no thrill to the taste buds...." Even when passion is not as great as at the beginning of a relationship, the tender and affectionate aspects of sex can be very fulfilling.

You still can keep the romantic spark alive if you make good sex a priority, and add some romance and surprise. You have to deliberately break the routine. Here's some ideas for how:

▶ Make love in a room outside of the bedroom

▶ Make love in the morning if you usually do at nighttime (or visa versa)

▶ Eat dinner together by candlelight

▶ Send your partner a suggestive note

▶ Kidnap your partner for an overnight or a distraction-free weekend (don't tell your partner where you're going)

- Trade houses with another couple just for a change
- Spend time apart periodically to increase tension and longing: it makes for a hot reunion

Anything that breaks the routine gives you greater opportunity for romance and more enjoyable sex.

℞ Think Sex

Key Point *Some people might feel that sex is only worthwhile when it involves actually touching a partner, but your body responds sexually to fantasies as well as to physical contact.* Many people find great enjoyment in imagined sexual encounters (📖 see page 97).

And although many men and women believe that feeling sexually excited must lead to sexual intercourse if it is to be worthwhile, sexual fantasies themselves can be a real turn on. They can add to arousal, and give variety and spice to your sexuality.

Any sexual feeling can be enjoyed for its own sake; you need not feel that it must be acted upon. Many of the most exciting relationships exist only in the mind; they're never realized.

Some people feel guilty or disloyal if they have romantic fantasies about someone other than their mate. Such fantasies are normal, though, and need not stir up guilt.

But you also want to be careful—sometimes fantasy gives rise to inflated expectations. Your real partner might not compare favorably to your dream lover. You may find diminishing sexual satisfaction if you regularly fire up your imagination with explicit photos or videos of nubile, hard bodies.

👁 WATCH OUT

CARELESS LOVEMAKING

Healthy sex is safe sex. Careless lovemaking can bring unwanted pregnancies, suffering, and deadly diseases. It's important to:

- Learn about birth control options
- Consider the benefits of abstinence and monogamy
- Use condoms
- Choose partners carefully
- Not mix drugs or alcohol and sex
- Avoid high-risk sex

Be aware that for some people:

- Sex can become an obsession
- Sex can become a substitute for achieving other things
- Sex is used to control or coerce others
- Sexually transmitted diseases, some life-threatening, can occur with unsafe sexual practices

Play safe when it comes to sex.

℞ Satisfy Yourself

To masturbate or not to masturbate, that is the question. The answer depends mostly on your personal preferences.

In some folklore, masturbation is seen as a cause of illness and suffering. It's not true. What little scientific information we have on the subject suggests that self-stimulation is common, natural, and healthy.

Many people find that masturbation is a welcome and pleasurable release of sexual

FOCUS ON ALL YOUR SENSES

Maximizing the pleasure of sex involves appreciating all our senses—yet many find it difficult to focus on the full range of pleasurable physical sensations. One technique that has been used successfully to reawaken whole body sexual feelings is called *sensate focusing*. It involves sensual touch which enables you to relearn how to give and receive pleasure. Here's what to do:

▶ First, you and your partner must agree to just experience and enjoy touching without proceeding to sexual intercourse. During this time it is important that you focus exclusively on pleasurable sensations without anticipating (or worrying about) intercourse.

▶ Have your partner lie naked on his or her stomach on a bed. Then begin lightly touching, caressing, and massaging your partner. Concentrate solely on the pleasures of touch, and sense your partner's enjoyment.

▶ Experiment with different kinds of stroking from head to toe. Your partner may wish to let you know (verbally or nonverbally) what he or she especially enjoys.

▶ Avoid genital touching for the first few times you try this exercise. Remember, the aim is not arousal, but to become more fluent in the language of touch, and to heighten all the senses and express your love. This allows you to communicate in deeper ways, as well as gain genuine intimacy. It also empowers you with greater expression of love.

▶ At the end of about fifteen minutes, briefly discuss the experience. Then switch places. This time your partner slowly, gently touches and explores your entire body. Don't be concerned with the outcome, just lose yourself in the sea of sensation.

At later sessions, you can begin to include genital touching, but again, it's best to start without a goal of intercourse. In time, when you both feel ready, you can let it happen.

tension. Others find it a means to self-discovery and exploration. From it they learn what does and does not turn them on. And self-stimulation also takes some of the pressure off the search for a willing partner. You may be surprised to learn that 47% of men and 23% of women report that they masturbate on a daily or weekly basis, and two-thirds of people see it as a natural, healthy part of life. The choice is yours.

℞ Focus on All Your Senses

Key Point

Sexual satisfaction depends to a great extent on sensual arousal. Sensual arousal is physical excitement in all areas of the body, not just the genitals. Sensuality involves all five senses: the taste of a kiss, the scent of a lover, the sight of an arching body, the sound of quickening breath, and the glorious sensation of skin to skin contact. All these delicious sensations are lost when the focus of sex is solely on genital contact, intercourse, and the rush to orgasm. Don't miss out on them (📖 see box page 78).

℞ Sex and Exercise

If you have trouble getting motivated to do regular physical exercise, consider a better sex life. You can add it to the list of benefits from physical activity. Several studies show that people who are more physically active report more sexual activity, and more satisfying sexual relations. During one nine-month study, people in a vigorous aerobic program said they had more sexual activity and satisfying orgasms.

Exercise may also raise testosterone levels to fuel sexual desire. But as sexuality is as much in the mind as it is in the hormones, increased self-esteem and sense of mastery may also contribute to better sex. Keep in mind that exercise helps the whole body stay in a better state of health, and sexual functioning is a whole-body response. Excessive exercise regimens can backfire, however, undermining relationships and deflating libido (desire). So easy does it (📖 see page 115).

℞ When a Partner is Not Available

Although the optimal dose for sexual activity has not been established, some people seem to do just fine without sexual intimacy. Others are as powerfully driven to seek out sex as they are to find food, air,

sleep, and exercise. Remember that sex satisfies many kinds of needs: being touched, caressed, feeling close to others.

When a sexual partner is not available, substitute other forms of intimacy and pleasure:

▶ Get a massage, or give one

▶ Masturbate

▶ Take a warm, aromatic bath

▶ Express your feelings to a close friend

▶ Listen to your favorite music

▶ Treat yourself to a movie or sporting event

▶ Personally volunteer to help someone else in need

These things won't replace sex, but they will help more than you think. They'll put you in a better mood and help you to feel better about yourself, and you'll feel less lonely.

If you feel your sex life is still not all it could be after exploring some of the suggestions above, consult some of the resources on page 273, or consider sex therapy. There are very effective behavioral techniques and medical treatments to help with such problems as premature ejaculation, impotence, decreased sexual desire, difficulty reaching orgasm, or painful intercourse. Don't let these problems stand in the way of a more satisfying sex life. Get professional help.

📖 *For more information, see page 273*

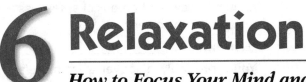

6 Relaxation

How to Focus Your Mind and Relax Your Body

"Happiness cannot be found through great effort and will power, but is already there, in relaxation and letting go."

— *Lama Gendün Rinpoche*

"Within you there is a stillness and a sanctuary to which you can retreat at any time and be yourself."

— *Hermann Hesse*

Your body has two powerful systems to help protect your health: a stress response and a relaxation response. Your stress response—also known as the "fight-or-flight response" or "emergency reaction"—is triggered by a real or imagined threat, and a feeling of not being able to cope with it. Whether the threat is real or unreal, your body responds automatically. It mobilizes for a physical struggle or a quick retreat.

If you are a terrified zebra running for your life, a hungry lion sprinting for a meal, or a warrior preparing for battle, your body's stress mechanisms are brilliantly adapted for the task:

▶ Surging hormones and nerve signals prepare you for flight or fight—the right response for survival

▶ Your sympathetic nervous system leaps into action

▶ Your heart rate speeds up

▶ Breathing increases for more oxygen

▶ Blood pressure surges

▶ Blood rushes to your muscles preparing you for action

▶ Body metabolism shifts into high gear

▶ Blood clotting mechanisms are readied

▶ Digestion is placed temporarily on hold

All this is great if you need it to survive.

The Inappropriate Stress Response

But to an alarming extent, the same stress response turns on when people face mortgages, criticism, traffic jams, insecurities, or thoughts of their own mortality—hardly the kind of challenges facing zebras, lions, or our own early ancestors.

The fight-or-flight response continues to be essential to help us survive in emergency situations. *But when our response to stress is repeatedly and chronically provoked, especially by mental fears rather than physical threats, the results can be disastrous to our health.* Prolonged, repeated stress can produce physiological changes that can contribute to digestive and sleeping

Key Point

81

Be Aware of Stress in Yourself

Many people find it difficult to focus inwardly, even for a few moments. They aren't aware of the tension in their bodies. *Muscle tension or discomfort is often your body's way of letting you know that you are under stress.* Yet you may fail to notice the link between external events and your body tension. A first step to reducing stress is to become more aware of your thoughts, feelings and bodily sensations, and the messages they are giving you.

Key Point

Listen to Your Body

First, focus your attention on the *outside world.* For example, you may be aware of the traffic noise, the hum of a fan, the smell of coffee, the chilliness of the room. Ask yourself what you see, hear, and smell. Say to yourself:

"I am aware of _____"

Now shift your awareness to the *internal world* of your feelings and physical sensations. For example, you may be aware of a tightness in your neck and shoulders, your stomach gurgling, an itchy nose, and an anxious, restless feeling. Say to yourself:

"I am aware of _____"

You'll probably discover a lot more's going on than you thought. Is it easier for you to focus on the external or internal world?

Do a Body Scan

Sit or preferably lie down on your back. Allow your attention to slowly and systematically move through your body. Note any physical sensations you feel from moment to moment.

Start with awareness of your breathing. Observe the different sensations in your body as the air moves in and out of your nostrils, and fills your chest and abdomen. *Just observe the sensations without judging them or trying to change them.*

Key Point

Next shift your attention to your toes. Scan for any sensations in your toes. If your mind wanders off, gently bring your attention back to the feeling in your toes. Concentrate on them; then move slowly up, through your whole body, becoming

Continued on next page

problems, cardiovascular disease, reproductive disorders, diminished immunity, and a host of other illnesses and symptoms.

The Relaxation Response

But just as we have an emergency stress response, we also have a relaxation response, first described by Herbert Benson, M.D. It is a powerful built-in healing mechanism for rest and recovery. The relaxation response is a natural set of physiological changes that offset the stress response:

▶ Your heart rate slows down

▶ Breathing declines

▶ Blood pressure decreases

▶ Body metabolism lowers

▶ Muscles relax

aware of your feet, ankles, lower legs, and knees, until you get to your face and head.

Pause at each body part, and notice any tension or other sensations. Are certain areas more tense than others? Which parts of your body can you easily feel, and which parts have little sensation? You can do a quick body scan in just a few minutes to pinpoint areas of tension. Or you can take 30 minutes or more moving very slowly through your body, as you practice the skill of focusing inwardly.

Keep a Stress Diary

Developing an inner awareness of your body and feelings is very helpful in identifying your sources of stress. To help determine how you respond physically and mentally, you might want to write down your reactions to a recent stressful event. Here are some examples:

▶ *I have trouble getting to work on time, so today I tried a short cut and got lost. I was frustrated, and the longer I drove, the more I kept picturing my boss chewing me out for being late.*

▶ *The sewer backed up into the basement this morning and my mother-in-law was coming to visit at noon. The plumber said he'd be here by 10 a.m., but at 11 o'clock, he hadn't shown up. I had a terrible headache and a pain in my lower back.*

You may find it especially helpful to keep a "stress log" for a week or so. Describe the stressful events or situations in your life, and how you respond to them (thoughts, feelings, and body sensations and symptoms). You might start to notice some patterns. For example, you might find that whenever someone asks you to do something, you think, "I'm too busy and way behind already." You begin to feel anxious and notice the energy drain out of your body.

You can also record positive events such as a compliment, a hug, or some physical activity, and the thoughts, feelings and bodily sensations they set off. *The skill to observe the reactions of your own body and mind is a way to help you learn to relax and manage stress.*

Key Point

Take advantage of your relaxation response. Try methods described below such as deep muscle relaxation, meditation, and breathing exercises, or the imagery and self-hypnosis techniques in Chapter 7 (see page 99). You can learn to refocus your mind and relax your body. It will help you to reduce senseless fight or flight responses from worry or imaginary lions.

How Do You Relax Best?

When you think of relaxing, what images come to mind? Sitting quietly, reading? Meditating? Contemplating a sunset? Not everyone associates relaxing with calm situations. For some people, thrilling stimulation relaxes them much more than sitting quietly. Playing a competitive game of basketball, driving a race car at high speed, or jumping out of an airplane

THE VALUE OF RELAXATION

Relaxation can help you to:

▶ Reduce anxiety, fear, and panic

▶ Decrease chronic tension

▶ Decrease pain and need for pain medications

▶ Reduce blood pressure in stress-related hypertension

▶ Decrease heart disease risk

▶ Improve comfort during medical, surgical, and dental procedures

▶ Reduce the length of labor and discomfort of childbirth

▶ Lessen the stress of infertility, and improve the chances of conception

▶ Speed healing and recovery from surgery, injury, or skin problems

▶ Boost immune function

▶ Ease sleep problems

▶ Improve management of chronic illnesses such as diabetes, asthma, lung, and heart disease

can bring relaxation for some people.

Because there are so many different types of tension, anxiety, fear, and fatigue, there are many different ways to relax.

Body Reactors: Some people tend to experience stress more in their bodies. For instance, if you often feel jittery, tight muscles, aches and pains, a nervous stomach, or a racing heartbeat, you're probably more of a "body reactor."

Mind Reactors: On the other hand, if you suffer more from excessive worrying, anxiety-provoking images, a racing mind, or difficulty concentrating, you may experience stress more as a "mind reactor." Most of us react to stress with both body and mind.

By matching your relaxation strategy to the type of tension you are experiencing (body or mind), you may be able to relax more easily. For example, if you are feeling more body tension, you might try muscle relaxation, walking, deep breathing, or a hot bath or sauna.

If worrying and mental fatigue is your problem, you might try a mind-focusing approach like meditation, visualization and imagery (see page 99), watching television or going to the movies, listening to music, reading, or absorbing yourself (and your tension) in a hobby or game.

After hours of writing, number crunching, or talking with customers, you may feel mentally fatigued. You can become revived by switching to another activity—even if it is physically strenuous. Vigorous exercise and competitive sports are usually good for relaxing both physical and mental tension.

If one relaxation method makes you *more* tense rather than less, try another. Sometimes a mental relaxer works better for body tension, and a physical relaxer relieves your mind. So experiment.

Try to choose leisure activities that balance the stresses of your job. If you sit all day, consider aerobic exercise, or walking at least part of the way to work. If your job involves mindless activity, take up an intellectually challenging hobby such as playing chess or learning a foreign language. If your days are highly structured, weekend hikes in nature can provide a restorative balance. If your work requires you to respond to others' demands, take the time for some solitary activity you enjoy.

CHECK SYMPTOMS FIRST

Relaxation is generally a very safe and useful addition to regular medical care, but it is not a substitute for it. Symptoms such as pain, nervousness, diarrhea, dizziness, or depression can be caused by an underlying medical problem. Make sure you first have appropriate medical evaluation and diagnosis for persistent symptoms before undertaking relaxation techniques. Otherwise you may end up using relaxation for an illness or condition that requires a different sort of treatment.

Medications

If you have certain medical conditions, relaxation can change your need for medications. For example, patients with diabetes or high blood pressure may find their need for insulin or blood pressure medication lessened with regular relaxation practice. Check with your physician before making any adjustments in your medication. Relaxation itself can be a powerful medicine.

Relaxation

Most of the techniques described in this chapter are designed to decrease arousal. Don't practice deep relaxation exercises while driving a car or in any situation where your safety requires full alertness and quick responses.

Seizure Disorders

If you have a seizure disorder, practice these relaxation exercises while lying down. Many patients report a greater sense of control over their seizures with relaxation. However, some types of seizures may be triggered by a change in level of arousal, such as with sleep-onset seizure disorders.

Relaxation-Induced Anxiety

Not everyone finds "relaxing" relaxing. For example, in one study of anxious patients who started to meditate, nearly half reported feeling *more* anxious. When attempting a method of deep muscle relaxation, nearly a third suffered increased restlessness, sweating, pounding heart, and rapid breathing. Many people are so used to feeling "wired" or tense that feeling relaxed may at first feel odd to them.

One cause of relaxation-induced anxiety may be a reaction to the new sensations: floating, heaviness, tingling, or muscle twitches. These sometimes accompany states of relaxation. Other causes may be fear of loss of control or reluctance to observe inner sensations. Sometimes just practicing a relaxation exercise with your eyes open can prevent this.

Strange or unpleasant sensations usually subside with regular practice, or by switching to a different relaxation technique. If your strange or unusual sensations are very intense or distressing, stop the practice and get professional help. If you have a history of psychiatric disorders, it may be wise to consult a professional before beginning any regular relaxation practice.

6 Relaxation

85

RELAX—IT'S GOOD MEDICINE

Relaxation, meditation, breathing exercises, self-hypnosis, imagery and other mind/body medicine approaches have been used for thousands of years. Although there's new interest in these strategies, they are still greatly underused in medical care and daily life today.

Mounting research shows that relaxation helps manage a wide variety of psychological symptoms and disorders, from anxiety and stage fright to panic and phobias. These techniques can also be used to lessen medical conditions and bodily symptoms.

Hypertension

In patients with hypertension, particularly those with stress-related high blood pressure, relaxation lowers it. In some patients it may be sufficient to decrease or eliminate (under a physician's supervision) the need for antihypertensive medications. A relaxation technique can be especially helpful for patients with "whitecoat hypertension"—those whose blood pressure is high only when they are in the doctor's office or a similarly stressful situation.

Heart Disease

A program combining yoga, relaxation, low-fat diet, exercise, and group support slowed the progression and even reduced the blockage of the coronary arteries. Relaxation techniques have been used to reduce anxiety, anger, hostility, and depression (all associated with increased risk of heart disease). In one study, men who took afternoon siestas in order to relax had a 30% to 50% less risk of having a heart attack.

Chronic Pain

In patients with chronic pain, relaxation and mindfulness meditation techniques have been used as part of comprehensive pain management programs. While the pain was not eliminated completely, many patients reported reductions in:

▶ Medication use

▶ Pain severity

▶ Anxiety

▶ Depression

▶ Interference with daily activities

Patients with recurrent headaches have also been helped with imagery, relaxation, and hypnosis.

Insomnia

Patients taught methods of relaxing, along with other behavioral techniques, learned to fall asleep more easily. On average, these patients fell asleep four times faster after treatment (📖 see page 192).

Infertility

Couples dealing with infertility often feel that they have lost control over their lives. They become angry, anxious, and depressed. High levels of stress can contribute to infertility by causing:

▶ Irregular ovulation

Continued on next page

- Hormonal changes
- Sexual problems
- A possible decrease in sperm production

In one study, women were enrolled in a behavioral program in which they practiced relaxation techniques on a daily basis. The program reduced anxiety, depression, and the associated distress of infertility. Thirty-four percent of the women became pregnant within six months of completing the program. This rate is higher than expected for women receiving medical treatment alone for infertility.

Immune Function

Certain types of stress depress immune function. But can people learn to voluntarily *boost* their immunity? A review of studies suggests that relaxation, self-hypnosis, and imagery (both with and without music) can enhance immune function. For example, healthy people using self-hypnosis and imagery have learned to voluntarily increase antibodies which fight infection. They have also learned to change the activity of disease-fighting white blood cells. Whether such changes in immune function can actually prevent or treat disease is not yet known.

Medical Procedures

Relaxation and imagery can lessen pain and discomfort when undergoing diagnostic tests, medical treatment, and surgery. Relaxation techniques have successfully been used to lessen the nausea and vomiting associated with chemotherapy for cancer and AIDS patients.

Relaxation can also significantly reduce pain during medical, surgical and dental procedures. Many surgical procedures have been performed under hypnosis without any medication or other anesthesia. And relaxation and breathing exercises can reduce the length and discomfort of women during labor and delivery.

Other Conditions

Relaxation and imagery techniques have been used to help a number of other conditions. For example:

- Relaxation has helped regulate blood sugar in diabetics, and reduced the severity of asthma attacks

- Some skin conditions also respond to mindfulness meditation and imagery: they appear to speed the clearing of skin in patients with psoriasis who are also undergoing ultraviolet light phototherapy

- Hypnosis has proved a safe, painless and effective treatment for warts

- In people suffering from emphysema and chronic obstructive lung disease, breathing relaxation exercises and mindfulness techniques appear to reduce the frequency and severity of breathlessness and panic

- Studies of patients with irritable bowel syndrome suggest that hypnosis, imagery, and relaxation can reduce abdominal pain, bloating, and diarrhea or constipation

How to Use Relaxation Techniques to Focus Your Mind and Relax Your Body

Relaxation techniques, of course, can't eliminate all the stress in your life. Sometimes it's necessary to take action to change the demands of an intolerable job or an unreasonable partner, child, or friend. But by learning how to relax, you can think through positive ways to make the necessary changes more effectively.

Everyday Relaxation

Take advantage of the attainable pleasures in life whenever you can—good films, baseball games, autumn foliage, summer sunsets. Indulging in personal pleasures does a lot to keep you relaxed, happy and healthy (📖 see page 57). Relaxation doesn't always require twenty minutes of meditation or muscle relaxation, as useful though they may be. Look for quick and easy opportunities in your everyday life to rapidly relax and refresh yourself (📖 see box page 89).

Preparing for Relaxation

Some relaxation techniques take only seconds and can be done just about any place. But to learn some of the deeper relaxation methods takes practice, and a quiet, comfortable place.

You may need to put up a "Do Not Disturb" sign and turn your telephone off to insure no interruptions (you deserve 10 to 20 minutes of private, undisturbed time). Wear loose, comfortable clothing. Sit in a comfortable chair or lie on a pad or carpeted floor with a pillow under your head. Do whatever you can to enhance your comfort: dim the lights, put on soft music, or use a relaxation or imagery audiotape (📖 see page 273).

Try to view your practice time as a reward and time for yourself, not as a task. Don't push yourself to do it "right." And don't expect miracles. Some relief may come immediately, but often these techniques take time to acquire the necessary skill. Sometimes it takes three to four weeks of practice before you really start to notice benefits. If you have difficulty finding time for regular practice, consider the tips for making and maintaining healthy changes (📖 see page 17). Below we provide instructions for

▶ Quick and Easy Relaxation

▶ Breathing Exercises

▶ Muscle Relaxation

▶ Mindfulness

▶ Meditation

Also see Chapter 7, *Imagery* for instructions on:

▶ Self-Hyponosis

▶ Autogenic Training

▶ Guided Imagery and Visualization

▶ Affirmations

Key Point

RELAX—QUICK AND EASY

Pleasurable everyday experiences can help you relax. Here are some to try:

▶ Take a nap, or a hot, soothing bath

▶ Curl up and read a good book

▶ Watch a funny movie

▶ Make a paper airplane and sail it across the room

▶ Get a massage

▶ Enjoy an occasional glass of wine

▶ Start a small garden or grow a beautiful plant indoors

▶ Do some arts or crafts like knitting, pottery, or woodworking

▶ Watch a favorite TV show

▶ Go for a walk

▶ Start a collection (coins, folk art, shells, or something in miniature)

▶ Listen to your favorite music

▶ Crumble paper into a ball; use a wastebasket as a basketball hoop

▶ Look at water (ocean waves, a lake or a fountain)

▶ Watch the clouds in the sky

▶ Put your head down on your desk and close your eyes for 5 minutes

▶ Rub your hands together until they're warm; cup them over your closed eyes

▶ Vigorously shake your hands and arms for ten seconds

▶ Call up a friend or family member to chat

▶ Play with a pet

▶ Go to a vacation spot in your mind

▶ Make up a mini-relaxation exercise

SIX SECOND MINI-RELAXATION

The *quieting reflex* is a six-second mini-relaxation technique that is designed to counteract emergency stress reactions. It relieves muscle tightening, jaw-clenching, breath holding, and activation of the sympathetic nervous system.

To be effective, it should be practiced frequently throughout the day, and at the moment a stressful situation arises. It can be done with your eyes opened or closed.

Step 1

Become aware of what is annoying you: a ringing phone, a sarcastic comment, the urge to smoke, a worrisome thought— whatever. This becomes the cue to start the quieting reflex.

Step 2

Repeat the phrase, "Alert mind, calm body" to yourself.

Step 3

Smile inwardly with your eyes and your mouth. This stops facial muscles from making a fearful or angry expression. The inward smile is more a feeling than something obvious to anyone observing you.

Step 4

Inhale slowly to the count of three, imagining that the breath comes in through the bottom of your feet. Then exhale slowly. Feel your breath move back down your legs and out through your feet. Let your jaw, tongue, and shoulder muscles go limp.

With several months' practice the quieting reflex becomes an automatic skill.

BREATHING EXERCISES

Tune in to Your Breathing

Focusing your awareness on breathing is an excellent way to settle your mind and relax. Just as we gasp with amazement, choke with sadness, or sigh with relief, breathing often mirrors our emotions. Breathing becomes irregular and ragged with anger; it stops with fear.

Changing your breathing can shift your attention and your mood. Breathing patterns can both reflect and redirect your emotions.

Alter Your Feelings

Most of the time we take our breathing for granted. But becoming aware of the link between your breathing and your emotional states can help put you more in control. Try this:

▶ Make a tight fist or pinch your leg hard enough to cause mild pain. Observe what happens to your breathing. Does your breathing stop or become shallow?

▶ Now relax for a moment. Make another tight fist or pinch yourself again, but this time, continue to breathe slowly and deeply. What happens to the tension in your fist or your sensation of pain? With slow, deep breathing, it should be reduced.

Key Point

It is difficult to maintain tension, pain, anxiety, or anger while breathing in a relaxed way. The next time you feel particularly stressed or in a bad mood, notice your breathing. Awareness and control of your breathing can be a powerful way to gain control over stress

and emotions, as shown in the exercises below. These exercises are designed to help you feel more relaxed. If you feel light-headed, dizzy, anxious, or faint while doing them, you may be breathing too quickly or too deeply. Just stop practicing for a few moments, and breathe normally until the symptoms pass.

Relax with Belly Breathing

We all start out in life by using abdominal (belly or diaphragmatic) breathing. Here our belly rises with in-breaths, and falls with out-breaths (just watch childrens' bellies as they breathe). As adults, many of us replace belly breathing with chest breathing—a shallow, rapid breathing pattern associated with tension and anxiety. Many take on an unhealthy, chest-breathing pattern in pursuit of a flat abdomen ("stomach in, chest out"). How do you breathe?

▶ Close your eyes. Place one of your hands gently on your abdomen over the belly button. Rest your other hand on the center of your chest over the breastbone.

▶ Without changing your normal breathing pattern, just observe your body as you inhale normally. Which hand rises the most—the one on your chest, or the one on your belly?

One way to relax is to relearn natural belly breathing. Here's how:

▶ Lie down on your back on a comfortable surface. You may wish to bend your knees, keeping your feet slightly apart. Loosen your belt or any restrictive clothing.

Continued on next page

- Place your hands gently just below your belly button. Close your eyes, and imagine a balloon inside your abdomen.
- Each time you breathe in, imagine the balloon filling with air. Your hands will gently rise. Each time you breathe out, imagine the balloon deflating. Your hands will gently settle lower down.
- Focus on the sound and sensation of breathing as you become more and more relaxed.

Or you can take a posture that restricts your chest breathing and exaggerates abdominal breathing. For example:

- Lie on your stomach with your head resting on your folded forearms. As you take in a breath, feel your abdomen pressing against the floor.
- Or sit in a chair and clasp your hands behind your head. Point your elbows out to the side. With each deep breath, feel the air inflate your belly.

At first belly breathing may feel unusual. But with practice, it becomes second nature again, and you'll discover its relaxing benefits.

Get Quick Tension Relief

If you are yawning or sighing, you may not be getting enough oxygen. Here are some ways to use breathing to quickly release your tension and increase your alertness.

- Try reaching for the sky as you inhale deeply and fully. Then exhale forcefully as you bend forward at your waist. Inhale again deeply as you straighten up and reach for the sky. Repeat several times.
- Stand up with your arms straight in front of you. As you inhale, make several large backward circles with your arms like a windmill. Then as you exhale, reverse the direction of the circles, bringing your arms forward. Or try alternately swinging your left and right arm backwards, as if you were doing the backstroke.

Use Breathing with Imagery

As you breathe, try using mental images like warmth, coolness, vitality, or peacefulness. Imagine that the breath you inhale is charged with that particular quality. Then, while you exhale, let your breath carry that quality throughout your whole body as though you were exhaling it through the entire surface of your skin. For instance:

- Imagine inhaling warm, soothing air on your in-breath, and sending this soothing sensation into all parts of your body as you exhale.
- Or on a hot day, imagine a few deep cool, blue breaths.
- See how you feel after trying several sparkling, energizing breaths.
- Breaths saturated with heaviness may help settle and relax you.
- If a particular part of your body is tense or injured, try directing the energy of your breath to relax and heal that area (□ see page 104).

Experiment with your own images.

MUSCLE RELAXATION

People often carry a lot of unnecessary tension in their muscles, but it feels "normal" or "relaxed" to them. Progressive relaxation helps you learn the difference between how it feels when your muscles are tense and when they're relaxed. *It is based on the idea that whatever relaxes your muscles will also relax your mind.*

Begin by getting comfortable in a chair that supports your head and neck or, preferably, lie down on your back on a soft surface. You are going to tense and relax muscle groups one at a time.

▶ Tense each muscle group for about five seconds, and concentrate on what the tension feels like.

▶ Then breathe deeply.

▶ As you exhale, *instantly* let go of all the tension as though an electrical current was suddenly turned off, so the muscle goes completely limp.

▶ For ten to twenty seconds, observe the difference between muscles that are tense and ones that are fully relaxed.

▶ Go through your body tensing and relaxing each muscle group twice.

▶ Leave time to notice the difference during the relaxation phase.

You can read the following instructions to someone else, or have someone read them to you. Or you can read them into a tape recorder, to play for yourself. Now let's go through each group:

Hands and Arms

▶ Clench your right fist very tight. Now even tighter. As you keep it tensed for several seconds, notice the feeling in all the muscles of your fingers, your hand, and forearm.

▶ Now relax your hand and arm. Feel the looseness in your right hand, and notice the contrast between loose muscles and tense ones.

▶ Repeat the process once more; then do the same exercise twice with your left hand.

▶ Now clench and relax both fists. As you relax, straighten out your fingers, and let the relaxation flow into your hands. Repeat once.

▶ Now bend your arms, and tighten your biceps muscles in your upper arms.

▶ Relax, and let your arms straighten. Notice how a tense, taut muscle feels different from a loose, relaxed one.

Legs and Feet

▶ Straighten your legs, tighten your thigh muscles, and press your heels down against the surface beneath you. Hold tight—then let it go.

▶ Point your toes down and curl them, making your calf muscle tense and

Continued on next page

taut. Study the tension. Then release them, and compare the feeling.

▶ Now bend your toes up toward your head, creating tension in your shins. Hold, and relax again.

Abdomen and Buttocks

▶ Pull your stomach muscles in and hold them tight. Then release them.

▶ Squeeze your buttocks together. Hold—then let go.

Chest, Back, and Shoulders

▶ Take a deep breath, hold it, then exhale and relax.

▶ Shrug your shoulders up, bringing them as close to your ears as you can. Hold—then drop them.

▶ Press your shoulder blades toward each other. Hold—then release.

▶ Arch your back. Hold—then relax.

Neck and Throat

▶ Press your head back as far as it can comfortably go. Hold—then relax.

▶ Next pull your chin down as if trying to touch your chest. Hold—then relax.

Head and Face

▶ Wrinkle your forehead as tight as you can. Hold—then release the tension.

▶ Now frown and "knit" your eyebrows together. Hold—then let go.

▶ Close your eyes tightly, and wrinkle your nose. Hold—then relax.

▶ Clench your jaws, biting your teeth together. Hold—then relax.

▶ Press your tongue hard against the roof of your mouth. Hold—then let go.

▶ Purse your lips, pressing them together tighter and tighter. Hold—then relax.

Your Whole Body

▶ Now let yourself relax even more, all over your body. Let go of more and more tension.

▶ Feel the relaxation deepening.

▶ Feel your face calm and soft; your arms and shoulders limp and relaxed; your chest and abdomen free and at ease; your legs and feet loose. Let your whole body be relaxed and peaceful.

▶ Enjoy the feeling of relaxation throughout your whole body.

▶ When you are ready to get up, take several long, deep breaths, and get up very slowly.

▶ Savor the relaxed, refreshed, wide-awake feeling.

Daily practice with this exercise will help you learn quickly how to scan your body and pinpoint any tight areas. You can then tense and then relax them.

PRACTICING MINDFULNESS

Most of us spend much of our waking hours on "automatic pilot," or "asleep at the wheel." We're preoccupied with thinking about the past or anticipating the future. Meanwhile, the present moment slips by barely noticed.

Key Point

Mindfulness involves simply keeping your attention in the present moment, without judging it as happy or sad, good or bad. It encourages living each moment—even painful ones—as fully and as mindfully as possible. Mindfulness is more than a relaxation technique; it is an attitude toward living. It is a way of calmly and consciously observing and accepting whatever is happening, moment to moment.

This may sound simple enough, but our restless, judging minds make it surprisingly difficult. As a restless monkey jumps from branch to branch, our mind jumps from thought to thought.

In mindfulness meditation, you focus the mind on the present moment. This 2500-year-old Buddhist meditation tradition is thoroughly modern and relevant to our present-day lives. You don't have to be a Buddhist to practice it. Mindfulness doesn't conflict with any beliefs or traditions, either religious or scientific.

The only moment we really have is this one. And living this moment as fully aware as possible is what mindfulness practice is about. It nurtures an inner balance of mind that enables you to respond to all life situations with greater composure, clarity, and compassion. It reduces our tendency to react automatically to any circumstances. For example, the sound of someone's voice (your mother's, teenager's, or boss') might automatically trigger tension, anger, or fear. You can learn to just mindfully *observe* the reaction their voice sets off in you without responding to it or judging it.

The "goal" of mindfulness is simply to observe—with no intention of changing or improving anything. But people are positively changed by the practice. Observing and accepting life just as it is, with all its pleasures, pains, frustrations, disappointments, and insecurities, often enables you to become calmer, more confident, and better able to cope with whatever comes along.

To develop your capacity for mindfulness, try the following exercises.

Single Focus Mindfulness

Sit comfortably on the floor or on a chair with your back, neck and head straight, but not stiff. Then:

▶ Concentrate on a single object, such as your breathing. Focus your attention on the feeling of the air as it passes in and out of your nostrils with each breath. Don't try to control your breathing by speeding it up or slowing it down. Just observe it as it is.

▶ Even when you resolve to keep your attention on your breathing, your mind will quickly wander off. When this occurs, *observe where your mind*

Continued on next page

went: perhaps to a memory, a worry about the future, a bodily ache, or a feeling of impatience. Then gently return your attention to your breathing.

▶ Use your breath as an anchor. Each time a thought or feeling arises, momentarily acknowledge it. Don't analyze it or judge it. Just observe it, and return to your breathing.

▶ Abandon all thought of getting somewhere, or having anything special happen. Just keep stringing moments of mindfulness together, breath by breath.

▶ Practice this for just five minutes at a time at first. You may wish to gradually extend the time to ten, twenty or thirty minutes.

Your thoughts are like waves on the surface of the ocean. Don't try to stop the waves completely so that the water is flat, peaceful, and still—that's impossible. But you'll find relief from constant turbulence when you learn to observe and ride the waves.

Mindfulness in Daily Life

Because the practice of mindfulness is simply the practice of moment-to-moment awareness, you can apply it to anything: eating, showering, working, talking, running errands, or playing with your children. Mindfulness takes no extra time. All that is required is that you take yourself off "automatic pilot," and stay tuned. Are you fully aware of your experience at this moment?

This is not as simple as it sounds. For example, think about your last meal. Do you remember what you ate? Did you pay attention to the taste sensations? Or was your mind elsewhere: engaged in thoughts, conversation, planning, and plotting, and nearly everything else but the experience of eating?

Try observing what you are about to eat.

▶ How does it look?

▶ Where does it come from?

▶ How do you feel about putting this particular food into your body?

▶ Feel the food in your mouth.

▶ Chew slowly. Focus on taste; texture.

▶ Notice the impulse to rush through this mouthful to get to the next. Stay present with the mouthful you already have.

▶ Before swallowing, be aware of your intention to swallow. Then feel the actual sensation of swallowing.

Continue with each mouthful in the same way, noting how fast and how much you eat, how your body feels, and whether you are eating in response to hunger, other events in your life, or a feeling such as anxiety or depression.

Or observe walking. Focus on the sensations in your legs and feet. Notice how your weight shifts from foot to foot. Feel the pressure on the balls of your feet.

How do your knees feel as they bend? Is the ground hard or soft? When other thoughts arise, note them. Then return to your focus on walking.

MEDITATION

Meditation can elicit the relaxation response. It has two essential components:

1. Focusing your mind by concentrating on your breathing or a repetitive word, phrase, image, or prayer.

2. Taking a detached, nonjudging observer's view of the thoughts that go through your mind. To meditate:

▶ Find a quiet place where you will not be disturbed.

▶ Sitting upright in a comfortable chair, close your eyes.

▶ Relax your muscles and breathe in and out, slowly and naturally.

▶ Focus on any object you are comfortable with (your breath, a word, or whatever). You might repeat "one" or "peace." A Christian might choose the first words of Psalm 23, *The Lord is My Shepherd.* A Jew might use the word *Shalom.*

▶ Breathe in, and with each out breath, repeat your word or phrase.

Some people find it easier to focus their minds by looking at an object or a picture. Others do a walking meditation and repeat "left, right, left, right," to themselves as they move along.

Keep a detached, nonjudging observer's attitude. Don't worry about how well you are doing. All kinds of thoughts will dart through your mind: "Will my boss approve my raise?" "Did I choose the right color sofa?" "What am I having for dinner tonight?" This is normal. Simply observe the thought, and gently return to your focus.

Don't be discouraged if you can't control your thoughts for more than a few seconds at a time. Just keep bringing your mind back to your focus.

Key Point

It's not necessary to feel that you are relaxing as you practice meditation. If you are struggling to make yourself relax, stop. Do something else for awhile, and try again later. Even if you find yourself continuously distracted by a thousand different thoughts, just accept each interruption and return to your focus. *Meditation helps you develop an attitude of relaxed tolerance and acceptance toward whatever happens.*

Key Point

Continue meditating for 10 to 20 minutes. You may open your eyes to check the time, but don't set an alarm (it is too jarring). When the time's up, sit quietly for a minute before rising.

Practice meditation once every day. Lasting psychological and physiological changes may take several weeks or months, so be patient. Though the instructions are quite simple, the practice of meditation takes practice and support. Sometimes it helps to meditate with a group, or find a teacher to guide you.

Adapted from the work of Herbert Benson, M.D., author of The Relaxation Response *and* The Wellness Book

📖 *For more information, see page 273*

7 Imagery

How to Use Your Imagination to Improve Your Health

"The greatest discovery of my generation is that human beings, by changing the inner attitudes of their minds, can change the outer aspects of their lives."

— *William James (1842-1910)*

"If you dream it, you can do it."

— *Walt Disney*

You may assume that "imagination" means "not real." But the thoughts, words, and images that flow from your imagination can have very real physiological consequences on your body. *Your brain often cannot distinguish whether you are imagining something or actually experiencing it* (📖 see box page 98). Perhaps you've had a racing heartbeat, rapid breathing, or tension in your neck muscles while watching a movie thriller. These sensations were all produced by images and sounds on a film. During a dream, maybe your body responded with fear, joy, anger, or sadness—all triggered by your imagination. If you close your eyes and vividly imagine yourself by a still, quiet pool or relaxing on a warm beach, your body responds to some degree as though you are actually there. Your imagination can be a very powerful resource in relieving stress, pain, and other unwanted symptoms.

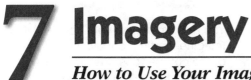

You can learn to use the power of your imagination to produce calming, energizing, or healing responses in your body. This chapter will show you how. It includes techniques to help you focus your attention on healing thoughts, images, and suggestions. They include:

▶ Self-hypnosis

▶ Autogenic training

▶ Guided imagery and visualization

▶ Affirmations

▶ Imagining yourself well

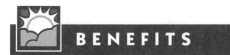

THE VALUE OF IMAGERY

Use imagery and hypnosis to:

▶ Reduce anxiety, fear, and panic

▶ Decrease chronic muscle tension

▶ Decrease pain and need for pain medications

▶ Improve comfort during medical, surgical, and dental procedures

▶ Reduce the length of labor and discomfort of childbirth

▶ Control bleeding

▶ Speed healing and recovery from surgery, injury, or skin conditions such as warts and psoriasis

▶ Ease sleep problems

▶ Improve management of chronic illnesses such as diabetes, asthma, lung, and heart disease

▶ Boost your immune function

▶ Increase sense of control and mastery

▶ Change bad habits successfully, and maintain healthy ones

Since most of the imagery techniques involve relaxation, the research findings on the benefits of imagery are discussed in the section on relaxation (📖 see page 86).

THE PLUMP, JUICY ORANGE

▶ You are standing in your kitchen. Imagine the time of day, the color of the countertops, the appliances, the cupboards. You hear the hum of the refrigerator. You notice a large, plump, juicy orange lying on the cutting board. You pick it up and feel its weight. You feel the texture of its dimpled, glossy skin. With a sharp knife, you carefully cut a large slice of the orange.

▶ As you cut into the orange you notice the rich, sweet, fragrant juice trickle onto the counter top. You see the bright whiteness of the pulp in contrast with the dazzling orange flesh. You see the small drops of orange juice forming on the cut surface. Now imagine lifting this dripping slice of orange to your mouth, and smelling its sweet fresh scent. Your mouth begins to water as you slowly bite into the orange. It releases a flood of sweet, tangy juice into your mouth.

This juicy orange imagery exercise causes most people to salivate. Just the words and multi-sensory images are enough to trigger a physiological response. In this case it's the flow of saliva. You can learn to use the power of your imagination to control other body functions.

WATCH OUT

▶ Imagery techniques are generally very safe. However, if you have symptoms such as pain, diarrhea, dizziness, nervousness, or depression, make sure you first have an appropriate medical evaluation. These imagery techniques may also change your need for certain medications, so be sure to check with your doctor.

▶ Don't practice imagery or self-hypnosis while in a car or in any situation where your safety requires full alertness and quick responses.

▶ If you experience very distressing sensations or feelings while practicing these techniques, stop and get professional help (📖 see page 85).

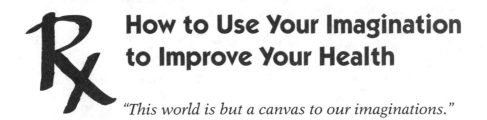

How to Use Your Imagination to Improve Your Health

"This world is but a canvas to our imaginations."

—*Thoreau*

"The mind is its own place, and in itself, can make heaven of hell or a hell of heaven"

—*John Milton*

℞ Skill, Not Magic

To practice the imagery and self-hypnosis exercises you will need 10 to 30 minutes of quiet, undisturbed time. You may need to put up a "Do Not Disturb" sign and turn off the telephone. Wear loose, comfortable clothing. Sit in a comfortable chair or lie on a pad or carpeted floor with a pillow under your head. Do whatever you can to enhance your comfort. Dim the lights. Put on soft music if you like. You may wish to use a guided imagery audiotape (📖 see page 274). You may also like to begin with one of the relaxation exercises from Chapter 6 to help relax your mind and body (📖 see page 89).

Don't expect miracles. Some relief may come immediately, but often these skills take time to acquire—sometimes several weeks of practice before you really start to notice benefits. Ideally, practice the techniques once or twice a day. If that's not possible, do them at least three to four times a week.

Key Point

SELF-HYPNOSIS

Hypnosis typically brings to mind an image of a stage performer casting a spell over a volunteer obediently carrying out the hypnotist's suggestions. But in fact, hypnosis is not some mysterious or magical force. It is a natural, relaxing state of mind that you can put to work for the benefit of your health. It is a state of attentive, focused concentration that can make it easier for you to relax, and to control your body and mind.

Hypnosis allows your body and mind to respond to your thoughts as though they were real. With self-hypnosis you are always fully in control. You choose what you want to think about, imagine, feel, and do. Self-hypnosis allows you to be relaxed and receptive, do more, and to think, evaluate and judge less. It enables you to control your attention and filter out painful or unpleasant thoughts, feelings, and sensations.

You've probably already experienced hypnosis in daily life—perhaps as a state of focused concentration while driving a car, listening to music, reading a book, or daydreaming. With self-hypnosis, you can capitalize on your natural ability to concentrate to reduce anxiety, relax muscles, control fears, diminish pain, improve mood, boost creativity, and help change unwanted habits.

Although some people seem to have a greater ability to focus their attention using self-hypnosis than others, most people can markedly increase this ability with practice.

There are hundreds of ways to ease yourself into the pleasant state of self-hypnotic focused awareness. You may want to record the instructions on tape in your own voice so that you can just relax and listen. You can also get help from a professional trained in hypnotherapy, or from books and tapes on self-hypnosis (📖 see page 274).

To get the full benefits of self-hypnosis may take 20 minutes. Don't get frustrated if at first you aren't able to maintain the focused concentration. Within a week or two of daily practice, self-hypnosis will get easier and more effective. Here's what to do:

▶ Get into a relaxed position.

▶ Take several slow, deep breaths.

▶ Fix your eyes on an object—a candle, a picture, or anything fixed.

▶ At the same time, say to yourself, *"My eyelids are feeling very heavy, very heavy; little weights are dragging them down. They feel so heavy they want to close."*

▶ Allow your eyes to roll up towards the top of your head while your eyelids gently close.

▶ As your eyes close say to yourself, *"Relax. I will count backwards slowly from 10 to 1. With each number, I will become more and more deeply relaxed and at peace."*

▶ After you say each number, add a phrase such as, *"My body is becoming much more relaxed and calm,"* or *"With every number I feel more at ease mentally and physically."*

Continued on next page

> **Key Point**

- You may wish to count backwards from 10 to 1 several times. With each cycle, you will become more and more deeply relaxed.

- Now envision going down in a slow-moving escalator. Count from 10 to 1 as you descend deeper into a state of warmth and relaxation. Repeat to yourself, *"Drifting down, down, down, into total relaxation. Drifting deeper, deeper, deeper, and deeper."*

Take advantage of this state of relaxed, focused awareness by deliberately offering yourself suggestions to improve some mental or physical aspect of yourself. Set a clear goal and give yourself specific suggestions to achieve your goals. You can repeat suggestions to yourself such as, *"Each time I use self-hypnosis I will find it easier and more effective."*

Also develop suggestions to yourself for managing specific problems such as insomnia, chronic pain, low self-esteem, excessive worry, specific fears, smoking, chronic anger or chronic illness. You can adapt the following examples by making them more specific to your needs and situation:

To Boost Motivation

"I am confident that I will achieve my goals. As I work toward them my enthusiasm and confidence grows."

To Communicate Better

"I feel relaxed and at ease with other people. I state clearly how I feel, and what I need. My point of view and needs are important."

To Stop Smoking

"I can stop smoking. The taste of a cigarette is extremely unpleasant. If I get an urge to smoke, I can watch it rise and then fade away. My body thanks me for not smoking."

Repeat each self-suggestion at least three times. Take the time to write a careful script, using positive words. If, for example, you are anxious about a deadline, you might say, *"'I can work steadily and calmly. My concentration will improve as I become more relaxed,"* rather than, *"I won't feel anxious anymore."*

Permissive suggestions usually meet with less resistance *("I can do well on my exam")*, but *some people respond better to commands ("I will do well on my exam"). In any case, be sure to avoid the word "try." It implies doubt, and the possibility of failure.* And keep your suggestions realistic. Don't promise yourself a pain-free, hassle-free life.

It helps to add a key phrase or action to your suggestions such as, "Whenever I hear the telephone ring, I take a deep breath and relax," or "Whenever I fold my hands together, I feel secure and confident." Or simply repeat a phrase like "breathe deep" or "calm and clear." This will reinforce the suggestion after your hypnotic session.

When you have finished your suggestions, say, *"Now I am going to wake up. I will feel alert and refreshed."* Count back up from 1 to 10. Pause a moment after each number and repeat to yourself "more alert, refreshed, and wide awake."

Key Point

AUTOGENIC TRAINING

Autogenic Training is a type of self-hypnosis. It uses simple phrases to cue your body to relax. Each of the phrases is thought to be linked to a specific physiological response. For example, the sensation of heaviness corresponds to a relaxation of the skeletal muscles of the body. The suggestion of warmth evokes relaxation of the blood vessel muscles to increase the flow of blood.

If you would like to try autogenic training, here's how to go about it:

▶ Get in a comfortable position either by sitting or lying down. Let your eyes close. Repeat to yourself the simple phrases given below, and notice the corresponding sensations in your body.

▶ If your mind wanders, gently bring it back to repeating the phrase.

▶ Start by slowly repeating each phrase at least five times. At your own pace, gradually build up to several minutes with each phrase. You may wish to linger longer on some of the phrases.

Breathing

First, focus on your breathing. Repeat, *"My breath is calm and regular"* quietly to yourself as you imagine waves of relaxation flowing through your body with each breath.

Heaviness

Focus on your hands and legs. Repeat quietly to yourself several times, *"My arms are heavy"* as you feel the relaxing sensation of heaviness in your arms and hands. Then concentrate on your legs as you repeat, *"My legs are heavy."* Finally, repeat several times, *"My arms and legs are heavy."*

Warmth

Now concentrate on your arms again, this time repeating to yourself, *"My arms are warm."* Next focus on your legs with the phrase, *"My legs are warm."* Finally end with, *"My arms and legs are warm."*

Heart

Place your attention on the area of your heart as you repeat slowly, *"My heartbeat is calm and regular."*

Solar Plexus

Put your attention at the area just below your breastbone and think to yourself: *"My solar plexus is warm."*

Forehead

Finally, concentrate on your forehead as you slowly repeat, *"My forehead is cool."*

When you are ready to stop the relaxation session, take a deep breath and say to yourself, *"When I open my eyes, I will feel refreshed and alert."* Stretch, and get up very slowly.

AFFIRMATIONS

Creating your own affirmations help make it clear what you really want. Affirmations are strong, positive statements. They are short, simple, and unconditional. Affirmations refer to something that is already true in the present, not something that will happen in the future. For example, "I forgive myself" is a stronger affirmation than "I will let go of past mistakes and forgive myself." Affirmations can help clarify your intentions, and replace negative self-statements that float endlessly around in your mind.

Put your affirmations in writing. Make a short list (no more than two or three). During your relaxation or guided imagery exercise, repeat your affirmations several times to yourself. You can also put them on individual cards and place them around the house so you can see them throughout the day. Here are some examples of affirmations:

▶ *I have a calm mind and a calm body.*

▶ *My body knows how to heal itself.*

▶ *I let go of tension.*

▶ *Peace is within me.*

▶ *At this moment, right now, everything is as it should be.*

▶ *I love and accept myself unconditionally.*

▶ *My relationship with _____ is more and more satisfying.*

▶ *I am a good friend.*

▶ *Tension flows out of my body.*

▶ *I can relax at will.*

▶ *I am in harmony with my life.*

▶ *I deserve to be treated well.*

▶ *I can accept my feelings.*

▶ *I have confidence in myself.*

▶ *I decisively create what I want.*

▶ *I am doing the best I can.*

> I am doing the
> very best I can.

> My body knows
> how to heal itself.

> I have confidence
> in my abilities.

> I let go of tension
> very easily.

7 Imagery

IMAGERY AND VISUALIZATION

With guided imagery, you deliberately focus your mind on a particular image. You do so in order to relax, manage stress, or alleviate a specific symptom. While imagery most often uses your sense of sight with visual images, you can also include the rich experiences of your mind's other senses. Adding smells, tastes, sounds, and other sensations makes the guided imagery experience more vivid and powerful.

Some people are very visual, and easily see images with their "mind's eye." But if your images aren't as vivid as a really great movie, don't worry. It's normal for imagery to vary in intensity. The important thing is to focus on as much detail as possible, and strengthen the images by using all your senses. Adding real background music can also increase the impact of guided imagery.

Remember, with guided imagery, you are always completely in control. You're the movie director. You can project whatever thought or feeling you want onto your mental screen. If you don't like a particular image, thought, or feeling, you can:

Key Point

▶ Redirect your mind to something more comfortable.

▶ Use other images to get rid of unpleasant thoughts (you might put them on a raft and watch them float away on a river, sweep them away with a large broom, or erase them with a giant eraser).

▶ Open your eyes and stop the exercise.

We have included a basic script for an imagery exercise below, and scores of other scripts and tapes are available (📖 see page 274). You may want to tape record yourself (or someone else) reading the script so that you can concentrate fully on the imagery. Feel free to change, modify, and personalize the script any way you please. Make it your own.

Creating Your Special Place

The purpose of this guided imagery exercise is to help you imagine a special place where you feel safe, comfortable, and relaxed. This place can be anywhere. It might be somewhere you have been, or a place you know well. It could be a place you create from scratch, or by taking bits and pieces from places you know. You may choose to put a dwelling in your landscape: a cabin, a castle, or a cave. Here's what to do:

▶ Begin by closing your eyes (or if you prefer, keep your eyes open). Take several slow, deep breaths, exhaling completely after each.

▶ Now see if you can imagine a place where you feel completely comfortable and peaceful. It might be real or imaginary, one from your past, or someplace you've always wanted to go (it doesn't really matter, just so long as this place feels very safe and peaceful to you).

▶ Allow that special place to take shape slowly (there's no rush).

As your place begins to take shape, look around. Look to your left, to your right, and all around you. What do you see?

Continued on next page

- Enjoy the scenery: the colors, the textures, the shapes.
- Listen to the sounds of your special place—perhaps waves gently lapping at the shore, the call of a distant bird, the sound of the wind in the trees.

Now just listen to the sounds of this wonderful place—a place that is so comfortable and peaceful to you.

- Perhaps you feel a breeze touch your face, or warm sun gently soothing your skin.
- You may feel the crunch of gravel or soft sand beneath your feet, or the comforting support of a favorite chair.
- Now touch or pick up some favorite object from your special place. Allow your fingertips to gently explore its surface (Is it smooth or rough? Wet or dry? Warm or cold?).
- Now take in a deep breath through your nose, and notice all the rich fragrances around you. Perhaps your favorite flower is in bloom. Or you may smell the pungent scent of a pine forest, or the tangy salt sea air, or the aroma of your favorite food.
- Relax and enjoy the peace, comfort and safety of your special place.

This is your place, and nothing can harm you here. Relax, feeling thankful and happy to be here, in your special place, at this moment.

- Begin to sense that something wonderful is about to happen. Feel the tingling sensation of expecting something good.
- Know the sense of certainty. Everything is right, just as it should be.

- Now notice a soft glow of golden light from above. It begins to bathe your body. A tingling, shimmering, vibrant energy surrounds you, energizes you, soothes you, heals you.
- You are washed in bright goodness, and draw everything you need to you, as a powerful magnet. Good wishes and kind thoughts come. This goodness and healing energy seeps into your body, infusing you with a generous, boundless energy and sense of well-being.
- Feel it move through the layers of your body, deeper and deeper into each and every organ, down to the bone.
- Feel it in each and every cell, dissolving any blockages, correcting any imbalances. Enjoy this free flowing, healthy energy sweeping through your body. Now you are relaxing; healing.
- Your body remembers how to be well, and savors this feeling of well-being. You feel peaceful and easy in your special place—a healing place—one that is always here. You know it's a place you can visit anytime, and feel this healing energy and peace.
- When you are ready to return, take a deep breath and exhale fully.

Open your eyes and spend a few moments savoring this relaxed, healthy, comfortable feeling.

You may want to explore different special places each time you do this exercise, or one special place may emerge as your favorite. Remember, you can visit this place any time you want to, in your mind.

Script adapted from Belleruth Naparstek

IMAGINE YOURSELF WELL

You have the ability to create special imagery to alleviate specific symptoms or illnesses. Use any image that is strong and vivid for you (this often involves using all your senses to create the image), and one that is meaningful to you. The image does not have to be physiologically accurate for it to work. Just use your imagination and trust yourself. Here are examples of images that some people have found useful:

For Tension and Stress

▶ A tight, twisted rope slowly untwists

▶ Wax softens and melts

▶ Tension swirls out of your body and down the drain

For Healing of Cuts and Injuries

▶ Plaster covers over a crack in a wall

▶ Cells and fibers stick together with superglue

▶ A shoe is laced up tight

▶ Jigsaw puzzle pieces come together

For Arteries and Heart Disease

▶ A miniature Roto Rooter truck speeds through your arteries and cleans out the clogged pipes

▶ Water flows freely through a wide, open river

▶ A crew in a small boat all row together, easily and efficiently pulling the slender boat across the smooth water surface

For Asthma and Lung Disease

▶ The tiny elastic rubber bands that constrict your airways pop open

▶ A vacuum cleaner gently sucks the mucus from your airways

▶ Waves calmly rise and fall on the ocean surface

For Diabetes

▶ Small insulin keys unlock doors to hungry cells, and allow nourishing blood sugar in

▶ An alarm goes off and a sleeping pancreas gland awakens to the smell of freshly brewed coffee

For Cancer

▶ A shark gobbles up the cancer cells

▶ Tumors shrivel up like raisins in the hot sun, and then evaporate completely into the air

▶ The faucet that controls the blood supply to the tumor is turned off, and the cancer cells starve

▶ Radiation or chemotherapy enter your body like healing rays of light; they destroy cancer cells

Continued on next page

For Infections

▶ White blood cells with flashing red sirens arrest and imprison harmful germs

▶ An army equipped with powerful anti-biotic missiles attacks enemy germs

▶ A hot flame chases germs out of your entire body

For a Weak Immune System
(Immune deficiency disorders: HIV, AIDS, and others)

▶ Sluggish, sleepy white blood cells awaken, put on protective armor, and enter the fight against the virus

▶ White blood cells rapidly multiply like millions of seeds bursting from a single, ripe seed pod

For an Immune System that is Overactive

(Allergies, asthma, arthritis, etc.)

▶ Hyperalert immune cells in the fire station are reassured that the allergens have triggered a false alarm, and they can go back to playing their game of poker

▶ The civil war ends with the warring sides agreeing not to attack their fellow citizens

For Pain

▶ All of the pain is placed in a large, strong metal box, closed, sealed tightly and locked with a huge, strong padlock

▶ You grasp the TV remote control and slowly turn down the pain volume until you can barely hear it; then it disappears entirely

▶ The pain is washed away by a cool, calm river flowing through your entire body

For Depression

▶ Your troubles and feelings of sadness are attached to big colorful helium balloons, and are floating off into a clear blue sky

▶ A strong, warm sun breaks through dark clouds

▶ You feel a sense of detachment and lightness, enabling you to float easily through your day

For Behavior Change

▶ If you are somewhat shy, imagine a vivid, detailed picture of yourself walking up to people and chatting with them confidently

▶ If you want to be more physically active, see yourself walking in the park, riding a bike, taking a dance class, or joining a sports team

Use any of these images, or make up your own. Remember, the best ones are vivid and have meaning to you. Use your imagination for health and healing.

Key Point

CONSULT YOUR INNER ADVISOR

You can use this type of imagery to explore the meaning of your symptoms or illness, and what you can do to improve your health. This imagery is a means of two-way communication between your mind and your body.

Begin with a general imagery exercise such as *Creating a Special Place* (see box page 104). Once you have entered your special place, invite an inner advisor to come and visit you.

Use all your senses to watch for your advisor, as the advisor may take any shape or form. Or you may have several inner advisors. They may be a person, a voice, an object, or a symbol. If you are not comfortable with what emerges, send him/her/it away, and invite another advisor.

Once you are comfortable with your advisor, ask questions. Feel free to ask anything, such as:

▶ *Are you my inner advisor?*

▶ *How can I relax?*

▶ *What is causing my tension? Pain? Symptom?*

▶ *What do I need to do to feel better?*

▶ *Who can help me?*

Then wait for the answers. Be patient. They may come in any form: a picture, image, sound, word, phrase, feeling. They can come at any time. Think about what they mean to you.

Sometimes you may be surprised at the directness and clarity of an answer. In response to "What is causing my anger?" one person heard back, "You need to learn to say no." If the meaning or usefulness is not clear to you right away, don't worry. It may become clearer in the days or weeks ahead.

You can use a similar technique to have an inner dialogue with a symptom you are having. For example, if you are in pain, give it a color, shape or form. Then ask your pain questions:

▶ *Why are you here?*

▶ *What can I learn from you?*

▶ *When will you go away?*

▶ *How can we live more peaceably together?*

▶ *How can I get better?*

Wait for responses. This dialogue can be done with any symptom or problem.

You have untapped knowledge, insight, and wisdom which is often drowned out by the incessant chatter of a busy mind. You can use imagery techniques to give voice to your inner wisdom, and consult your own inner advisor. There is nothing mysterious or magical about it. Simply by quieting down and bringing your mind into a focused and receptive state, valuable insights can emerge. These include suggestions on how to improve your health and well-being.

Adapted from Martin Rossman, M.D. and the Academy for Guided Imagery

Key Point

📖 *For more information, see page 274*

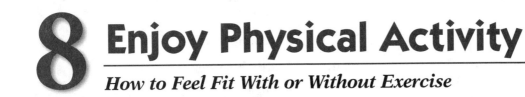

8 Enjoy Physical Activity

How to Feel Fit With or Without Exercise

Imagine a world without cars . . . or planes, or trains, or bicycles, or elevators. Think of a world without labor-saving devices: no washing machines, no power tools, no farm machinery. And one without televisions, remote controls, or even couches.

This was the world of our ancestors. They had no need for exercycles, aerobics classes, fitness clubs, or personal trainers. Their day-to-day survival *required* mild to moderate physical activity. This is the world to which our bodies and minds are most well adapted. To get food, our ancestors needed to run down prey or scour the bush for fruits and berries. Later, they had to plant, sow, and harvest the crops. Today, we jump in the car and make a quick run to the supermarket or a fast food restaurant. No sweat.

The modern world is dramatically different from the one our ancestors knew. Some people avoid physical activity at every turn, while others have joined the "Fitness Revolution" with the battle cry, "no pain, no gain." And they all are suffering. The couch potatoes get denied the pleasures and health benefits of gentle physical activity, while the "fit-fanatics" are prone to suffer the frequent aches and pains of overuse and abuse.

Humans didn't evolve to inhabit the couch, but neither did we evolve to run marathons or bench press hundreds of pounds. We evolved to walk, hunt, gather, and partake in other moderately strenuous physical activities.

The New Prescription

Now you really don't have to knock yourself out to keep yourself healthy. **Key Point** *New research emphasizes the bodily and mental benefits of modest, enjoyable physical activity.* Remember the life of our ancestors. It will help us live healthier (and easier) lives in our modern world.

When you hear the word "exercise," what comes to mind? For some who are already physically active, it brings images of pleasurable exertion, competition, and challenge. For others who are sedentary, the word "exercise" conjures up images of sweat-soaked athletes, exhaustion, huffing and puffing, and, too often, feelings of guilt, failure, and hopelessness.

Unfortunately, there is an epidemic of physical inactivity in this country today.

Twenty-five percent of adult Americans are completely sedentary, and another fifty percent would benefit from being more active.

Part of the problem is due to a misunderstanding of what really is healthful physical activity. For the past twenty years authorities have over-emphasized the importance of high-intensity exercise. So many people think the only way to reap health benefits from exercise is through prolonged bouts of vigorous exercise. It's understandable to see how this perception has turned off so many people.

Physical activity shouldn't be an exclusive club for youthful, attractive, lean, hard-bodied athletes. Exercise is for every body: young, old, fat, thin, well, and ill.

Physically active people, on average, outlive inactive people at any age. The greatest gains in health come to those who advance from outright couch potatoes to moderately active people.

Recent findings by leading health and fitness authorities are radically changing our ideas about physical activity. They offer good news for the sedentary: physical activity does not have to be torture to be beneficial.

Normal Activities Count

The old prescription for exercise was 15 to 60 minutes of continuous, vigorous exercise three to five times a week. The new recommendation from The US Centers for Disease Control and Prevention and the American College of Sports Medicine call for *"accumulating 30 minutes or more of moderate-intensity physical activity on most, preferably all, days of the week."* The differences between the old and the new recommendations are important.

Intense or vigorous effort is not required. Normal chores, activities, and pleasures count. These include such things as:

▶ Raking leaves

▶ Climbing steps

▶ Walking briskly

▶ Dancing

▶ Playing catch or ping pong

▶ General calisthenics

▶ Cycling for pleasure

▶ House cleaning

▶ Painting walls or fences

▶ Gardening

▶ Washing windows

▶ Washing the car

These qualify as moderate-intensity physical activity, and they produce significant health benefits. Carrying golf clubs or pushing a power lawn mower does count; riding on a golf cart or a power mower doesn't.

And the physical activity doesn't have to be done in one continuous bout. You can accumulate short spurts of activity—from walking several blocks to climbing a flight of stairs—so that it adds up to the recommended 30 minutes. Scientists now say that the benefits of accumulated periods of activity are probably equivalent to those of a sustained vigorous workout such as aerobics, swimming, tennis, or rowing. In fact, exercisers who divvy up their workouts into short chunks actually seem to get a greater boost in the ratio of "good" cholesterol to "bad."

Benefits of Moderate Exercise

Experts now admit they were mistaken in saying that exercise had to be intense and continuous to do any good. Not only is there clear evidence that moderate exercise is better than none, but there is also evidence that moderate exercise results in many of the same health benefits of vigorous exercise.

One study found that men who took part in even small amounts of light or moderate physical activity had lower rates of heart attacks and death than sedentary men. In fact, men with 30 minutes of moderate exercise were as protected from fatal heart attacks as those who exercised three times as much.

Another study found that men who walked as little as a mile a day had a 30% lower risk of stroke; those who walked more than a mile a day had a 50% lower risk.

Even the most sedentary people should know that every bit of activity—no matter how small—counts. Just standing instead of sitting can burn off up to 20 calories an hour. That's a pound a year if you stand instead of sit for one hour a day. If you move around a bit while you are standing, you'll get more benefit. Even energetic sex counts; it burns about as many calories per minute as mowing the lawn, scrubbing the walls, doubles tennis, halfcourt basketball, and gymnastics!

BENEFITS

Enjoying physical activity can:

▶ Reduce risk of coronary heart disease and stroke

▶ Raise "good" artery-clearing HDL cholesterol

▶ Help control blood pressure

▶ Decrease risk of osteoporosis and diabetes

▶ Help with weight maintenance

▶ Possibly protect against cancer of the colon, breast, ovaries, and cervix

But if you really want to "go for the burn," great. Many people enjoy a vigorous workout, the "high," the sleeker body, and the somewhat greater physical health benefits that come from more intense exercise. Just don't think that it is required for improved mental or physical health.

Remember, it doesn't matter how brief your periods of activity are—the benefits are cumulative. It's the total amount of activity that counts, not the manner in which you do it. You don't have to kill yourself to save your life.

Key Point

Our change to an inactive life is costly. More than 250,000 deaths per year in the United States (12% of the total) may be due to a lack of regular physical activity. This number is comparable to deaths from smoking, high blood pressure, and elevated cholesterol.

It's Never Too Late to Start

A Massachusetts geriatrician encouraged ten 86 to 96-year-olds to lift weights. They did so three times a week for 10 to 20 minutes, starting with just five pounds. After eight weeks, they had doubled their strength. Two of them no longer needed their canes, and one, for the first time in a long time, was able to get up from his chair.

Exercise Helps with Stress and Anxiety

Most people report that physical activity improves their mood and helps them manage anxiety, depression, and stress. It doesn't take much to make a difference. Short periods of gentle activity can make your problems seem less serious. It can also boost optimism, self-esteem, confidence, and give you a greater sense of control.

Exercise may be an outlet for the body's excess tension, providing a healthy way to release anger and anxiety. It appears to be a particularly potent buffer against stress. When people face a difficult problem or an insult, those who exercise regularly show less muscle tension, less anxiety, and lower blood pressure than those who don't. And although people who endure a lot of stress have more illness, regular exercise blocks the stress-illness link.

For those faced with a serious, life-threatening illness, regular physical activity can be a healthful coping strategy. After beginning an exercise program, patients infected with the HIV virus were less anxious and depressed, and their immune systems were stronger. In fact, the beneficial effects of exercise on mood and immunity are comparable to those of a stress-management course.

Exercise seems to have a tranquilizing effect that reduces anxiety even more effectively than many antianxiety medications or quiet rest. And exercise works fast: within five to ten minutes of finishing aerobic exercise, anxious feelings are significantly reduced. The effects last for four hours or more.

Regular physical activity throughout the day may be helpful in reducing chronic anxiety. In fact, exercise appears to produce a longer-lasting sense of relaxation than does an equal amount of time spent just resting or practicing a relaxation exercise.

And strenuous exercise may not be necessary to reap the antianxiety benefits. Several studies suggest that gentle and moderate-intensity physical activity such as walking a mile or two, lifting light weights, stretching, and relaxation exercises decrease anxiety just as effectively as vigorous jogging.

Continued on next page

Exercise Improves Mood

Exercise can also help depression. A group of mildly to moderately depressed patients were divided randomly into two groups. One would walk or jog; the other would receive psychotherapy. Within a week most of those doing the exercises reported feeling better, and within three weeks they were "virtually well." The exercisers did as well as those who received short-term psychotherapy, and they did better than the patients who underwent long-term therapy. After one year, those treated with exercise were essentially free of depression, while nearly half of those receiving psychotherapy had to return for additional treatment.

Similar results were found in a follow-up study of depressed patients. They were treated with exercise, meditation training, and group psychotherapy. At first, patients improved equally. But after nine months the exercisers and meditators stayed better while the psychotherapy patients slipped back into depression. Regular physical activity appears to reduce recurrent depression.

How Exercise Improves Mood

How does physical activity work its mental wonders? Changes in body and brain chemistry associated with exercise may help explain some of the psychological benefits.

But improvement in physical fitness is not needed to improve mental health. Some of the psychological benefits of exercise may come more from positive expectation than from physiological changes.

In one study, healthy young men and women were divided into two groups. Both were supervised and met three times a week for 10 weeks. Group activities included jogging, aerobic dancing, swimming pool games, and soccer. Both groups had the same enthusiastic instructors. Participants in group A were told repeatedly that their program was designed to improve *both* psychological well-being and aerobic capacity. The instructors reinforced this positive expectation by encouraging the participants to notice any improvements in their mood and feelings of well-being. Participants in group B were led to expect *only* physical benefits.

Both groups reported about the same levels of enjoyment and experienced similar fitness benefits. They were unanimous in recommending the programs to their friends. The only major difference between the groups was that Group A participants scored higher in self-esteem and well-being. This suggests that some of the psychological benefits of aerobic exercise may be more related to how you *expect* to feel rather than to the increased aerobic activity itself.

Capitalize on these findings. Look for improvements in your mood and well-being both during and after exercise, and enjoy them!

How to Make Exercise More Enjoyable

"If exercise could be packed into a pill, it would be the single most widely prescribed and beneficial medicine in the nation."
—Robert Butler, M.D.

Choose Exercise That's Fun

During an interview with her doctor, a patient was asked if she ever exercised. She replied "No" without hesitation. Later in the interview she mentioned that she went square dancing three times a week. The doctor responded somewhat surprised, "I thought you said you never did any exercise!" She smiled and said, "Square dancing isn't exercise, it's fun!"

The best way to ensure that you get regular exercise is by choosing activities that you enjoy. Instead of going through a joyless exercise program, why not have fun? You'll do your body good and lift your mood by doing something that gives you satisfaction.

Replace sedentary leisure activities with active, enjoyable ones: go dancing instead of to the movies, have a gardening or work party rather than a brunch, toss a football with a neighbor rather than tossing down some beers in front of the TV.

Take an Exercise Break

For many, exercise provides the only break in an otherwise harried day. As little as ten minutes of brisk walking can increase your energy level and reduce tension for an hour or more. Taking the time to work on your tennis game or notice the trees on a morning walk distracts you from your troubles. It provides a restorative "time-out," and takes you away from work and personal problems. Think of it as a coffee break without the caffeine, or a mini-vacation without the expense.

Take a Walk

Walking 15 to 20 minutes four to five days a week is all that you need to markedly improve your health. Walking is easy, free, and you need no special training or equipment. You can burn up almost as many calories walking briskly as you do when you run at a moderate pace. Even walking slowly (about two miles per hour) will give you considerable physical and psychological benefits.

Don't Be Too Competitive

Some people thoroughly enjoy competing against others, and that may be what attracts them to sports such as tennis or soccer in the first place. A little competitiveness may be healthy; a lot is not. Some competitive players find themselves fighting the urge to storm off the court or field because they can't stand the thought of losing. Getting hung up on winning may counter many of the benefits of exercise. And putting that pressure on yourself often increases psychological stress.

Even if you are not involved in a particularly competitive sport, you may still make unreasonable demands on yourself. Resist the temptation. Remember, you'll get the most out of exercise by

Too Much Vigorous Exercise

With light or moderate physical activity the risk of injury is minimal. In contrast, nearly 20 percent of all 10-mile-per-week joggers are forced to cut back at some point each year due to injuries. Injury rates are even higher for those who:

▶ Exercise vigorously every day

▶ Spend longer than 30 minutes per session in strenuous exercise

▶ Work out at 90 percent of their capacity

Extremely high levels of vigorous exercise can cause problems with women's hormones interfering with:

▶ Ovulation

▶ Menstrual cycles

▶ The risk of osteoporosis (thin and fragile bones)

Research on laboratory animals suggests that the benefits of moderate exercise on reducing cancer rates may disappear at very high levels of physical activity. So easy does it.

Check With Your Doctor

Before increasing your physical activity, consult with your doctor if you have any of the following:

▶ Concerns related to a medical condition, especially a heart condition or diabetes

▶ Any symptoms such as chest pains, extreme shortness of breath with exertion, wheezing, faintness, dizziness, or joint pains

If you are currently a very sedentary person, remember to *start slowly* and increase your activity *gradually.* If you develop symptoms, consult your doctor.

---

doing it in moderation, and by enjoying it. Focus on the activity, not on the outcome.

℞ What You Tell Yourself Matters

Preoccupation with one's own performance may also be counterproductive. We all know the feeling of being mad at ourselves for dropping a ball, missing a shot, or otherwise falling flat on our faces. Self-sabotaging thoughts are damaging. The tennis player who thinks, for example, "my backhand is lousy," or "I'll never catch up," or "I'm so clumsy," is not getting the full benefit of the exercise. Learn to encourage yourself with positive self-talk (📖 see page 149).

℞ How to Overcome Your Excuses

If you're still hearing reasons for not exercising in your head, examine these common excuses and myths. It's often the first step to overcoming them.

1. *"Exercise bores me."* Incorporate physical activities into your normal day (for example, take the stairs, not the elevator), and seek out physical leisure activities you actually enjoy. Be creative: figure out ways to add fun to your exercise. Listen to a cassette, watch TV, or read while you pedal away on a stationary bicycle. If you jog or go for a walk, take along a radio, cassette player, or a friend to talk to. Vary your routes and routines regularly. Try doing something different each day or alternate activities: Monday and Wednesdays on the exercycle, Tuesdays a brisk walk, Saturday mow the lawn and garden, Sundays a game of tennis.

2. "Exercise is painful." Well, it shouldn't be. The old saying "no pain, no gain" is simply wrong and outdated. You're probably exercising improperly or over doing it if you hurt during or afterwards. Slow down. Go for "all gain, no pain."

3. "I don't have time." We all have exactly the same amount of time. Making more of it available for physical activity involves resetting priorities and changing the way you see your daily activities (see page 183). You can think of household chores as a burden or as an opportunity for exercise. Your trip to work can be a boring bus ride or an interesting walk. Create more time by doubling up on activities: schedule a "walking meeting" to discuss business or personal matters. Keep in mind that any physical activity, even for just a minute, is better than none.

4. "I'm too tired." Often you'll feel tired because of a *lack* of physical activity. When you're out of shape, you feel tired, weak, and listless. These feelings lead to more inactivity, and the vicious cycle continues. But as you become more active, your energy level and stamina will gradually increase, and you'll feel less tired.

5. "I might hurt myself." In most cases, the risk of heart attack is much greater for those who are *not* physically active. With moderate-intensity activities such as walking and swimming, the risk of injury is extremely low. Choose activities you are comfortable with. The more you do them, the more proficient and resilient you will become.

6. "I already get enough exercise." This may be true, for some. Just be sure that your activities add up to at least 30 minutes of moderate physical activity a day.

7. "My neighborhood isn't safe." It's true, some areas are more dangerous than others for walking or jogging. Examine the evidence in your neighborhood. If your neighborhood isn't safe, think about walking in another one or at a shopping center. Or exercise in the house. Use an exercycle, treadmill, or videotape program. Or turn on music and dance as you clean up the kitchen. Find a partner or group to exercise with.

8. "I feel guilty taking time for myself." Your friends, family, and work associates need you to be healthy, and you deserve good health. Stick to your plans for exercise even if others consciously (or unconsciously) make you feel guilty. Let family members know you still care about them, and that by taking time to exercise now, you'll have more energy for them later. And you'll also probably be in a better mood.

Do not let other excuses or barriers stand in your way to becoming more fit. Challenge them! (see page 42)

℞ Work In Your Workout

Matthew was going to a gym twice a week after work and on weekends to lift weights or ride the exercise bike. He hated going but believed it was doing him good, even with the stressful, smoggy, traffic-jammed trip to the gym and the mad rush home in time to see his children before they went to bed.

Then it occurred to Matthew that if he spent a few hours a week mowing the lawn, raking leaves, weeding, and doing all the repairs that needed doing around the house, he would be getting just as much exercise. He'd save money on the gardener and health club, do something useful and satisfying, and he'd have more time at home with his family.

Exercise should be a regular part of your life, like eating and sleeping. There are two broad approaches to it:

▶ You can schedule specific blocks of time for doing a particular type of activity ("working out").

▶ You can grab every small opportunity to be more active throughout the day ("working in").

Although you can certainly combine both approaches, most peoples' lifestyles lend themselves more easily to one than the other. "Working out" at a precise time every day requires a set schedule and a stick-to-it attitude. "Working in" your exercise requires a flexible schedule and lots of creativity. If you go the "working in" route, think of as many ways as possible to build physical activity into your day. Here are some possibilities:

▶ Climb stairs instead of taking the elevator. Climbing stairs demands an intensity level similar to cross-country skiing and mountain-climbing.

▶ Garden. Gardening activities such as hoeing, digging, and pulling weeds can boost your heart rate by 20 to 25 percent.

▶ Mow the lawn. Mowing the lawn with a hand mower can burn a healthy 400 calories an hour.

▶ Walk to work or to shops instead of

taking the car or the bus. If it's too far to walk, park the car or get off the bus and walk part way.

▶ Go on foot to visit colleagues or neighbors instead of calling them on the phone.

▶ Pace up and down in your office as you read reports or memos.

▶ Do brief neck and shoulder exercises periodically if you sit all day.

▶ Turn on the radio and dance as you clean up the house.

▶ Throughout the day, fit in additional physical activity by avoiding labor-saving devices such as leaf blowers, chain saws, or remote controls.

Seize every opportunity you can to get up and move around! You'll be surprised to discover how much exercise you can get just by doing what needs to be done. Short burst exercise is easier to incorporate into busy lives, and for many people it is easier to keep up than 30 minutes of non-stop exercise. This is an effective and efficient way to improve your health.

℞ Make Exercise a Social Event

Are you having difficulty getting started? Try making plans for a regular activity with a friend. Arrange to have lunch on the weekend at a favorite restaurant a mile away, and walk there and back together. Or set up a regular Saturday morning tennis game. Or schedule a walk after dinner twice a week with your friends or family.

Some people prefer solo exercise, but for others, much of the pleasure comes from getting together to play a sport, plant a garden, or clean a house with someone else. This social side of exercise can boost your enjoyment of the activity as well as help you stick with it.

℞ Include Your Children

If you are concerned that regular exercise will give you less time with your children, do something active *with them*. You might, for example:

▶ Walk to the local park

▶ Visit the zoo

▶ Play ball

▶ Ride on bicycle trails

▶ Take them canoeing or rowing

▶ Get them involved in gardening

▶ Jump rope together

▶ Teach them how to dance

By enjoying physical activities with your children, you'll encourage them to see it as a normal part of everyday life and an alternative to flopping in front of the television. These times together may also give you the chance to talk in depth with your children and find out what is really on their minds.

℞ Your Pulse: Take It or Leave It

Some people, especially those with heart disease, may be advised by their doctor to take their pulse before, during, and after exercise. This is one way to be sure that you are exercising hard enough, but not too hard.

 Fortunately, most people don't need to measure their pulse to find out if their exercise is boosting their heart rate enough. Just do what feels right and use your own judgment. Before the fitness craze, that's what we always did anyway. We took a breather or stopped when we got too tired, hot, or sweaty. You should

feel like you are working a little bit hard, but are in no way near exhaustion or putting in your full effort.

Remember to listen to your body. If you still want to monitor the intensity of your exercise, pay attention to how hard you are working. You can imagine a scale from 0 to 10: 0 is lying down doing nothing; 10 is the equivalent of exerting yourself as hard as possible (something you should *not* do). A good level of exertion is generally between 3 and 6 on this scale. At this level, you should:

▶ Feel a bit warmer

▶ Breathe somewhat deeper and faster

▶ Have a faster heart beat

But at this rate you won't feel uncomfortable or strained.

You can also monitor the intensity of your activity with a simple "talk test." With moderate intensity activity you should still be able to talk comfortably without gasping. Or try one of the fitness self-tests (📖 see box page 119).

℞ How to Keep Yourself Motivated

Sometimes it's difficult to find the inspiration to keep exercising. On those days, remind yourself of its pleasures, and ask yourself:

▶ Does exercise make me feel or look more fit, strong, and toned?

▶ Do I have more energy?

▶ Am I feeling less physically vulnerable?

▶ Do I enjoy looking at gardens or window shopping on my walks?

▶ Am I improving my breaststroke?

▶ Am I getting better at playing basketball?

Sometimes linking your exercise with some

TRACK YOUR PROGRESS

Although some people are satisfied knowing they are feeling more fit in general, others may want a more precise measurement of their progress.

Diary. Keep an exercise diary or calendar of your physical activity. Record what you do, how much you do, and how you feel. You can also take one or both of the following fitness self-tests before you begin an exercise program, and repeat it every few weeks.

Time test. Choose an activity such as walking, bicycling, swimming, or water walking. After warming up, start timing your activity. Continue briskly but comfortably for five minutes. Stop and record how far you went (blocks, miles, laps, etc.), heart rate, and how hard you exerted yourself from 0 to 10. Then continue the activity at a slow pace for three to five minutes to cool down. The future goal for this test is to exercise for the same amount of time but to cover a greater distance, at a lower heart rate, or at a lower level of perceived exertion.

Distance test. Find a good place to walk, bicycle, or swim where you can measure distance. Estimate about how far you can go in about 5 minutes. After warming up, begin your activity and go briskly but comfortably to cover your estimated selected distance (e.g.: 10 blocks, 1 mile, 10 laps, etc.), moving at a steady pace. Then stop and note how much time it took. Immediately take your pulse, and rate how hard you exerted yourself from 0 to 10. Then continue the activity at a slow pace for three to five minutes to cool down. Your goal now is to cover the same distance in less time, or at a lower heart rate, or at a lower level of perceived exertion.

other activity or purpose can help keep you moving.

Angela arranged to take an elderly neighbor's dog for a walk after work, twice a week and once on weekends. "I'm not someone who can just walk without a purpose," she said. "Taking the dog gives me some much-needed exercise, and it helps my neighbor. Now I really like the dog and we always end up in the park playing fetch. I have the best of all worlds. I exercise, get to play with a nice dog without the responsibility of owning one, and I've become friends with my neighbor."

℞ Make the Most of a Setback

Everyone, even the most dedicated, will experience some setback which interferes with a usual exercise routine. It may be an illness, a job change, prolonged bad weather, or loss of an exercise partner.

Expect occasional bad days (or weeks), and don't get discouraged. It doesn't mean you have failed. Just rethink your goals and activities, and start again. If you can't do your usual exercise, maybe you can indulge yourself in a relaxing few minutes of stretching, or treat yourself to some new plants for the garden, or just walk to the corner store for a newspaper. There are skills you can develop to set specific goals and maintain healthy change (📖 see page 26).

℞ Stretch and Strengthen

If you really want to be fit, think about muscle strengthening and flexibility in addition to aerobic exercise. Stretching is good for everyone because it keeps the muscles flexible and helps prevent injury.

Do several minutes of stretching in the morning and throughout the day. It's easy to do simple stretches just about anywhere: in the car at traffic lights, at your desk, sitting in boring meetings, or at the hairdresser's. There are classes and books available to help you design a personal, balanced fitness program—from yoga to calisthenics, from Tai'Chi to weight training—whatever suits your interest.

There are very many fitness options available today. The trick is to keep trying new ones until you find one that's just right for you. Not only will you look better, feel better, and be stronger—you're also likely to discover a new form of pleasure you'll thoroughly enjoy.

📖 *For more information, see page 274*

9 Communicate Well

How to Speak and Listen Better to Improve Your Health

▶ *A wife says to her husband, "Did you pick up the package at the post office?" She's thinking that she's going to the post office later, and can save him a trip. He's thinking that she's saying he is irresponsible and not doing his share.*

▶ *Sally notices her friend Roberta is unusually quiet and asks, "What's wrong?" Roberta turns away and mumbles, "Nothing."*

▶ *The boss asks Mark to work overtime. Mark says "yes" because he's too intimidated to say "no," and cancels his date.*

We all do it. We say yes when we really want to say no. We don't make our meaning clear. We hedge or we're vague. We misinterpret what someone else is saying. We hog conversations.

How you communicate has a very real impact on your happiness and your health. When you communicate effectively, you feel understood. Life is joyful and satisfying, and you feel in control of events. You feel connected, valued at work, and people trust and respect you. Even sex can be more fulfilling.

Words can be like surgeons' scalpels: they can harm or heal. Imagine that someone says something that embarrasses you. You may blush and feel a warm sensation in your face. Words trigger a specific reaction in your body.

Or say you fail to communicate, and feel unappreciated and misunderstood. Not communicating well can also make you feel defensive, hostile, frustrated, or distressed.

We've been communicating since we were small children so you'd think we'd have it down—especially considering its impact on our happiness and well-being!

Why We Don't Communicate Better

There are several reasons why many of us find it difficult to communicate:

▶ We learn from less than perfect role models: our parents, teachers, bosses, and friends. They themselves may not know how to communicate effectively.

▶ Few of us have studied basic techniques for really good communication. We often assume we already know just about all there is to know about how to communicate well. It doesn't occur to us that there's more to learn.

1 Ask for Clarification

Asking friendly questions when something is unclear allows you to get more information. It also demonstrates your interest and concern. You might say "Please tell me more about that?" or "Can you give me an example?" Even "I don't understand" or a simple "mmm mm" will encourage the speaker. Some people feel threatened by questions, so make your probing gentle and supportive. Be especially careful with "why" questions. Instead of asking, "Why do you say it like that?" try instead, "Are you angry at me for something?" Instead of "Why didn't you call me?" try "Was there something that held you up?"

2 Say Back What You Hear

Paraphrasing (saying back what you hear) is not the same as parroting. It's repeating, in your own words, what you think the other person is saying. Here are some examples:

▶ "So even though it's expensive, you think a night course in desktop publishing will help your career."

▶ "If I understand you correctly, you are unhappy with the teacher's handling of the children."

▶ "It sounds like you want help with the project. Is that correct?"

Your summary may be off base, but the purpose of paraphrasing is to correct such misunderstandings.

Paraphrasing sometimes works best as a question.

More skillful: "Are you saying that you'd rather stay home than go to the party with me?"

Less skillful: "Obviously you're telling me you don't want to go to the party with me."

3 Say What You Think the Other Person is Feeling

Let him or her know that you heard the emotional content. Listen between the lines. What is the person feeling but not saying? Asking for, but not directly? Be empathetic. Say to yourself: "If I were having this experience, what would I be feeling?"

Body language gives you clues: posture, facial expression, and gestures often reveal underlying emotions. Then check out your guesses. Say, "You seem very disappointed. Is that true?"

4 Interpret the Meaning

As you listen attentively, you may begin to sense links between feelings and facts. Offer your tentative interpretations as feedback in an accepting, nonjudgmental way. Use the word *because* to link feelings and facts. For example, "You feel scared because this is something you've never done before. Does that make sense?" This type of communication helps you gain both understanding and insight.

- Our egos and self-esteem are very much involved: we're often afraid our requests will be turned down.
- If we are put off we take it as a personal rejection.
- We may be preoccupied, wrongly motivated, or just not listening.
- Often we are simply not aware that different people have very different communication styles.

Whatever the reason effective communication may be difficult for us, it involves skills that can be learned. And there's increasing evidence that improving those skills may be one of the most important health-enhancing steps we can take.

BENEFITS

COMMUNICATING WELL

There are many advantages of communicating well. Communicating well is a skill that can:

- Improve your mood and sense of well-being
- Decrease your conflicts and stress
- Improve your social support
- Reduce hostility and possibly the associated risks of heart disease, high blood pressure, and a weak immune system

How to Communicate Well

The following techniques can help you be a better communicator. With practice, you can learn to say what you feel, think, and want clearly and comfortably. You'll be able to express your likes and dislikes more effectively, accept compliments more graciously, deal with criticism, and say no—all without putting extra stress on your body. And because you are communicating more directly, other people are likely to be more responsive to your needs.

Learn to Listen

"Just listen and smile, and people will say what a marvelous conversationalist you are."

— Anonymous

This may be good folk wisdom, but good listening is more than keeping quiet, smiling, and hearing someone else's words. It's a process that requires your active participation, openness, and receptivity. When someone really listens to you with their full attention, it feels different. Attention is itself a vital nutrient. Attentive listening is one way we can nourish those around us. The next time you are in a conversation with someone, notice if the person is really paying attention and listening to you.

Poor Communication is Bad for Your Health

New evidence suggests that communicating effectively enhances our health and self-esteem, nurtures our relationships, and helps us cope with stress. Healthy communication is the life-blood of relationships, and relationships are a lifeline to health. Those who have close relationships in which they can share their feelings and feel supported tend to live longer lives.

Those who don't communicate effectively are more vulnerable to disease, and may be at an increased risk of death. Several studies suggest that hostile, confrontational people have an increased risk of heart disease. And those who feel misunderstood report more of a kind of depression that weakens the immune system.

When communication breaks down, heart rate speeds up. Cholesterol and blood sugar levels rise. We become susceptible to headaches, backaches, and digestive problems. We are more sensitive to pain. At work, worry over conflict and misunderstandings can make us irritable, unable to concentrate, and increase the risk of accidents.

Unhealthy Conflict Between Husbands and Wives

Marital conflict is especially harmful. One recent study looked at how hostile communication would affect happy newlyweds. The couples were asked to discuss sensitive topics for 30-minutes. Their conversations were monitored for:

▶ Criticism

▶ Put-downs

▶ Denying responsibility

▶ Making excuses

▶ Interrupting

▶ Trying to force one partner into accepting the other's point of view

Expressing hostility elevated the couples' blood pressure and heart rates, and resulted in a significant decline in the strength of their immune systems. The more hostile the communication, the greater the weakness in immune function. And since arguments in the laboratory are usually milder than the ones at home, the impact of marital conflict on health is probably greater than these results show.

Reach Out and Touch Someone

One study showed that when people are touched, even casually, and even if they are not consciously aware of it, they respond more positively. For example, if a librarian gently makes physical contact with someone she is helping, the person tends to be more satisfied with the interchange. Touching someone while talking with them can have a big impact. If the situation permits, put your hand on his (her) shoulder and say the person's name.

Anger and disagreement in themselves are not harmful to a marriage, but marriages with heavy doses of criticism, contempt, defensiveness, and withdrawal most often end in separation and divorce. One nasty put-down can erase many positive acts of kindness.

While a conflict-free relationship is unrealistic, healthy relationships tend to accentuate the positive and minimize the negative. Even minor improvements in communication skills can lessen the negative aspects and enhance health and well-being.

Being a good listener is not so easy. It takes practice. Our minds are filled with a continuous stream of reactions, responses, judgments, questions, and ideas. Instead of listening to the speaker, we're often thinking about what we're going to say next (📖 see box this page and page 122).

℞ Watch Your Body Language

Research shows that more than half of what we communicate is not conveyed by our words but by our body language. When we smile, frown, sigh, touch, drum our fingers, or blush, we send powerful messages. Even when we are saying nothing, our bodies are still communicating.

For good communication, your body language and tone of voice should match what you are saying. If you are making an assertive statement, for example, look straight at the other person and keep your expression friendly. Watch out for sneers or lip biting. Relax your arms and legs. Breathe. Stand tall and confident, and lean forward to show your interest. Arching away suggests you'd rather be somewhere else. Slouching communicates uncertainty.

When you detect a mismatch between body and words in others, point it out in a friendly way. You might say, "I appreciate your saying you want to go dancing, but you look tired and your voice is flat. Would you rather go tomorrow?"

℞ Notice Conversational Styles

Maria complains that her husband, Hector, doesn't pay attention to her when she talks. But, in fact, Hector can usually recount every word Maria says. Hector listens quietly whereas Maria gives a lot of feedback: nodding, changing facial expressions, and saying "uh huh."

TRY THIS

LISTENING

Try this simple exercise with a partner: You each get to talk for three full minutes about anything you want. When it is your turn to listen, give the other person your total attention.

Just listen. Lean forward toward the speaker. Make eye contact occasionally, but don't stare. Try not to judge what the other person is saying. Don't interrupt. Don't respond except to say such things as: "Could you explain that more?" "Go on...." or just a simple "Ah-ha" or nod.

When three minutes are up, reverse roles. Then discuss how it feels to be the listener, and how it feels to be listened to.

Kim pauses longer than Michael between sentences. Michael thinks Kim is finished talking and interrupts. Kim feels hurt that Michael is always interrupting her, or she accuses him of being arrogant and rude.

Studies show that styles of conversing play a major role in misunderstandings. For example, women ask more personal questions because they believe "it shows I care." Men think "if there's something she wants me to know, she'll tell me."

Men are more likely to interrupt. This is something they learned as boys. A high value was placed on status and dominance among males. In general, women learned to use conversation in order to

HOW ASSERTIVE ARE YOU?

Check the letter next to the way you'd most likely respond.

1 **Your neighbor plays his stereo full blast late at night.**

❑ **A.** You resolve to say something if you ever run into him. Meanwhile you buy earplugs.

❑ **B.** You knock on his door and tell him you are trying to sleep and the noise disturbs you. Ask him to turn it down.

❑ **C.** You pound angrily on his door, call him an inconsiderate creep, and threaten to call the police if he doesn't stop the racket.

2 **A good friend has started to criticize you in small ways.** He says things like: "You jiggle the steering wheel when you drive" or "You always look tired" or "You seem to be eating a lot of ice cream lately."

❑ **A.** You grin and bear it, reminding yourself that no one is perfect.

❑ **B.** You tell your friend, "You've been commenting a lot on my behavior lately, and your criticisms made me feel bad. I wish you'd stop."

❑ **C.** You retaliate, looking for ways to find fault with your friend. Or you get sarcastic: "Who put you in charge of my life?"

3 **A relative calls and says she wants to visit next weekend.** You respond by saying:

❑ **A.** "Well, we did have some plans, but I guess we can work around them somehow."

❑ **B.** "Next weekend is not a good time. With more advanced notice, I'm sure we could arrange a time that would work."

❑ **C.** "Look, you just can't come and visit whenever you feel like it. I've got my own plans, you know."

The "A" answers are passive responses. The "C"s indicate aggressiveness. The "B" answers are properly assertive statements. You speak up for your rights, and at the same time respect the rights of others.

---

form and maintain friendships. Men more often give opinions and make declarations of fact than women. Men tend to discuss problems just to seek solutions, whereas women want to share their feelings and experiences. Other factors that influence conversational style include: where people are born and how they're raised, the size of their family, their occupation, and their cultural background.

Just recognize that others express themselves differently. It can reduce a lot of misunderstanding, frustration, and resentment.

Key Point

℞ Know Your Legitimate Rights

There are basically three ways we communicate with other people: aggressively, passively, or assertively. Effective communication is usually **assertive** communication. When you communicate assertively, you stand up for your rights in a friendly way, without being aggressive.

Many of us carry unhelpful assumptions about ourselves, our rights to express ourselves, and to be respected. These assumptions make it more likely that we'll respond in either an aggressive or a passive manner rather than in an assertive one.

Our ability to communicate well often depends on examining—and sometimes challenging—our assumptions about our own legitimate rights. Consider the following:

❑ Do you believe it is selfish to put your needs before others' needs, or do you have a legitimate right to sometimes put yourself first?

❑ Do you assume that other people's views should win out over your own opinions and convictions?

❑ Do you think you should always be flexible and adjust to others, or do you think it's better to negotiate a mutually acceptable solution?

❑ Do you feel that you shouldn't take up other people's valuable time with your problems, or do you have a legitimate right to ask for help and support?

❑ Do you assume that when someone is in trouble you should always help them, or do you have the right not to take responsibility for someone else's problem sometimes?

1. Aggressive Responses

The assumption underlying aggressive responses is "I'm superior and right, and you're inferior and wrong." Aggressive responses often set off retaliation and defensiveness, and increase tension. This kind of response is also less likely to resolve problems.

2. Passive Responses

Underlying passive responses is the belief that "I'm weak and inferior, and you're powerful and right." Passive responses usually lead to a lot of bottled-up anger, resentment, and hurt feelings. Like aggressive responses, they are less likely to resolve problems.

3. Assertive Responses

Assertive responses are based on the attitude that although you and the other person may have your differences, you are equally entitled to express yourselves. You are communicating assertively when you can stand up for your rights without violating the rights of others. You can express your personal needs and opinions, you can disagree openly, and you can say no. Assertive responses usually result in improved self-esteem, less tension, and, often, the resolution of problems. It is not selfish to assertively express your beliefs, communicate your feelings, and stand up for your values.

Key Point

℞ Learn to Be More Assertive

You can learn to express yourself more effectively. To communicate assertively:

1. **State Your Observations.** Explain your thoughts or perception of the situation in as objective and nonjudgmental way as you can.

2. **State Your Thoughts.** This is your opportunity to express your opinions, your beliefs, your interpretations, and/or your interpretation of the other person's observations.

3. **State Your Feelings.** Use "I" statements. For example, say "I get really upset when I'm late. It's important for me to be on time," instead of "You're always making me late." Focus on your own emotional

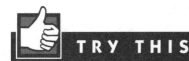

ASSERTIVENESS EXERCISE

Practice being assertive with a friend. Choose a specific situation. Then make your case using the following statements:

▶ *I observe* (state just the facts)

▶ *I think* (state your opinions)

▶ *I feel* (say what your feelings are)

▶ *I want* (state exactly what you'd like the other person to do)

For example, you make a special bread to bring as a gift to a friend. Somebody comes along in the kitchen, sees it on the counter, and cuts out a large slice. You're upset because, with a piece missing, the gift is ruined. Rather than sulking (passively) or exploding (aggressively), you say to the bread eater: "You cut into my special bread (observation). You should have asked me about it first (opinion). I'm really upset and disappointed because I can't give it as a gift now (feeling). I'd like an apology, and for you to ask me first next time (want)."

Keep a log of your progress. Describe situations that required you to be assertive, what worked and what didn't, and what you'll say next time.

reaction to the situation rather than blaming the other person for making you feel this way. State only the impact of the situation or someone else's behavior on you.

4. **State Your Wants.** Make clear, specific requests of the other person.

Following are some examples of using these kinds of statements to communicate effectively:

Maggie and Her Husband

Maggie wants to talk to her husband, Joe, about sharing the housework. She says, "Our house is a mess, and I'm the one who usually cleans it up. I don't have time to do all the cleaning (she's stating an observation). I think you should help out (thought). I feel frustrated when it isn't clean (feeling), and I would like us to share the responsibility (want)."

Joe doesn't respond the way Maggie would like. He says, "I'm reading the paper now."

If Maggie were a passive person she would probably say, "Okay," and retreat. If she were aggressive she might yell, "You never want to talk about cleaning the house. You don't even care about me." Instead Maggie remains friendly, but assertive. "It won't take long," she insists in a pleasant tone.

Joe stays friendly but firm too. "But I just want to finish this paper now." Maggie holds her ground. "Okay, we'll talk about it later. How about after dinner?" Joe says, "Okay." Maggie says, "Good." In this exchange, both partners show respect for the other's wishes, and move toward a resolution.

Linda and Her Daughter

Or consider this exchange between Linda and her daughter Mindy. Mindy complains, "You're always hassling me about what clothes to put on. You're mean. I hate you." How could Mindy communicate better?

What if Mindy said, "You often tell me

what clothes to put on (observation). I think I should be able to make my own decisions (thought). I feel angry when my opinion isn't considered (feeling). I'd like you to let me choose my own clothes for a week and see how it goes (want)."

℞ Watch "Always" and "Never"

When you describe your observations, stick to the facts. Try to avoid words like "always" and "never." These words rarely are true and they often make people react defensively.

So instead of saying, "You never clean up the dishes after dinner," you might say, "After dinner the dishes collect in the sink (observation). I'm angry about this because I feel like you are not doing your share (feeling). I'd like us to alternate doing the dishes (wants). How does that sound to you?"

Or instead of saying, "You're always selfish and inconsiderate," try something like, "I'm angry because you didn't tell me you'd be home late."

℞ Make Your Requests Specific

When you state your wants, make them specific. Help the other person know exactly what you are requesting. If you want your son to mow the lawn, tell him "I would like you to mow the lawn some time this afternoon. Will you agree to that?" Communicating a specific request is more likely to accomplish the goal than complaining: "Look at the lawn. It hasn't been mowed in weeks. Why don't you ever mow it?"

℞ How to Say "No"

Learning how to decline a request is an essential life skill. Many of us have a hard time saying no, even when we're overwhelmed with things to do. We may say yes from an exaggerated desire to please, but in the end we often feel resentful, frustrated, disappointed, and angry with ourself. Remember, you have a legitimate right to decline any request, even if it's a reasonable request. Here are some tips on how to say no:

▶ Take some time before you answer. Say you have to think it over or check with your family or boss.

▶ Think of how you want to respond, and rehearse your answer.

▶ Separate the person who is asking from the task you are being asked to do; say no to the request without rejecting the requester. Acknowledge the importance of the request to the other person. You can say, "Thanks for calling. I appreciate your asking me, but I can't take on any more tasks."

▶ Offer no further explanation. Give no details of your busy schedule.

- If the person is persistent, use the "broken record" strategy. Say, "I understand you need special help, but I just can't take on any more tasks," or "I'd help out if I could, but I can't take on any more tasks."

- Make a counter offer along these lines: "I won't be able to drive tonight. Perhaps you can ask Anna for a ride. I can drive next week."

And how do you respond when someone says no to your request? Remember, it's not necessarily a rejection of you as a person; it's merely an honest decline of that specific request.

℞ Check Out Your Assumptions

Communication is sometimes blocked by incorrect assumptions or fantasies about what the other person means. For example, Sarah has just quit her job at an art gallery. She wants to tell Julia about it but she is afraid Julia will disapprove of her action, so she says nothing. The truth of the matter is, Julia may or may not disapprove. Sarah will never know what Julia really thinks, since she has made an assumption about Julia's response.

Sarah could share the reasons she quit her job with Julia. She could also tell Julia exactly how she feels: that she fears Julia's moral judgment or disapproval. Checking out our assumptions and fantasies through direct communication is the best antidote to misunderstanding. People can't read your mind, and you can't reliably read theirs.

> **Key Point**
> *If you can't check out someone else's intentions or thoughts directly, at least give them the benefit of the doubt.*
Assume that their intentions are good unless you have strong evidence to the contrary.

℞ Nip Conflict in the Bud

Minor communication problems can escalate into major conflicts. An employee might think, for example, that his perfectionistic boss is out to get him; partners might accuse each other of nagging or being too defensive. To minimize conflict before it gets worse:

- **Use "I" statements instead of "you" statements.** "I" statements are direct, assertive expressions of your views and feelings, whereas "you" sentences are accusative and confrontational. For example: "I try very hard to do the best work I can," not, "You always criticize me." Or "I appreciate it when you turn down the television while I talk," not, "You never pay attention." Notice that "I feel that you are not treating me fairly" is actually a disguised "you" statement. A true "I" statement really would be, "I feel angry and hurt" (📖 see page 127).

- **Shift the perspective** from what is being talked about to what is going on between you. For example: "We're both getting upset and drifting away from the topic we agreed to discuss."

- **Buy time.** For example: "I think I understand your concerns. I would like a little time to think about it and gather more information before I respond."

- **Make sure you understand** each other's concerns, positions, or feelings by summarizing what you heard. For example: "Before I say what I think, let me repeat what I think you said..."

- **Reverse roles.** Try arguing each other's position as thoroughly and thoughtfully as you can. Try to win the debate for the other side. You'll find this is a great way to understand all sides of an issue, and the validity of different points of view. This tactic will also help you develop empathy and tolerance for diversity.

▶ **Look for a workable compromise.** In a conflict it is usually not possible to satisfy everyone. Look for something you all can agree to try for awhile. Here are three possibilities:

1. Do it your way this time; the other person's next time.

2. Agree to part of what you want, and part of what the other person wants.

3. Compromise. Decide what you'll do, and what the other person will do in return.

℞ Change How You Talk to Yourself

The way we talk with others is often determined by the way we talk to ourselves. Let's say your boss asks you if the report you just handed in was the final version. You think to yourself, "Oh, no. He thinks it's lousy. I probably need to revise it for the tenth time. I can't write very well." But in fact your boss is quite pleased, and is wondering about what assignment to give you next.

Be aware of the difference between what you say to yourself and what is actually said by others. Learn to hear what you tell yourself, and change your pessimistic self-talk (📖 see page 42). If, for example, you hear in your head, "I'm a lousy actor," challenge your own inner assumptions. Ask yourself, "If I write a script and rehearse my lines, why would I make a fool of myself? And even if I messed up, so what? Everybody makes mistakes. I'll do better next time."

℞ Practice Praising

You can dramatically shift the mood of a conversation just by letting someone know you appreciate their effort or achievement. Compliments and thank-yous are all vital nutrients. Watch for the hundreds of opportunities to practice praising.

You may be surprised at the power of praise. You can also dramatically shift the mood of hostile, distant people with just a few kind words.

Offer general praise like, "I am really happy to see you." But your praise will be more effective if you link it to a specific quality of activity such as, "I really liked the way you stood up for yourself in that meeting." The next time you see someone doing something well, say so. Watch their reaction. They seem a bit embarrassed, but inside they're feeling good.

Tell co-workers that you appreciate the good job they're doing on a project, for example, or compliment your mother on how nice she looks. Or tell your doctor how much you appreciate the way he or she listens to you or explains the treatment.

You can also ask for praise for yourself. When someone offers you a compliment, just say "thank you," or return the compliment by saying how good it made you feel. When you give criticism, balance it with praise. Say, "I really appreciate your writing," for example, "but I wondered if you could tighten it up a bit." Criticize the performance, but praise the performer.

℞ How to Cope with Criticism

We assume that receiving criticism must automatically be uncomfortable. But the impact of criticism on us depends more on how we describe the criticism to ourselves and interpret it rather than on what our critic actually says.

Think about a specific time when you were criticized. Did you get angry? Depressed? Did the comments trigger a barrage of negative self-talk and self-criticism? Did you turn to medications, alcohol, smoking, or food to soothe your hurt feelings?

There are a whole range of healthier ways to respond. Here are some questions to ask yourself when you're criticized:

▶ Does the criticism seem reasonable?

▶ Is it fact or opinion?

▶ Does the critic have the authority, credentials, or knowledge to add validity and value to his or her view?

▶ Are there others who might confirm this view? Dispute it?

▶ Does it concern an unimportant area, or is it one in which you don't expect to be skilled or competent?

▶ Were there unusual or special circumstances?

▶ How would others have behaved in a similar situation?

In some circumstances, it is perfectly reasonable to say, "I can see why you might think that, but I see it differently." Or buy time, think it over, and collect more information. Or decide to accept the criticism without feeling bad, and take action to modify your behavior.

℞ Say You're Sorry

We have all said or done things that have, intentionally or unintentionally, hurt others. Many relationships are hurt—sometimes for years—because people have not learned the powerful social skill of apologizing. *Often all it takes is a simple, sincere apology to restore a relationship.*

Key Point

Rather than a sign of weak character, an apology shows great strength. To be effective, an apology must:

▶ Admit the specific mistake, and accept responsibility for it. You must name the offense; no glossing over with just, "I'm sorry for what I did." Be specific. You might say, for example, "I'm very sorry that I spoke behind your back."

▶ An effective apology points out that what you did does not represent how you see yourself, or how you want to be. Explain the particular circumstances that led you to do what you did. Don't offer excuses or sidestep responsibility.

▶ Express your sadness, guilt, and shame. A genuine, heart-felt apology involves some suffering. Sadness shows that the relationship matters to you. Guilt conveys that you are truly upset about hurting another person. And shame communicates your disappointment with yourself over the incident.

▶ Acknowledge the impact of wrong-doing. You might say, "I know that I hurt you and that my behavior cost you a lot. For that I am very sorry."

▶ Offer to make amends. Ask what you can do to make the situation better, or volunteer specific suggestions.

Making an apology is not fun, but it is an act of courage, generosity, and healing. It brings the possibility of a renewed and stronger relationship, and it can also bring peace within yourself.

📖 *For more information, see page 274*

10 Healthy Helping

How Helping Others Improves Your Own Health

▶ *"When I signed up to be a reading tutor, my life went from being two-dimensional to three-dimensional. It was terrific. I got to be close friends with the young man—really connected—and I felt good about how I was spending my time."*

▶ *"At first it was really difficult and sad, but now going to the hospital every week and cuddling those AIDS babies means everything in the world to me. It gives me a chance to forget myself. I feel so great afterward—energetic, and somehow lighter—and I can't wait until next time. It's now what gives my life meaning."*

▶ *"A lot of people can't understand why I continue to counsel other women with breast cancer. It's not all roses, but the pleasure I get from helping others go through what I went through far outweighs the downside. If I can make it easier for someone else, it means my having had cancer wasn't all for nothing."*

Clearly, doing good feels good. And the act of helping itself may indeed improve health. More and more studies show that helping, caring relationships can improve the health of the helper and, truly, may be part of our own innate nature. Paradoxically, *sometimes one of the best ways to promote your own health or to cope with a health problem is to forget yourself, and concentrate on caring for someone else.*

Key Point

The benefits of healthy helping certainly extend beyond the person being helped. More and more people are realizing that self-centered concentration on exercise, nutrition, and getting more money is not enough to take care of the body or soul. In fact, excessive preoccupation with our own comfort and discomfort can lead to depression, poor health, and a life without much meaning.

True well-being is achieved only when we feel connected to something beyond ourselves, whether it's other people, a pet, a plant, or the planet. Evidence suggests that a regular regimen of helping may be as important to our health as regular exercise and proper nutrition. Helping not

133

only improves the health of the helper, it also aids the health of our entire society and our world.

Altruism, generosity, kindness, and service are more than moral virtues. They are part of what it means to be truly human, and they may be key to breaking the deadly cycle of fear and tension now gripping our self-centered society. While more volunteering may not solve all the problems in our society, it could be a powerful antidote to the reluctance to "get involved." Volunteering forms bonds. It changes our experience of "us" and "them" to "we," and it also strengthens our sense of community.

Now almost half of all American adults volunteer. The average volunteer offers nearly five hours a week for a total of nearly 19.5 billion hours a year. This is roughly equivalent to a work force of 10 million full-time employees.

Volunteer activities are not just for the rich—in fact, people with less money do more than their share. Families earning less than $10,000 a year give proportionately more of their income to charity than people earning $100,000.

The actions of just one individual can have a significant impact. Once you become involved in helping, the positive experience often motivates you to do more helping. The growing awareness of the emotional and physical benefits of helping can create a ripple effect, spreading healthy altruism in its wake.

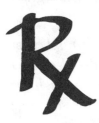

Helping Yourself by Helping Others

Fortunately, helping others doesn't require a huge time commitment, a change in careers, or a move to the inner city. It can range from planned work with a volunteer organization to spontaneous acts of kindness. Here are some pointers to help you get the most out of helping.

℞ Go for the Personal Contact

Any kind of helping helps. But hands-on activities that require personal contact—such as tutoring kids, reading to the blind, or visiting the elderly—seem to be more beneficial to the helper than the less personally engaging ones.

Volunteers who have a one-to-one personal relationship with the person they are helping are more likely to experience "helper's high," increased self-esteem, and reduced signs of stress. For example, among volunteers surveyed, those who helped face-to-face had a more improved self-concept than those who did adminis-

trative work. But even those who served as administrators fared better than those who didn't help at all!

So the more you have contact with others, the better. You need to meet those you help, see their lives, and feel connected with them. Seeing the responses of the person you are helping is important. The powerful feelings of personal connection with another human being increases our understanding and sympathy for that person's situation. It also reduces your sense of isolation, and reaffirms your link to the larger human community.

This is not to say that less personal

forms of helping are not worthwhile. Collecting clothes, baking cookies, stuffing envelopes, or donating money are all certainly better than not helping. But getting close to someone else makes the helping more personally rewarding.

℞ Finding Your Way To Help

Pick an activity you're interested in—one you do well. You're more likely to have a positive effect on the person you're helping if you feel at ease and useful, so find some activity that is comfortable for you. If you help someone who is facing something you've gone through yourself, you'll feel closer to the person and more empathic.

Most people who join support groups originally do so to get help for themselves, but they often find they are helping other group members deal with their problems too. This adds to their feelings of self-worth, and they also get the related health benefits.

It's important to understand your motivation for helping, and monitor your reactions. Some cancer patients, for example, find helping others with cancer simply too emotionally taxing. It may arouse unpleasant memories, and it may block the helper's own recovery. But for others with cancer, this work is emotionally rewarding.

People's responses to volunteer work are highly individual. It is important to find out what works for you. Learn all you can about a volunteer activity first, and talk with other helpers. Then give it a try.

℞ Working with an Organization

Some people prefer to find their own way of helping; others prefer to work through an organization. Volunteering through an

established organization can provide you with support, training, and a regular schedule. The connection and teamwork with fellow helpers can be a powerful bonus. Volunteer organizations can also put you in touch with strangers who need help, so you can reach beyond your own family and friends. Nearly every community has volunteer organizations to support your efforts and interests (see page 275).

℞ Avoid Over-Helping

Perhaps the greatest mistake that caregivers make is to provide too much help. Don't confuse "doing for" with "caring about." Too often we take on the role of rescuer, expecting to be rewarded with thanks or praise. Meanwhile the other person becomes more and more helpless,

People Need Help

New evidence supports what we feel instinctively: people need people. Inadequate social support is as dangerous to your health as smoking, lack of exercise, and obesity. Consider the facts:

▶ Single, separated, divorced, or widowed people are two to three times more likely to die prematurely than married people.

▶ People with weakened social connections have higher rates of cancer, heart disease, infections, depression, arthritis, and problems during pregnancy.

▶ Social support predicts death rates among the elderly, and in people with serious illness. For example, women with advanced metastatic breast cancer who attend weekly support groups (in addition to their medical treatment) live twice as long as those who receive medical treatment alone.

Strong social ties and being connected with others appear to protect health.

Helping Helps the Helper

Social support takes many forms. Relationships with family, friends, neighbors, casual acquaintances, memberships in groups and organizations, contacts at work—these all together make up the general mix of social support. But there is a specific ingredient in social contact that involves personal helping—one that appears to have health benefits all its own. Helping helps the helper.

In a study of 2,700 residents in Tecumseh, Michigan, for example, men who volunteered for community organizations were two and a half times less likely to die from all causes of disease than the men who didn't.

A national survey involving 3,300 volunteers from all fields (helpers of AIDS patients, homeless families, shut-ins, crime victims, runaway youths, hospital patients) provides further evidence that helping helps the helper:

▶ Nearly 95% of the volunteers reported that personal helping on a regular basis gives them an immediate pleasurable sensation. This phenomenon is called "helper's high." It consists of physical and emotional sensations that include a sudden warmth, a surge of energy, and a feeling of euphoria immediately after helping.

▶ "Helper's high" is often followed by a longer-lasting state that involves feelings of increased self-worth, calm, and relaxation. Nearly 80% of those surveyed reported that some of the good feelings returned when they remembered helping.

▶ People who experienced "helper's high" said they felt their health was better. Nine out of ten said that they were healthier than others their own age. Other studies indicate that this perception of good health is one of the strongest predictors of a person's future health and longevity.

Continued on next page

Many helpers also reported fewer colds, headaches, and backaches, and improved eating and sleeping habits. Even relief from the pain of chronic diseases such as ulcers, asthma, arthritis, and lupus was reported.

The "Helping Gene"

The powerful urge to help and take care of someone stems at least in part from the helpless human infant's long and total dependency on a caretaker. As adults, we continue to depend on each other for basics like food, protection, and love. It's not surprising that more and more studies show that helping, caring relationships are mutually beneficial to survival, and may be encoded in our genetic makeup.

So it appears that we have an inborn tendency to care about other people. Studies found that even newborns show signs of empathy by crying more intensely when they hear another baby cry than when they hear other equally loud noises.

How Helping Keeps Us Healthy

A variety of mechanisms are possible to explain the link between helping and your health:

▶ You might pity yourself for not having as much money or as good a job as your neighbor, but by working with people less fortunate than you are, you may become more content with what you have.

▶ Since we tend to assess our own situation by comparing ourselves to a select group, helping others can expand our feelings of confidence and competence. Teaching someone to read, for example, reminds you of your own skills and strengths.

▶ You may relieve your own distress at the sight of pain or misfortune by helping others, and prevent feelings of guilt.

▶ Focusing on others can free you from the gridlock of your own family, work, or money hassles.

▶ We have a limited capacity to pay attention to several things at once. Concentrating on something outside yourself can distract you from your own troubles and pain.

▶ We also get a special kind of attention from those we help. Most of us need to feel that we matter to someone, and sincere gratitude can be very nourishing.

▶ Our bodies also appear to be positively affected by helping. One study showed that just by watching a film of Mother Teresa at work, students' immune systems got a temporary boost.

▶ Numerous studies have found that the lethal culprits of Type A behavior seem to be hostility, cynicism, and aggression. Hostile people do not enjoy the company of others. They see themselves as separate. So helping others may break the stranglehold of hostile self-centeredness on their heart.

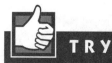

TRY THIS

HOW MUCH HELP TO GIVE

Here's a good rule of thumb: the optimal dose of healthy helping may be the same as for other healthy habits like exercise or relaxation —about two hours a week. The more frequently you help, the more likely you are to experience positive feelings and better health.

In one survey, those who volunteered once a week were ten times more likely to report good health than those who were once-a-year helpers. But as with exercise, any time spent helping is better than none.

and may lose both the skills and the will to do things for him or herself. Instead of rescuing, try empowering:

▶ Help the person gain as much control over his or her life as possible

▶ Encourage independence

▶ Allow him or her to make decisions, even about simple matters

▶ Give clear responsibilities—even for things you know you could do better or faster

▶ Break down complicated tasks into small, easy steps

▶ Allow for mistakes and reward efforts, even if the results fall short (small successes build a sense of confidence, pride, and independence)

▶ Try not to shield or protect another person from bad news or problems

▶ Beware of unrelenting optimism— forced cheerfulness that doesn't allow the other person to express their anger, disappointment, or sadness

Sometimes the best way to help is not to help. Limit your availability.

The importance of responsibility and sense of control is well illustrated in a study of nursing home patients. The first group of residents was told they were competent and capable people. They were then asked to choose a house plant from a large box and told that they would be responsible for caring for it.

The second group of residents were given a plant and told that the staff would take care of it as they did the patients. The patients who were given responsibility became more physically and socially active, and surprisingly, lived longer. Eighteen months later, the responsibility-enhanced group showed a death rate only half that of the control group (15% versus 30%). No data were available on how well the plants in the two groups fared!

℞ Adopt a Healthy Attitude

Our helping efforts may seem hopeless in the face of overwhelming poverty or illness. If you concentrate your efforts on changing someone or making a measurable difference in the world, you are setting yourself up for a "helper's low" rather than a "helper's high."

We can't always know for sure what the results of our actions will be. *We do better by focusing on the process of helping rather than the outcomes. Take satisfaction in knowing you're doing your best, and enjoy the feelings of closeness as you go along.* If good does result from your efforts, celebrate the achievements, both big and small.

HELPING WHEN YOU "HAVE TO"

Instead of the joyful spontaneity that enhances well-being, helping because you have to can result in increased stress, and sometimes even illness. We are more likely to have positive feelings and a sense of meaningful connection when we help from free choice rather than from obligation or necessity. Though helping family and friends is important, it's often not done with the same free spirit as helping strangers.

"Have-to" helping situations, such as taking care of a loved one who is ill for a long time, can be a generous expression of love, and it can create strong bonds. But it can also be an unbearable burden—especially when you do it alone, or if you feel unappreciated. In this case, the act of helping then becomes a source of stress rather than good health.

One study of family members caring for relatives with Alzheimer's disease showed a decrease in the caregivers' immune system strength. A year later, many of them were ill.

If you find yourself in an obligatory helping situation—even a very loving one—follow the safeguards against burnout (📖 see page 140).

℞ Put Kindness into Practice

This world is plagued by violence. When something bad happens, it's front-page news. As an antidote to this misery, despair and cynicism, practice acts of kindness. Look for opportunities to give without expecting anything in return. You might:

▶ Hold the door open for the person behind you

▶ Offer an unrequested neck rub

▶ Give an unexpected gift of movie or concert tickets

▶ Send an anonymous gift to a friend who needs cheering up

▶ Send a thank-you note to someone who made a difference in your life

▶ Help someone with a heavy load

▶ Tell positive stories you know of helping and kindness

▶ Cultivate an attitude of gratefulness for the kindness you have received

▶ Plant a tree

▶ Write a thank-you note to the boss of an employee who has helped you

▶ Smile and let people cut in ahead of you in line or on the freeway

▶ Pick up litter

▶ Give another driver your parking space

Be creative. Such kindness is contagious, and it has a ripple effect. In one study, the people who were given an unexpected treat (cookies) were later more likely to help others.

BEWARE OF BURNOUT

The condition called "burnout" was first recognized among the helping professions. Dedicated workers who pushed too hard for too long suffered physical ills, depression, anger, exhaustion, and hostility. They felt like giving up and withdrawing.

When used as prescribed, helping others is generally safe and effective. But burnout can happen to anyone. Taking on too much is not healthy, either for you or the person you are helping. In spite of your good intentions, you feel lousy instead of good, and can suffer a prolonged state of stress and exhaustion. For ways on how to prevent burnout, see below.

℞ Prevent Burnout

Here are some suggestions for preventing helper's burnout:

▶ **Monitor yourself.** Watch out for feelings of being overwhelmed by the needs of another person. They can make you feel helpless, out of control, resentful, guilty, and stressed. These are signs of burnout.

▶ **Pay attention to your own needs.** Take a break when you need it, eat nutritious foods that you like, get adequate rest and exercise, and have fun yourself.

▶ **Recognize your limits.** Learn to set boundaries on your availability.

▶ **Get help.** Get plenty of support and encouragement from team members, support groups, the director of volunteers, or friends. If you are a caregiver for a family member, don't try to do it all alone. Locate other family or community resources to fill in for you, and take time regularly for yourself.

Attend a support group for friends and families of those who are suffering from a similar disease or disorder. At the very least, share the emotional burden by talking about it with friends.

Don't be afraid to ask them to do some small favors for you so you feel less overwhelmed and alone (📖 see page 142).

▶ **Pace yourself.** Don't try to do everything. Ease into helping gradually, especially if the work is emotionally draining. Have realistic expectations about what you can accomplish.

▶ **Move on.** If things just aren't working out, find another helping situation that's better for you.

▶ **Cancel guilt trips.** Consider giving up on a particular effort when it isn't right for you. Though it may be difficult, guilt is not a healthy reason to help. Nobody is really indispensable. We just think we are.

▶ **Give yourself a pat on the back.** Tell yourself you are doing a very good job at what may be a very difficult task. Take pride in being a caregiver or volunteer. It is not always an easy job, and those who do it are special.

℞ Make Your Money Count

You can help both others and yourself by investing your money as well as your time and attention. We're not speaking here of charitable contributions, but ways to invest your personal savings to create a better world. While safety and favorable returns are the prime considerations in most financial investments, many people want their money to support their values and convictions.

How much do you really know about the companies your money is invested in? Are their business practices compatible with your values, or do they contradict your ethical or moral beliefs?

Why donate to saving the whales if your pension is invested in companies that are killing them? Why complain about pollution if the companies you're investing in routinely dump toxic waste into the environment? Why invest in tobacco companies (directly or indirectly) if you are concerned about the health impact of smoking?

Many people are now trying "socially responsible" investment strategies by directing their money to companies that provide safe and useful products or services; ones that treat their employees and customers fairly, respect the environment, and make a positive contribution to the community. This is capitalism with a social conscience.

It is possible to do well while doing good. Several socially responsible stock mutual funds have outperformed Standard and Poor's blue chip stocks. They also outperformed top mutual funds that focus exclusively on investor returns. Your money can yield high returns *and* help build a better world for you and your children. In the long run, the way companies treat their employees, their customers, and their communities—not just their stockholders—has an impact on the bottom line.

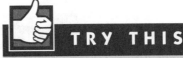

TRY THIS

HELP A PET

The health benefits we get from helping others extend even to caring for our pets. Several studies suggest that pet owners enjoy better health.

▶ One year after a heart attack, patients who have pets have one-fifth the death rate as the petless.

▶ Petting a dog has been shown to lower blood pressure.

▶ Bringing a pet into a nursing home or hospital can boost peoples' moods and enhance their social interaction.

The relationship between pets and health can be explained in several ways. Pet owners often feel needed and responsible, which may stimulate the survival incentive. They feel they need to survive to take care of their pets. Stroking a dog, watching a kitten tumble, or observing the hypnotic explorations of fish can be an antidote to a foul mood or a frazzling day.

Pets can also be a source of unconditional, nonjudgmental love and affection. This may be easier to appreciate in cats and dogs than in fish, reptiles, or even people! And pets can shift our narrow focus beyond ourselves, helping us to feel connected to a larger world.

A trip to the pet store or animal shelter could improve your health and happiness even more than a trip to the doctor or pharmacy.

KINDS OF SUPPORT YOU NEED

You'll be able to help others better if you get the support you need; it's critical to everyone's good health. There are several types of social support:

▶ **Emotional support:** An expression of caring that lets another person feel liked, loved, and valued

▶ **Positive regard:** Acceptance of another person's beliefs and feelings

▶ **Information:** Providing knowledge that might be helpful to someone

▶ **Physical support:** Providing physical aid or an opportunity to work

▶ **Financial support:** Providing money

When you seek support, first identify what type you really need. Then decide who might be able to provide it. Some friends might be great at providing emotional support, but not very good at offering practical advice.

Try answering the following questions to identify your sources of support:

▶ *When you are feeling upset, who can you share your most private fears and worries with?*

_____

▶ *Is there someone who takes pride in your accomplishments and thinks highly of you?*

_____

▶ *When you have a problem, who would you go to for practical advice or information?*

_____

▶ *If you needed a loan of $100 for an emergency, who would you go to?*

_____

▶ *Who would bring you dinner if you were sick (or even if you weren't sick)?*

_____

The *number* of people in your social support network is not as important as the *quality* of support you're likely to receive, and how well you use your network. *Having a strong social support network doesn't just happen. You have to build, cultivate and maintain it.* And you need to learn how to make clear, specific requests for help and support (📖 see page 128).

Key Point

📖 *For more information, see page 275*

11 Anxiety

How to Overcome Excessive Worry, Panic, and Phobias

"My life has been full of terrible misfortunes, most of which never happened."

—Montaigne

Sylvia is waiting to give her first paper at a conference. Her heart is racing and she feels a flash of terror. She starts to breathe quickly and her hands sweat and shake.

Sylvia climbs up to the podium, takes a deep breath, and plunges in. The audience laughs at her first joke. She feels encouraged. Her hands are still shaky, but she can cope. When the applause at the end is over and she sits down, her heart is still pounding from the excitement. Sylvia feels great.

Philip is in the bank. He is depositing some checks when he finds, to his horror, that he hasn't endorsed one. Ever since his hand shook and his teacher couldn't read what he had written, he has found it almost impossible to write in front of other people. The cashier pushes the check across to him, asking him to sign it now. Philip's heart beats faster and he starts to shake and sweat. He can't breathe and he's getting dizzy. He can't possibly sign the check! He runs out of the bank. Philip feels awful.

Sylvia and Philip were both anxious, and their bodies were geared up to deal with a challenge. But their responses to their anxiety were quite different. Sylvia saw her symptoms as excitement; Philip reacted with terror. Sylvia felt positive about what she was going to do; Philip felt out of control. Sylvia's talk was rewarded, and that reinforced her courage. Philip was so panicked that he ran away, which reinforced his belief that he couldn't cope.

Some fear is normal and healthy. It alerts us to specific threats and dangers, and readies our body for action. It helps us respond to crises, and it prepares us to meet new challenges. Worrying allows us to plan, search for alternatives, rehearse actions, and prepare for negative outcomes. The problem arises when there's too much of a good thing.

Key Point

Destructive Anxiety

How do you know when your anxiety is healthy and normal, and when it's not? Here are three signs of excessive anxiety:

1. Anxious feelings are extremely intense, far out of proportion to the real danger.

HEALTHY AND UNHEALTHY STRESS

Anxiety is a generalized fear. It is accompanied by bodily responses that prepare you to run or fight to protect yourself. Your heart rate and blood pressure rise; blood sugar increases; blood flow is reduced to the head, gut, skin, hands and feet. You sweat and your muscles tense up. This response to a threat is deeply programmed into your physiology. Our ancestors lived in a world of physical threats. Failure to run from a lion could mean death.

But we also fear abstract situations, not just physical threats. We worry about the future. We fear loss of life, health, love, status, and belonging. *These modern-day "lions" trigger the same responses that were helpful when we needed to fight or flee, but they are often inappropriate in dealing with psychological threats.*

Key Point

Occasional anxiety, even when pro- voked by imaginary threats, is not harmful. *But prolonged anxiety is both unpleasant and damaging to health. While the body is built for short bursts of stress, frequent physiological arousal can undermine the immune and cardiovascular systems.* People often get sick after episodes of uncertainty and worry. "Stress hormones" raise blood pressure and heart rate. They can increase blood cholesterol and result in the breakdown of muscle tissue.

Key Point

Over time, this may increase the risk of heart and blood vessel disease. High blood pressure is more common in chronic worriers. High anxiety is also strongly associated with the risk of sudden death from heart disease. Chronically nervous, tense, and anxious people are more likely to have abnormal heart rhythms, and they are 2 to 6 times more likely to die of a heart attack. And anxiety can also trigger asthma attacks in susceptible people.

2. Anxiety interferes with your work, pleasure, and relationships.

3. Anxiety undermines effective problem-solving.

Anxiety is at the same time both destructive and useful. Healthy fear keeps you from walking through a dangerous part of town. Sylvia's worry energizes her to rise to a challenge. But misplaced fear stops Phil from signing a check in front of a bank teller. Students' anxieties over exams can motivate them to work harder, or can interfere with their test performance.

Anxiety has a way of robbing us of daily pleasures. Everyday fears may be related to unrealistic and unexamined assumptions you hold. You may respond to them by being unproductive, and prolong the anxiety unnecessarily. This can take a toll on your health and happiness. We can all benefit from learning to deal with anxiety more effectively.

Three Kinds of Anxiety

1. Generalized Anxiety

When worrying gets out of hand, psychologists refer to it as *generalized anxiety disorder*—a chronic anxiety state that has lasted for more than six months, and is not accompanied by panic attacks, phobias, or obsessive behavior. It often derives from one or two major areas of concern, and spills over into all aspects of life. People with generalized anxiety disorder are worried and on edge continually. They can't relax and enjoy life, and may have difficulty sleeping. They may be too anxious to concentrate on anything. The anxious feelings become overwhelming and life-disrupting.

2. Phobias

Phobias are intense fears of a specific object or situation. They are usually out of proportion to any real risk. People can develop phobias for almost anything: spiders, snakes, heights, or the sight of blood. We seem to have an inborn tendency to develop some of these phobias. They may have originally provided an evolutionary advantage to keep us safe. It may also be possible to *learn* a phobia, especially from a parent.

Sometimes a traumatic experience—such as being stuck in an airplane bathroom—can trigger an ongoing fear of enclosed spaces (claustrophobia). Nearly any social situation can become feared: public speaking, blushing, writing in public, eating in restaurants, or using public toilets. Sufferers often worry continuously about whether the situation they fear is going to occur.

3. Panic Attacks

Panic attacks overcome some people, even when there's no real danger. These attacks seem to come out of the blue. They're usually intense for a few minutes, and then subside. Bodily symptoms include:

- Chest pains
- Heart pounding
- Sweating
- Nausea
- Dizziness
- Sensation of choking or smothering
- Numbness or tingling

These symptoms are often accompanied by feelings of unreality and overwhelming fears of dying, going crazy, or losing control. In the absence of a real cause, the sufferer often invents one, such as, "I must be having a heart attack."

In some cases, only a single panic attack occurs; in others, panic episodes come back repeatedly. Bodily sensations that accompany the anxiety are seen by the victim as symptoms of impending death. This heightens and magnifies the anxiety, and accelerates the panic. Sufferers may live in constant fear of their next attack. They may avoid driving, being alone, or leaving the house.

Causes of Anxiety

Usually a combination of factors contribute to the feelings of anxiety. These include:

- Personality and attitudes
- Childhood environment and experiences
- Heredity and biology
- Medical conditions
- Use of stimulant medications and caffeine
- Current life stresses
- Lack of confidence and security
- A lack of skills for relaxation and mood management

Sometimes the problem starts with a particular event or life change. Being ignored as a child, for example, may lead to a fear of abandonment. A significant life change such as a death in the family may precede the first anxiety attack. But even when a triggering event can be identified, ongoing anxiety usually has more to do with other contributing factors than with the event itself.

TREATMENT OPTIONS

Medications

Many people drink alcohol to lessen feelings of anxiety, but research shows that dependency on alcohol makes anxiety worse. Antianxiety medications such as benzodiazepines (Valium, Xanax, Ativan, Klonopin, for example) and other medications may help with severe symptoms, especially in the short run. But they have side effects such as drowsiness, lethargy, interference with learning, disturbed sleep patterns, and dependence.

Sometimes it's difficult to stop anti-anxiety medications after you've been taking them regularly. So drugs should be used sparingly for chronic anxiety. First consider possible adverse consequences, as well as alternative non-drug treatments. Sometimes just cutting back or eliminating stimulants such as caffeine (in over-the-counter medications and sodas as well as coffee) may be all that is required to lessen feelings of anxiety.

Behavioral management

Key Point

In treating anxiety disorders, there are studies that show that *learning a better response to stressful*

situations can often be more effective than medications.

And learning how to respond better to anxiety doesn't have the negative side effects of drugs. Also, you don't have to dig up past causes of your anxiety to lessen its hold over you.

Behavioral techniques can help you:

▶ Change your *body symptoms* such as heart pounding, sweating, cold hands, stomach butterflies, and tense muscles

▶ Change *thoughts* that trigger, sustain, or increase anxious feelings

▶ Change *actions* in response to anxiety

How to Calm Anxiety, Phobias, and Panic

Below are several techniques that you can practice on your own, with a self-help or therapy group, or with a professional. Most of this advice is useful for all types of anxiety, but some is specific for phobias and panic attacks. If your anxiety is associated with a traumatic experience such as the death of a loved one or abuse, advice in Chapter 16, Surviving Trauma, may also be helpful (📖 see page 201).

Learn to Relax

Chronic anxiety can keep your body unnecessarily mobilized for action. You can learn to become calm by practicing various techniques designed to relax your muscles or still your mind (📖 see page 86). With 15 to 30 minutes of regular practice, the effects can last the whole day. Or you can use brief relaxation techniques frequently throughout the day for a calm feeling in just a few seconds or minutes. Focusing on body sensations such as progressive muscle relaxation (📖 see page 92) and breathing (page 90) is sometimes more effective for managing anxiety than purely mental techniques. Experiment to find what works for you.

Sometimes the best way to relax is to indulge in a healthy pleasure that involves one of your five senses (📖 see page 57). Listen to your favorite music. Get or give a massage. Smell sweet fragrances, savor delicious food, or pet your cat or dog. Body-focused experiences can help take your mind off your worries.

Exercise Reduces Anxiety

Exercise often has a "tranquilizer effect" that is even more effective than anti-anxiety medications or quiet relaxation

(📖 see page 112). Aerobic exercise can lessen anxious feelings for up to four hours. Regular physical exercise throughout the day may help reduce chronic anxiety. Strenuous exercise may not be necessary. Gentle exercise such as walking a mile or two decreases anxiety just as effectively as vigorous jogging. In one study, exercise produced longer-lasting relaxation than equal amounts of time spent resting or doing a relaxation exercise.

Another study compared the effects of eating a candy bar with taking a 10-minute walk on a person's mood. At first, both the candy bar and the walk improved people's moods. But an hour later, the candy eaters were more tired and tense than they had been before, whereas the walkers still felt good.

Move From Worry to Action

Jack lies awake in bed at night worrying. He worries about his work. He worries about being able to keep up with the expenses of a house and raising four children. He worries about whether his daughter Carolyn is happy at school, and whether his wife is feeling depressed. Yet Jack doesn't make plans to get a raise or a better paid job. He doesn't speak with

Carolyn's teachers. He doesn't ask his wife how she is feeling.

Anxiety can be a signal to take action. Don't accept or ignore it. Worrying is only worthwhile when:

▶ It prepares you for the inevitable

▶ It prompts you to take useful action

You could, for example, spend lots of time worrying about a suspicious lump. But it's more useful to get a check-up. Or if you're worried about a business report that's not right, rewrite it instead of imagining the terrible results if you hand it in as is. Move from worrying to action.

℞ Check the Facts

Look at your worries more objectively, and ask yourself if your fear is well-founded. *Worries have a way of becoming exaggerated. Most of the awful things we imagine never come to pass.* For instance, if you worry that you'll lose your voice when you address a meeting, ask yourself if this has happened before. Question what you assume will happen. You might think your wife will never forgive you if you're late. But she might be angry for a short while—or not at all—if you have a good reason.

Also be aware of which circumstances you can influence, and which ones you can't. If you are stuck in a traffic jam and miss an appointment, relax. There's nothing you can do. But if you're worried about your brakes, take the car to a mechanic.

℞ Deal with Uncertainty

Uncertainty is a major contributor to worry. Unclear, unpredictable situations in which you don't know how to act are highly stressful. Your body and mind go on constant alert. And worrisome, nagging "what-ifs" keep you perpetually on guard.

Knowing what you're worrying about is sometimes less frightening than not knowing. In a classic experiment, psychologists gave a group of rats electric shocks. Some were warned first with a buzzer; the others received no warning at all. All the rats were distressed, but the health of the ones who had no warning was most affected.

Hospital studies show that when procedures or treatments are thoroughly explained to patients, their stress is reduced. So get more information. When you find yourself worrying, make sure you have all the available facts. Instead of worrying about not paying your mortgage for three months in a row, find out what the consequences are. If you think someone is angry with you, ask the person directly.

Are you trying to decide which job to take or whether or not to get married? *Sometimes the only way to reduce uncertainty is to make a decision. Once you decide, you at least know what to do. But while you are uncertain, you are under constant stress with no obvious course of action.*

Ultimately, no matter how much control you develop over your thoughts, fears, behaviors, and outside events, you will need to accept that some uncertainty is just a fact of life for all of us.

℞ Distract Yourself

Sometimes it may be difficult to put anxious thoughts out of your mind. When you try to suppress any thought, you may end up thinking more about it. For example, try not thinking about a tiger charging at you. Whatever you do, don't

COUNTER ANXIOUS SELF-TALK

Anxious *thoughts* usually precede and trigger anxious *feelings.* You can learn to challenge negative, anxious thoughts. Try these steps:

Step 1

For a week, write down anxious thoughts that recur often in your mind. Watch for thoughts like:

▶ *They'll think badly of me if they see me in this state*

▶ *I'll never get out of here without humiliating myself*

▶ *I can't face it*

▶ *I'm so incompetent*

▶ *I'm such a coward*

▶ *I look stupid*

▶ *I always mess up*

▶ *I may as well not even bother*

Step 2

Then write a statement to counter each anxious thought:

▶ Make your responses more objective, positive, and confidence-promoting.

▶ Whenever your negative, anxiety-provoking self-talk arises, respond to it with your positive statements.

▶ If you find your negative self-talk undermining your self-esteem, challenge those thoughts by asking yourself what evidence you have for believing that. The answer may be that there is none; you always manage to cope.

Keep your thoughts in the present. Focus on what you can do now. Instead of telling yourself you'll be all right in a minute (future), say to yourself that you can breathe and relax right now (present).

Step 3

Make a list of the qualities you like in yourself. Keep it handy and repeat it often. Use self-esteem affirming phrases such as:

▶ *I am worthwhile, even if I'm having a difficult time*

▶ *I deserve to be respected and treated well*

▶ *At any given moment, I am doing the best that I can*

▶ *I know I can do better*

▶ *This too will pass*

For more suggestions on how to break patterns of negative thinking, look at Chapter 2, *Healthy Thinking* (see page 35), and Chapter 7, *Imagery* (page 97).

let the thought of the tiger enter your mind. You'll probably find it nearly impossible not to think about the tiger.

While you may not easily be able to stop thinking about some particular thing, you can distract yourself and redirect your attention elsewhere. For example, think about the tiger again. Now stand up suddenly, slam your hand on the table and shout "STOP!" What happened to the tiger? Gone. At least for the moment.

You can practice this technique whenever your mind endlessly repeats negative thoughts. With practice, you won't have to shout out loud. Just whispering "STOP" or tightening your vocal cords and moving your tongue as if saying "STOP" will often work. Some people imagine a large stop sign. Others put a rubber band on their wrist and snap it hard to break the chain of negative thought. Or you can just pinch yourself. Do anything that redirects your attention.

℞ Schedule Worry Time

Worrisome thoughts feed anxiety. Ignored problems have a way of thrusting themselves back into your mind. You'll find it easier to set aside worries if you set up a specific time deal with them.

Set aside a 20 to 30 minute period during each day as your "worry time." Whenever a worry pops into your mind, write it down and tell yourself that you'll deal with it during your worry time. Jot down the little things (Did Linda take her lunch to school?) along with the big ones (Will our children be able to find jobs in this society in the future?). During your scheduled "worry time," don't do anything else except worry, brainstorm, and write down possible solutions. For each of your worries you might ask yourself:

▶ What is the problem?

▶ How likely is it that the problem will occur?

▶ What's the worst that could happen?

▶ What's the best that could happen?

▶ How would I cope with the problem?

▶ What are possible solutions?

▶ What is my plan of action?

Be very specific. Instead of worrying about what might happen if you lose your job, ask yourself how likely it is that you will lose your job. And if you are laid off, ask yourself what you will do, with whom, and by when. Write a job-search plan.

If you're anxious about getting seasick on the ocean and not making it to the bathroom in time, imagine how you would manage the situation. Ask yourself if any of this is really unbearable. Tell yourself you might feel uncomfortable or embarrassed, but you'll survive.

Remember, if a new worry pops up during the rest of the day, jot it down. Then distract yourself by intently refocusing on whatever you are doing.

Scheduling a definite "worry time" cuts the amount of time spent worrying by at least a third. If you look at your list of worries later, you'll find that the vast majority of them never happened. Or they were not nearly as bad as you anticipated.

℞ Just Do It

Nervousness is normal the first time you do something new that's challenging or threatening. This is especially true if embarrassment or humiliation could be an outcome. Fear can provide positive energy to do your best. The trick is to *feel the fear,* and do it anyway.

The fear will probably decrease the second time you do something, but it may be just as strong when you try something new again. That's just how we're made. There is no reason to back away from challenge. *The things we fear most are also often the most exciting and satisfying. If you find yourself feeling fear, try relabeling the sensations as "excitement" or "anticipation."*

℞ Desensitize Fears and Phobias

A very effective way to eliminate anxiety connected to specific situations and objects is called *desensitization*. It is the method of getting accustomed to what you fear gradually, step-by-step. Before attempting desensitization, you should be experienced with:

1. A relaxation technique (📖 see Chapter 6: *Relaxation*, page 88 and Chapter 7: *Imagery*, page 99)

2. Ways to counter negative thoughts with constructive ones (📖 see Chapter 2: *Healthy Thinking*, page 35)

You can desensitize your fears and phobias by gradually exposing yourself to increasingly threatening situations—first in your imagination and then in real life. The easiest place to start lowering your sensitivity level is in your imagination. If you are worried about an upcoming event, for instance, imagine the worst and best case scenarios, and see yourself coping with both. If you want to overcome a phobia, imagine yourself in progressively more frightening circumstances. Here's how:

1. Make a list. List several situations associated with your fear. Then rank them from the least to the most fearful. If you have a fear of eating in a restaurant, the least anxiety-provoking thought might be to walk past a restaurant, but not enter it. The most fearful might be eating in a crowded restaurant with a large group of friends. Now think of five or six such situations between these extremes, such as eating in an empty restaurant with friends, eating at home with friends, or eating with one friend at their house.

If you have an elevator phobia, your steps might be:

1. Watch people getting on and off an elevator

2. Stand with a friend in an empty elevator with the door open

3. Stand in an empty elevator alone

4. Go up one floor with your friend

5. Ride an elevator alone

2. Imagine the scene. Then close your eyes, and relax completely. Imagine the least fearful situation. See yourself and your surroundings in great detail: what you're wearing, and what you can hear, smell, and see. You want to conjure up real anxiety, so you can learn to deal with it. Or you might choose to face the situations in real life with a trusted, supportive companion to accompany you.

3. Counter your anxious feelings and thoughts. Control your anxious feelings by breathing deeply and slowly. Notice any muscular tension and relax. Notice your thoughts, and counter negative ones with positive ones such as "I can cope with this" (📖 see box page 149). If you stick with the scene, your anxiety will start to decrease, and you will feel relief. *It is important not to run away from the image or scene. If you feel overwhelmed, you can briefly retreat by imagining a calming, peaceful scene or withdrawing from the situation temporarily. But keep returning to your challenging scene until you are no longer anxious.*

Key Point

4. Practice until the anxiety is all gone. Repeat this exercise every day for about 15 minutes. When you feel no more anxiety, even at the start, move on to your next challenge. Keep at it until you reach the most frightening situation, and have eliminated all anxiety associated with it.

Take it at your own speed. Set realistic standards, and expect some setbacks. If you start by facing your fears in your imagination, you will eventually need to use the procedure to face them in real life. Be prepared for the process to be somewhat unpleasant. You may do worse today than yesterday, but tomorrow you may progress far ahead.

℞ Flood Your Symptoms Away

If you want to quickly get rid of a phobia and are willing to go through some psychological pain, you can try "flooding." Immerse yourself in your feared situation, feel it to the max, and stick with it until the fear is completely gone. A person with a cat phobia, for example, might spend several hours in a room with cats. At first the anxiety is great. Then it usually subsides as the person experiences the harmlessness of cats.

Flooding is strong medicine. It should be used only if gentler methods fail, and with a trained person around. You may be scared (even panicky) for a while (perhaps as long as several hours), but if you persist, the anxiety will eventually pass.

Andrea was afraid of riding buses. She overcame this fear by spending three days riding buses. She was terrified when she boarded for the first time. As the bus pulled away from the stop, her fear increased. After about thirty minutes her fear peaked, and then it started to decrease. By the end of three hours, she was no longer panicky. The next day she again felt anxious at first. But her anxiety was less, and it decreased faster. By the third day, she experienced very little anxiety. She started using buses regularly, and had no further problems.

℞ Redefine Your Panic

A panic attack can be frightening and uncomfortable, but fortunately, it is completely harmless. Panic is an entirely natural bodily reaction triggered in response to an emergency or obvious threat. In a panic attack, the reaction occurs in the absence of any immediate or apparent danger. It is this inexplicable, unknown quality of these attacks that heightens the sense of fear. Since people experiencing panic don't know what its cause is, they usually invent an explanation. They think they are having a heart attack or they're suffocating. *It is this critical misinterpretation of bodily symptoms that sets off the escalating cycle of anxiety, and more symptoms.*

Key Point

What to do: If you feel a panic attack coming on, don't try to fight the symptoms. If you don't tense up, the symptoms will generally rise and subside within a few minutes. Try to let go and let it happen, *safe in the knowledge that no physical harm will come to you.* The sensations will pass more quickly if you don't resist them.

Try to control the thoughts running through your head. Challenge your negative thoughts and explanations (📖 see page 42). Instead of telling yourself you can't handle this or you're going to die, (thoughts which will increase your anxiety), repeat to yourself:

▶ *Okay, here it comes again*

▶ *I'll just watch my body respond*

▶ *I've done it before*

▶ *I always survive, this is not dangerous*

▶ *I can handle this even though it's unpleasant*

▶ *These feelings will pass; it's just anxiety*

WATCH OUT

DON'T OVERREACT

When you're having a panic attack, you must correct the misinterpretations that often accompanies it. Remind yourself of the true facts:

▶ You are not having a heart attack

▶ You will not stop breathing and suffocate

▶ You will not faint

▶ You are not "going crazy"

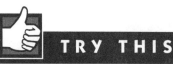

TRY THIS

BREATHING TO CALM PANIC

If you're feeling especially anxious or panicky, you may be breathing either too deeply or too rapidly (hyperventilating). Try calming yourself down by slowing your breathing down with counting, like this:

▶ Begin with a full exhalation

▶ Then count to four as you take in a slow breath through your nose

▶ Feel your belly rise and expand as it fills with air (📖 see page 90)

▶ Then exhale slowly as you count to eight

▶ You can slow your exhalation by breathing through your nose, or through tightened, pursed lips

Your uncomfortable symptoms may subside more quickly if you think about them as normal, harmless, and temporary. Feeling faint is a normal reaction to the perception of danger. Less blood goes to your brain, more goes to your muscles so you're ready for action. The feeling is misleading—you won't actually faint. Fainting is usually due to a heart rate that's too slow or blood pressure that's too low. During a panic attack your heart rate and blood pressure increase, so you're actually less likely to faint. Similarly, feelings of suffocation are due to over-breathing, not the inability to get air. Neither of these feelings causes serious harm. They will subside.

℞ Develop Your Social Skills

If shyness and fear of interacting with others are a source of anxiety for you, here are some suggestions:

Start small. Set up a non-threatening social interaction that can build your confidence. For example, you might write out prepared comments or questions, and call

an information line or a local talk show.

Just say "Hi." Practice saying "hello" or "good morning" to people you pass. Watch their reaction. If you make brief eye contact, smile.

Make small talk. Small talk communicates to others that you're interested in them. What you say is not as important as your carrying on a conversation. Rehearse some opening lines to start a conversation. They don't have to be profound, clever or cute. For example: "Can you give me some directions?" or "This elevator is so slow." or "Have you seen _____ (a particular movie)?"

Ask questions. Ask people about their work, hobbies, pets, or family. Most people love to talk about themselves. Encourage others to express their opinions. Ask questions that require explanations rather than simple yes-or-no answers. Practice your listening skills (📖 see page 122).

Give honest compliments. Complimenting others makes them feel good about themselves and about talking to you. Tell someone you like his clothing, for example, and ask him where he got it.

Share a common experience. Look for some common experience to comment on. You might say, for instance, "We both seem to be stuck in this long line," or "I see you have on a University of Michigan sweatshirt. I went there," or "Did you hear the results of the election?"

Focus on the other person. Concentrate all your attention on the person you are interacting with. Do not think about your own feelings. Help the other person feel comfortable and relaxed.

Develop positive self-talk. Rather than saying that being shy is part of your personality and you're not likely to change, try telling yourself it is natural to feel shy at times, and you can learn how to be more outgoing. Or tell yourself being rejected isn't fun, but it happens to everyone, and you'll survive (📖 see page 149).

℞ Make Yourself Useful

Find yourself plagued by daily hassles, minor aches and pains, and normal insecurities? Try focusing on someone else's worries, and help them. You might:

▶ Try teaching a child to read

▶ Care for someone with a life-threatening disease

▶ Volunteer at a soup kitchen

▶ Take on an environmental cause

By helping others, your life takes on a different perspective. You become more able to appreciate your own assets, and you spend less time worrying about your own concerns (📖 see page 133).

The advice given here can help you gain greater control over your anxiety. Don't be discouraged if it takes some time to feel better. But if these self-help strategies are not sufficient in themselves, please seek additional professional help from your physician or a mental health professional.

📖 *For more information, see page 275*

---

12 Depression

How to Lighten Depression and Bad Moods

▶ *Feeling persistently sad, blue, or down in the dumps?*

▶ *Lost interest in things you used to enjoy?*

▶ *Feeling anxious, worried, irritable, tearful, or hopeless?*

▶ *Feeling extremely guilty, worthless or helpless?*

▶ *Difficulty concentrating, remembering, or making decisions?*

▶ *Feeling tired all the time for no apparent reason?*

▶ *Has your appetite or weight increased or decreased?*

▶ *Problems sleeping or sleeping too much?*

▶ *Frequent aches and pains?*

▶ *Have thoughts of suicide, death, or harming yourself?* *

f these symptoms sound familiar, you may be depressed. If that's the case, you're not alone. At this moment, between 10 and 14 million Americans are depressed. According to World Health Organization (WHO) estimates, there are over 100 million depressed people worldwide.

Depression seems to be more common than it was fifty or a hundred years ago. It's so common it is called the mental health equivalent of a common cold, though it can be far more serious. The good news is that there are several very effective ways to treat and reverse depression. And the same self-help techniques can help just about anyone brighten a bad mood.

Depression and Bad Moods

Feeling sad is natural and inescapable. However, "normal" sadness is a temporary feeling, often linked with a specific event or loss. We sometimes loosely use the word "depressed" to describe feeling sad or disappointed: "I'm really depressed about losing my keys," or "I'm depressed because the basketball game (concert, chess match, play) I wanted to see is sold out." In these circumstances we feel sad, but we can still relate to others and find joy in other areas of our lives.

It is one thing to be saddened when a loved one dies, or you face the breakup of a marriage, or even when your raise is lower than you expected. But true

* *Contact health professional immediately.*

155

Depression Affects Mind & Body

Depression not only takes a heavy toll on mood and quality of life, it also has an impact on physical health.

Depression can be even more disabling than other chronic diseases such as high blood pressure, arthritis, diabetes, back problems, or gastro-intestinal disorders. Only advanced heart disease keeps people in bed more days than does depression, and only arthritis causes more pain. If you have a chronic disease, depression makes it worse—you function less well, visit the doctor more often, stay in the hospital longer, and recover more slowly from surgery.

Depression can depress immunity. Blood samples were taken from 26 people whose spouses were fatally injured or died from heart attacks, strokes, or cancer. The grieving spouses' immune systems were measurably weakened after their losses. Even mild swings in daily mood can depress immune function. For example, on days when mood is depressed, the levels of antibodies in saliva that defend against cold viruses drop.

Depressed people get sick more often than those who are not. They have more colds and more sleep problems.

Depression can also be deadly. Depressed people tend to die earlier due to suicide, failure to comply with medical treatment, and the negative impact depression has on the body. Hardly any body system or disease seems able to escape the physical toll of depression.

▶ One study found that the thinning of the bones (osteoporosis) is greater in depressed people.

▶ Rates of stroke are two times higher in depressed persons compared to those not depressed.

▶ Depressed patients with coronary heart disease are more likely to have heart attacks, undergo bypass surgery, and suffer other heart-related problems. In a study of patients who suffered a heart attack, depression more accurately predicted future heart problems than the severity of artery damage, high cholesterol levels, or cigarette smoking.

▶ Another study of heart attack survivors found that depression increased the risk of dying within six months by three to four times.

The good news is that most people's depression improves with appropriate treatment. And the relief of depression may prevent many of the associated health problems. The importance of these findings: don't ignore depression. Get treatment.

Key Point

depression is something else. It drains the pleasure out of life, leaving you feeling hopeless, helpless, and worthless. With severe depression feelings may become numb, and even crying brings no relief.

Depression affects everything. The way you think, the way you behave, the way you interact with others, and even the way your body functions. When your depressed or sad feelings are severe, long-lasting, and recurrent, you may be experiencing a true depression.

What Causes Depression?

Key Point *Depression is not caused by personal weakness, laziness, or lack of will power. The way you think helps produce and sustain a depressed mood.* Negative thoughts are automatic, recur endlessly, and are often not linked to any event or triggering cause.

Negative thoughts can undermine your feelings of self-worth and happiness. The future appears hopeless, and you attribute this to your own personal failure. You reinterpret your successes as failures, and highlight your shortcomings. Small obstacles seem like insurmountable barriers.

When you are depressed, pessimistic, negative thought patterns become even more pronounced, coloring your perceptions and reactions to life.

When bad events occur, as they do, pessimists explain the causes in permanent, general, and personal terms ("It's going to last forever; it's going to affect everything I do; it's all my fault"). But if something good happens to a pessimist, it's discounted as temporary, specific, and impersonal ("It won't last; it won't change my life; I was just lucky") (📖 see page 38).

People with pessimistic thought patterns get depressed more often, stay depressed, and relapse more often after treatment.

Heredity also may play an important role in certain types of depression. But in most instances, depression is triggered by a complex interaction of psychological, social and environmental factors including:

- Loneliness and lack of social support
- Boredom
- Recent traumatic experiences, major stressful life events, and grief
- Lack of childhood emotional support

MANIC DEPRESSION

One form of depression which is often inherited is called *bipolar disorder* or *manic-depressive disorder*. It is characterized by alternating episodes of terrible "lows" (depression) and inappropriate "highs" (mania) that can last from several days to months. Mania appears as:

- Unwarranted euphoria and positive feelings
- Excessively grand ideas and plans
- Frenzied, nonstop activity
- Little sleep for days on end
- Inflated self-esteem

- Parents who suffered from depression
- Medical illnesses and medications
- Lack of light (an environmental factor that has been linked to depression—see Seasonal Affective Disorder discussed below)
- Drinking too much alcohol or using drugs (when the drug and alcohol use is stopped, the depression usually improves)

All these factors, along with others, Key Point *can contribute to an imbalance in the chemicals in your brain (neurotransmitters). This imbalance can result in changes in the way you think, feel, and act. As you'll see below, changing the way you think and behave can be a powerful and effective way of changing your brain chemistry, lightening depression, and improving an ordinary bad mood.*

Fortunately, the treatments for depression, including antidepressant medications, counseling, and self-help, are highly effective in decreasing the frequency, length, and severity of depression.

Medications Can Help

A variety of antidepressant medications are available to help restore the balance of chemicals in your brain. They are highly effective and bring significant relief up to 60% to 70% of the time.

Key Point *Most antidepressant medications take from several days to several weeks before they begin to work. Don't be discouraged if you don't feel better immediately after starting a medication. Stick with it.* To get the maximum benefit of an antidepressant, you may need to take it for six months or more.

Depending upon the particular type of medication, you may experience one or more of these side effects:

▶ Dry mouth

▶ Blurred vision

▶ Constipation

▶ Drowsiness

▶ Nervousness

▶ Sleeplessness

▶ Dizziness

▶ Weight gain or loss

Side effects are usually most noticeable the first few weeks, and then lessen or go away. If the side effects are not especially severe, try to continue to take your medication. As your body gets used to the medication you will begin to feel better.

It is important to remember to continue taking your medication every day. If you

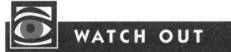

WATCH OUT

CHANGING BAD MOODS: WHAT DOESN'T WORK

Research has shown that some of the more popular ways people attempt to deal with bad moods and depression aren't very effective. They include:

▶ Being alone and isolating yourself

▶ Crying a lot

▶ Getting angry and yelling

▶ Blaming your failure or bad mood on others

▶ Accepting a bad mood without trying to change it

▶ Using alcohol or other drugs

These common strategies usually leave you feeling worse.

stop the medication because you're feeling better (or worse), you may relapse. Antidepressant medications are *not* addictive, but talk with your doctor before stopping or changing the dose.

Counseling Can Help

Several types of psychotherapy can also be highly effective, relieving symptoms up to 60% to 70% of the time. As with medications, counseling rarely has an immediate effect. It may be weeks (or longer) before you see improvement. Several types of psychotherapy help depression:

Cognitive therapy works on changing habitual negative thought patterns that underlie and sustain the depression. Automatic thoughts are monitored, challenged, and reinterpreted.

Interpersonal therapy helps people deal with problems of getting along with others. Current disputes, frustrations, anxieties, disappointments, and unresolved grief reactions are explored. The depressed person learns new ways of coping, communicating, and expressing emotions.

Both types of therapy are brief, usually involving one to two sessions a week for several months. By learning new skills for ways to think and relate, psychotherapy may also help reduce the risk of recurrent depression.

Self-Help Can Help

You can learn many successful psychotherapy techniques on your own. For mild to moderate depression, these self-help strategies can sometimes be very effective.

One study showed that reading and practicing self-help advice improved depression in nearly 70% of patients. You can learn strategies to change negative thinking, distract yourself with pleasurable activities, and develop an increasing sense of hope and self-worth.

As with most forms of treatment, the sooner you start, the better. It is much easier to prevent depression than it is to remedy it, but the same strategies can work in both situations. Even if you are receiving medications and/or counseling, self-help techniques can be used to improve your mood, and may help prevent a relapse.

Depression can be adequately treated with medications, psychotherapy, self-help, or a combination of these. Medications may be especially helpful for severe depression. Medications can provide the boost in mood that helps give you the energy to take new actions and learn new skills. But medications alone may not produce permanent changes in the way you think, feel, and experience the world; they don't change pessimists into optimists. Self-help and/or counseling can help you learn skills to manage your moods.

Get Help Early

Early treatment for depression is important. It may help keep the depression from becoming more severe, chronic, or recurrent. Keep in mind too that the risk of multiple episodes of depression is very high. A person is 50% more likely to be depressed again after the first time, and 70% after the second. After the third time the recurrence rate is 90%. The techniques described here may help avoid a first depression. If you've already had a depressive episode, they can help prevent a second or third occurrence.

Key Point

How to Lighten Depression and Bad Moods

The self-help advice below can sometimes be sufficient to prevent or relieve mild depression, sadness, or bad moods. Or these skills and strategies can be used to supplement medications and counseling.
Overcoming depression can become an opportunity to make positive and lasting changes in your life. If you practice these techniques, you can markedly shift your mood and the basic way you look at life, giving it new richness and meaning.

Women's Vulnerability

It is known that depression is more than twice as common in women than in men. Biological differences may contribute. But a major cause appears to lie in the way our society defines sex roles. It offers men and women different levels of power and control over their lives. A feeling of helplessness and the sense that one is not in control of one's own life is a powerful predictor of clinical depression.

Women of all ages are often taught to be helpless. Boys are trained for self-reliance and activity, girls for passivity and dependence. Women's roles as caregivers, mothers, and homemakers are often undervalued. Even when a woman works, her achievements are frequently credited less than men's.

Men still earn much more than women in the same job, and they currently occupy much higher status jobs than women do. The family moves when *his* job changes; *her* job is often seen as lesser than his. Many women have given up their work (or taken lesser jobs) for the sake of the man's. In times of crisis they have little to feel proud of, and little career security.

Men's Vulnerability

Women's traditional role in society does not place them at risk for all psychological disorders, however. On the contrary, men are more likely to abuse alcohol and drugs, more likely to be hyperactive, or have an antisocial personality disorder. Men suffer much more when their spouses die, since they more often have no one to discuss their feelings with. It's not that women suffer more than men, but women experience more despair and lack of control which makes them more vulnerable to depression.

Different Coping Styles

There is another way that women's social roles make them more susceptible to depression. Both men and women have down times, but they respond to them differently. Males typically cope with initial depressive experiences by doing things that distract them from their mood, whereas women focus on the mood itself and, in doing so, may amplify it. Men tend to lose themselves in other activities, and women tend to brood on their troubles.

Learning from Each Other

Both sexes have something to learn from the other. Distraction may help to insulate people from depression, but used excessively, it may place them at risk for other problems like alcoholism, aggression, or antisocial behavior. Similarly, focusing on feelings may help people survive the loss of a spouse, a job, or other life disappointment, but it can also lay the groundwork for depression.

℞ Plan for Pleasure

Our daily mood is based more on the small but pleasurable things that happen each day than on major events like marriage, job promotions, or traumatic experiences. Studies on happiness show that the number of small happy moments and accumulated time spent being happy is what contributes the most to our overall good mood and life satisfaction.

There are lots of opportunities to have a good time, and if you take them, you will be less at risk for getting depressed. Going for a walk, looking at a sunset, watching a funny movie, getting a massage, learning another language, taking a cooking class, or joining a social club can all help keep your spirits up, and keep you from falling into a situation where you can get depressed.

But sometimes having fun isn't such an easy prescription. You may have to **Key Point** *make a deliberate effort to plan pleasurable activities. Even if you don't feel like doing it, try to stick to the schedule.* You may find that the nature walk, cup of tea, or half hour of listening to music will improve your mood despite your initial misgivings. Don't leave good things to chance. You might want to make up a schedule for your free time during the week and what you'd like to do with it.

If you are feeling hardly any emotion and the world seems devoid of color, make an effort to put some sensation back into your life. Go to a bookstore and look through your favorite section. Listen or dance to some upbeat music. Exercise or ask someone to give you a massage so you can reconnect with your body. Eat some spicy food. Treat yourself to a very hot bath, or try a cold shower. Go to a garden center and smell all the flowers. Try these and other healthy pleasures (📖 see page 57).

℞ Take Action

You can momentarily boost your mood just by resolving to try harder in the future. But taking action to solve the problems immediately facing you provides the surest relief from a bad mood.

More important than *what* you change or *how much* you change is the **Key Point** confidence-building feelings that come from successfully changing *something—* anything! Taking action is the important thing. Incorporating some simple things into your life can boost your mood. You might decide to clean or reorganize a room, for instance, or a closet, or even a desk drawer. Or get a new magazine subscription or call an old friend.

If you keep telling yourself that you are useless, lazy, or inadequate, one way to prove yourself wrong (and help lift the depression) is to take action. Do something that will prove to yourself you can still be a good friend, run a home, work efficiently, or whatever. Once you start doing something you'll become absorbed in it, and your mood will improve. Even taking a moment to remember your past successes can help you feel better about yourself. Starting is the hardest part. Once you've begun, it gets easier and more satisfying.

Be careful not to set yourself difficult goals or take on a lot of responsibility. Break large tasks into small ones, set some priorities, and do what you can as best as you can. Learn some of the proven steps for taking successful action (📖 see page 21).

℞ Move Your Mood

Physical activity lifts depression and negative mood. One study compared walking or jogging with psychotherapy for depressed patients. Within a week most of

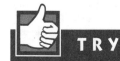

DISTRACT YOURSELF

The more you mull over your sad feelings, the greater hold they take on your mood. If you find yourself trapped in recycling negative thoughts, break the mood cycle by distracting yourself.

▶ Splash cold water on your face

▶ Pinch yourself

▶ Stand up suddenly, slam your hand on the table, and shout, "STOP!"

▶ Put a rubber band on your wrist and snap it hard whenever you want to break a chain of negative thoughts

▶ Try anything that will help you refocus your attention

Or use more pleasant distractions. Seek out any positive, absorbing activity that is unrelated to your sadness. Active distractions (such as hobbies that require your full attention) lift mood better than passive distractions such as watching TV.

Use your imagination to reconstruct the details of a happy moment or concentrate on something you're looking forward to. Distraction tends to work best for minor upsets. It also helps to clear your mind so you can take more effective action at solving a more serious problem.

the exercisers reported feeling better, and within three weeks they were "virtually well." The exercisers did as well as those receiving short-term psychotherapy, and did better than patients undergoing long-term, unlimited therapy. After one year, those treated with exercise were essentially free of depression, while nearly half of those people receiving psychotherapy alone had to return for additional treatment.

Another study tested the effect of eating a candy bar or taking a 10-minute walk on mood and depression. Both the candy and the walk improved mood, but, an hour later, the candy eaters were more tired and tense than they had been before, while the walkers still felt good.

So boost your mood and energy level with many pleasurable physical activities. Depressed people often complain that they feel too tired to exercise. But the feelings of fatigue associated with depression are not due to physical exhaustion. If you can get yourself moving, you may find you have more energy (📖 see page 114).

℞ Lighten Up

Are you more tired, depressed, and unable to cope as winter approaches? Perhaps you put on weight, sleep more, and scale down your social life. You may lack motivation and feel that your life is going to pieces. But when spring comes, your spirits lift.

We all feel brighter and more enthusiastic on sunny days, and moody on dull, gray days. But if the difference in your winter and summer moods is dramatic, you may be suffering from seasonal affective disorder (SAD). SAD people typically begin experiencing seasonal mood swings in their teens and twenties. The symptoms appear to be directly related to the amount of sunlight that reaches the brain. The brain responds to light (or the lack of it) by secreting various hormones—ones that control mood and internal body clocks.

So if you find yourself fantasizing in midwinter about a trip to a warm and sunny vacation spot, it may not be pure escapism. It may be your brain writing you a prescription for more light. People who live closer to the equator or spend some winter vacation time in sunny climates tend to be less affected by SAD.

If you can't take off to a sunnier place, you may be able to brighten your mood by increasing your exposure to light, especially in the early hours of the morning. Rise earlier in the morning and go outdoors when it's light, or at least sit near an open window. If possible, you may want to replace your current indoor lighting with bright, full-spectrum fluorescent light bulbs. The technique, called phototherapy, consists of exposing yourself to very bright lights (such as a light box with eight full-spectrum fluorescent bulbs). Consult a professional experienced in phototherapy (□ see page 276).

℞ Watch Out for Negative Thoughts

When you're feeling down, observe the negative, pessimistic thoughts that race through your mind. For example, you might find yourself thinking, "I'm really worthless because Sally didn't like the report I made." "The future looks quite hopeless." These automatic thoughts go almost unnoticed and unchallenged in our minds, yet they shape our moods, actions, and bodily symptoms. *Remember, by changing these negative thoughts, you can change your mood.*

Key Point

℞ Challenge Negative Thoughts

Many people tend to be excessively critical of themselves, especially when they're depressed. You may find yourself saying groundless, untrue things about yourself.

TRY THIS

Write down some of your negative thoughts. Look for patterns. How do you interpret the events in your life? Do your explanations tend to be:

▶ Permanent *("It's always going to be this way")*

▶ General *("It's going to undermine all aspects of my life")*

▶ Personal *("It's all my fault")*

Challenge those negative thoughts.
(□ see page 42)

(□ see page 42)

If these comments were made by someone else, you might dispute their assertions.

You need to do the same with your own self-talk. Learn how to constructively argue with yourself. Ask yourself what evidence there is to support your beliefs.

Almost nothing that happens has just one cause or explanation. If there are multiple explanations, why focus on the worst one? For example, if you are saying to yourself, "I'm just a terrible parent," look around for different evidence. You provide shelter and food. You taught your child to ride a bicycle. You took your children to an amusement park. And so on. Then the heavy, global judgment that you are a bad parent will lighten.

Check to see if your explanations, judgments, and criticisms are out of proportion:

❑ Are you exaggerating?

❑ Are you making a minor setback into a catastrophe?

❑ Are there alternative explanations for your behavior, or circumstances that don't lay the blame completely on you?

If you feel guilty about nearly everything, stop the next time this feeling arises, and assess exactly what the guilt is. If none of the guilt is really yours, don't assume it. If part of it is yours, then accept that, and do what is necessary. Apologize, make it right, or make an effort not to repeat it (but don't beat yourself up if you do accidentally make a mistake).

℞ Develop Positive Thoughts

As you challenge your automatic negative thoughts, begin to rescript the negative stories you tell yourself. For example, one of your underlying beliefs may be, "Unless I do everything perfectly, I'm a failure." This is a pretty tough standard for anyone to live up to. Perhaps this belief could be revised to, "Success is doing the best that I can in any situation."

When confronting a problem, try to focus on what is changeable, specific, and non-personal. You can learn special strategies to change your *negative* thinking in Chapter 2: *Healthy Thinking* (📖 see page 35), and develop positive *affirmations* in Chapter 7: *Imagery* (page 103). Remember that negative thinking (blaming yourself, feeling hopeless, expecting failure, and other such thoughts) is part of depression itself. As you change these pessimistic thought patterns, your depression will lift.

℞ Remember The Good Things

Suppose somebody asks you what you did over the weekend. *"Oh, it was awful,"* you say. *"Cliff and I had a fight. I burned the steaks on the barbecue. Angela fell and hurt her foot badly, so I had to take her to the emergency room."*

Try rethinking the weekend, but this time, concentrate on the positive. Ask yourself: Was it a nice day? *"Yes, it was glorious. We sat outside, went swimming, and I had a great conversation with my best friend."* Then examine your statements: Angela fell, but what was going on? *"Yes, I was playing with her. We were having a great time together, the first time we've had so much fun in weeks, and then she fell."* Was she okay after you went to the hospital? *"Yes, she was fine. Nothing was broken. She got lots of attention and rather seemed to enjoy the excitement of a trip to the hospital."* Actually, the weekend wasn't a total disaster. There were lots of good things in it.

When you are depressed, it's easy to forget that anything nice has happened at all. This is because you are so focused on the negative events. Keeping a diary can be a good idea at such a time. Make a definite effort to put down the positive events as well as the negative ones, and how you feel about them.

℞ Clear Up Your Communication

Think back over what was happening in your life in the months before you started feeling blue. Sometimes depression is triggered by a traumatic event like a divorce, death of a loved one, loss of a job, or a series of smaller, cumulative setbacks.

While sadness and grieving is normal, prolonged, pervasive feelings of despair and hopelessness indicate depression. There are many ways of dealing with trauma that can short-circuit depression. Try expressing your feelings by writing, confiding in others, or through assertive communication (📖 see page 207).

If you have not communicated fully what you feel about something that has occurred in a family or work relationship, try to clarify what you feel and why. Then approach that person and tell him or her.

Talking may clear the air for you and help lift your depression.

Remember to speak assertively rather than accusingly so you can get things off your chest in a constructive way, not one that puts anyone else down (📖 see page 128). If you cannot confront the person because he or she is no longer alive or will not see you, write out what you want to say, as though you were writing the person a letter. You don't have to send it, but this can help settle your feelings.

℞ Eliminate the Negative

Clearly, it isn't possible to avoid all unhappy events. But you can reduce bad news and bad company. Spending time with pessimistic people only strengthens your negative thoughts. Don't isolate yourself. Try to seek out positive, optimistic people who can lighten your heavy feelings.

If you are depressed, reading bad things in the newspapers or seeing upsetting things on television doesn't help. Studies show that when people watch negative news programs their level of sadness and anxiety climbs. News items that show war, poverty, murder, and crime induce viewers to dwell on the negative.

Exposure to the world's misery appears to affect the viewer in a broader way. Negative news encourages more worrisome thoughts about the viewer's own problems. So skip negative news when you're depressed.

℞ Do Something for Someone Else

Lending a helping hand to someone in need is one of the most effective ways to change a bad mood, but it is one of the least commonly used. When you're depressed, you may greet the advice of helping others with thoughts like, "I've got enough troubles of my own. I don't need anyone else's."

But if you can bring yourself to help someone else, even in a small way, you'll feel better about yourself. Feeling useful is good for self-esteem, and you will be temporarily distracted from your own problems.

There are many things you can do:

▶ Arrange to baby-sit for a friend

▶ Take someone's children to school

▶ Do some shopping for somebody who is house-bound

▶ Read a story to someone who is ill

▶ Do some physical chores for someone who needs help

If you arrange a specific time to offer your help, you are also assigning yourself a responsibility to meet.

And there's another psychological payoff. *Helping others more needy than yourself can help you appreciate your own assets and capabilities. By comparison, your problems and difficulties may not appear as overwhelming.* Sometimes helping others is the surest way to help yourself (📖 see page 134).

Key Point

Don't be discouraged if it takes some time to feel better. Recovering from depression can be a slow process. Remember that it took time for the depression to develop, and it will take time for it to go away. You can use the advice given here to gain greater control over your moods.

If these self-help strategies alone are not sufficient, seek help from your physician or a mental health professional.

📖 *For more information, see page 276*

13 Anger

How to Manage Your Anger and Hostility

"Anyone can get angry—that is easy...but to do this to the right person, to the right extent, at the right time, with the right motive, and in the right way, that is not for everyone, nor is it easy."

— *Aristotle*

Janet: *"I bought a new dress to wear to the party on Saturday."*

Paul *(glaring): "Another dress? I hope you picked the money off a tree."*

Janet *(eyes flaring): "You're the one who insisted on joining the damn club."*

Paul *(getting louder): "I'm sick of you blaming everything on me."*

Janet *(even louder): "It cost a fraction of what you spend on club dues. You're just like your father. Selfish."*

Paul *(face turning red): "Leave my father out of this!" (He's shouting and pounds his fist on the table). "I work hard all week. Playing tennis is my only fun."*

Janet *(now crying): "Well, that makes me feel just great. Thanks a lot."*

Paul *stalks off to the living room and puts a wall of newspapers in front of his face. Janet starts dinner, banging pots and pans and slamming cabinets.*

Janet and Paul are not headed for a great evening. But worse, they are among some 20% of Americans whose hostility is potentially harmful to their health, and perhaps life-threatening. In spite of the popular belief that suppressing anger is bad for you, "letting it out" may be worse.

Anger is not all bad. And without the "fight-or-flight" response prompting our early ancestors to defend themselves, we probably wouldn't be here at all. Without any anger, slaves might never rebel, workers might not stand up for their rights, and you might never express your distress about being mistreated.

The key issue is how often and how much we get angry, and what we do then. In today's world, the fight-or-flight response is too easily triggered, and is rarely useful. We overreact. We treat relatively minor frustrations and setbacks as though they were emergencies or serious threats. We generalize, and see everything as "black or white." *We get angry at one event and dredge up other unrelated anger-causing experiences and make it worse. The anger response floods our body with stress hormones, weakens our health,*

> **Key Point**

THE EFFECT OF ANGER

When you get angry, your body launches its fight-or-flight response to prepare for danger. The sympathetic nervous system is put on full alert. Stress hormones—adrenaline and cortisol—are released into the bloodstream. Heart rate and blood pressure surge upward, the blood clots more rapidly, and the immune system is temporarily suppressed. The body's fat stores discharge, causing cholesterol levels to rise. When this happens repeatedly, it can damage the arteries that feed the heart. As the arteries narrow and blood flow decreases, chest pains or heart attacks may result.

When we're feeling or acting hostile, the parasympathetic nervous system which calms and protects the body from the onslaught of stress hormones, is slow to activate. The bodies of those who are often angry take much longer to return to normal after stress than calmer, more relaxed people.

The people at greatest risk of heart disease score high on three dimensions of hostility (📖 see box page 170):

1. Cynical mistrust of others

2. Frequent angry feelings

3. Aggressive behavior

In one study, medical students with high hostility scores were four to five times more likely to develop coronary heart disease than those with low scores. They were also seven times more likely to die within 25 years *from any cause* than their cool-headed counterparts.

Hostility also appears to make the symptoms of heart disease worse. A study found that when heart disease patients remembered an incident that made them angry, their hearts received less blood flow and pumped less efficiently. Just the

Continued on next page

---

and usually doesn't even solve the problem!

Fortunately there is hope. We are not preprogrammed robots when it comes to anger. We can learn to see it coming, and choose how to respond. And we can make more creative uses for this important, natural human emotion.

"Blow up" or "Put up"

Should you express your anger and let it out, or should you suppress your feelings? *Research now suggests that people who vent their anger get more angry, not less.* But suppressing anger isn't the answer either. The angry feelings often smolder, only to flare up later at the slightest incident. But "blow up" or "put up" are not the only options we have. Here are two better ones:

1. You can raise your anger threshold—that is, allow fewer incidents to trigger your anger in the first place

2. When you get angry, you can *choose* how to react—without either denying your feelings or giving in to the situation

Sounds simple enough, but what gets in the way is our tendency to see anger as coming from outside ourselves—something over which we have little control.

Key Point

thought of anger or hostility can produce these potentially dangerous effects.

To make matters worse, chronic anger drives friends and family members away, so the angry person loses the stress-buffering benefits of social support. Hostile people report less social support, less marital satisfaction, and more family conflict.

Cynical, hostile people also tend to take more risks with their health. They're more likely to take up smoking, abuse drugs and alcohol, and overeat. All these things take a toll on health.

Angry Men, Angry Women

While the research on anger has mostly involved men, early research on women suggests some interesting findings. Men and women tend to get angry equally often, equally intensely, and usually for similar reasons. But the *expression* of anger often differs:

▶ Women are more likely to keep their anger to themselves, or express it in private to a spouse or close friend

▶ Women more often release tension and express anger by crying (tears of rage and frustration should not be confused with sadness or remorse)

▶ Men tend to yell, scream, pound the table, and publicly display their wrath

▶ Women often feel embarrassed and guilty about angry outbursts, while men feel their anger is justified and appropriate

Frequent expressions of anger appear to damage the hearts of both men and women, however it is expressed. But the good news is that by changing your response to anger—especially when it is combined with enhanced social support and relaxation skills—you are likely to have a positive effect on both your health and your own happiness.

We see ourselves as helpless victims. We blame others and we say, "You make me so angry!" We explode and then we say, "I couldn't help it." We see friends as selfish and insensitive, bosses as snobs or bullies, friends as unappreciative. So it seems that our only choice is an outburst of hostility. But with a little practice, even a seasoned hothead can master a new repertoire of healthy and more effective responses.

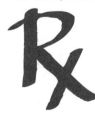

How to Defuse Anger and Hostility

Anger may seem like an automatic response to a person, event or situation. But your angry feelings are usually a response to your own thoughts.

TEST YOUR HOSTILITY

To measure your hostility, check the boxes that apply to you:

❏ When I'm in the express checkout line at the supermarket, I often count the items in the baskets of the people ahead of me to be sure they aren't over the limit.

❏ I am often irritated by other people's incompetence.

❏ When an elevator doesn't come as quickly as I think it should, I am likely to pound on the button, or think nasty thoughts about the people delaying the elevator on other floors.

❏ I tend to remember irritating incidents and get mad at them all over again.

❏ Little annoyances have a way of adding up during the day, and leave me frustrated and impatient.

❏ If my hair cutter trims off more hair than I wanted, I fume for days.

❏ When I get into an argument, I can feel my pulse quicken, my breathing change, or my jaws clench.

❏ When someone doesn't show up on time, I rehearse the angry words I'm going to say.

❏ I've been so angry at someone that I've thrown things or slammed doors.

❏ When someone cuts me off in traffic, I flash my lights, honk my horn, pound the steering wheel, curse, or shout.

❏ If someone mistreats me, I look for an opportunity to pay that person back, just for the principle of it.

Scoring

▶ If you checked three or less boxes, you have a pretty cool head.

▶ If your score is 4 to 8, take it as a warning. Hostility may be raising your risk of heart disease.

▶ A score of 9 or more puts you in the hot zone. This level of cynicism, anger, and aggression is probably high enough to endanger your health and your relationships.

Adapted from Redford Williams, author of Anger Kills.

℞ Reason with Yourself

How you interpret and explain a situation determines whether you will feel angry or not. A series of automatic thoughts and cynical interpretations of the situation flash through your mind before the angry feelings or hostile acts. "He's late on purpose." "If she really cared about me, she'd hang up her clothes. She knows I hate the mess." It is these automatic, hostile thoughts that trigger and sustain your angry feelings.

These thoughts and interpretations are often inaccurate and untrue. But you can learn to defuse anger by pausing and questioning your anger-producing thoughts. If you change your thoughts, you can change your response. You can decide whether or not to get angry, and then decide whether or not to act.

You don't have to wait until you find yourself in an angry situation—you can learn from a review of past experiences (📖 see box page 172). Or step deliberately into a personal hot spot for practice. For example, choose the longest, slowest line in the grocery store. At the first sign of anger, count to three and ask yourself the following questions:

1. Is this really important enough to get angry about?

▶ What's really going on?

▶ What's the worst that can happen?

▶ Is this incident serious enough to merit the time and energy I'm giving it?

▶ Will this issue make a big difference in my life in an hour? Next week? In a year?

▶ Is it an isolated incident, in which case I can probably forget it, or is this a recurring problem that I need to deal with?

Let's say somebody pushes ahead of you and takes the very last seat on the bus. You could think, "That selfish jerk," and seethe all the way to work.

Or you could say to yourself, "Boy, that certainly was inconsiderate. But what does it matter?" Or be empathetic: "Maybe he feels dizzy and needs to sit down." Then put the incident behind you. In time, you are likely to discover these two handy rules to live by:

▶ Don't sweat the small stuff.

▶ It's usually all small stuff.

2. Am I justified in getting angry?

Again, looking at the evidence, ask:

▶ Do I have just cause to be angry?

▶ Are my expectations realistic?

▶ Am I confusing my feelings now with something that happened in the past?

▶ Am I jumping to conclusions?

▶ Could this person have a reasonable explanation for his or her behavior?

▶ Do I really know what's going on?

▶ Am I misinterpreting?

If icy roads are causing traffic to slow down, it's ridiculous to assume that nature deliberately set out to thwart you.

You may need to question some of your most basic thoughts, beliefs, and assumptions—the ones that set off your angry responses (📖 see page 42). You may also need to gather more information to really understand the situation. Here's where good listening skills can also come into play (📖 see page 122). If you conclude that your angry thoughts and feelings are not justified, use the evidence to talk yourself out of being angry.

KEEP AN ANGER LOG

As with changing any habit, the first step is to become aware of it. When you're dealing with anger and hostility, it means learning to recognize your own "early-warning" symptoms. Also watch for the events, thoughts, and attitudes that are most likely to trigger your anger.

Think of a recent incident that made you angry, and write a description of it. Or keep an anger log, and record the following kinds of things:

▶ **The situation:** What provoked you?

▶ **Thoughts:** What were you thinking about just before you felt angry?

▶ **Feelings:** Did you feel angry, hurt, betrayed, mistrustful?

▶ **Physical Response:** What changes did you notice in your body?

▶ **Actions:** What did you do and say?

▶ **Outcome:** What were the results?

Jotting down entries like the examples on the next page will help you spot your regular patterns of anger. After a few days, review your log.

Remember, anger doesn't always mean that someone is yelling. Maybe you blow-up, simmer, or stew. Many people express their anger subtly, in indirect "passive-aggressive" ways such as:

▶ Procrastination

▶ Getting bored

▶ Becoming confused

▶ Making digs disguised as "jokes"

▶ Giving the cold shoulder or silent treatment

What are the consequences of how you express your angry feelings, thoughts, and actions?

ANGER LOG

Situation: _____

Thoughts: _____

Feelings: _____

Physical response: _____

Actions: _____

Outcome: _____

Continued on next page

ANGER LOG: EXAMPLES

Example 1

Situation: A person pulled into a parking spot I was waiting for.

Thoughts: That person deliberately stole my parking spot.

Feelings: Angry, betrayed.

Physical response: Rapid breathing, tense neck and jaw muscles.

Actions: Shouted at the other driver. Pounded my steering wheel.

Outcome: Other driver made an obscene gesture and yelled back that he hadn't seen me. I didn't get the parking space.

Example 2

Situation: I told my friend something that was supposed to be confidential, and she passed it on to another friend.

Thoughts: My friend doesn't care about me. She deliberately tried to get me in trouble.

Feelings: Angry, hurt, betrayed.

Physical response: Chest got tight, face felt flushed, stomach churned.

Actions: I didn't say anything.

Outcome: I now feel a wall has developed between us. We avoid each other.

3. Will getting angry make a difference? Sometimes you may decide that an issue is important enough to get angry about, and that you have valid reasons to be angry. For example, a co-worker is repeatedly late for meetings, and this disrupts your work. Should you get angry? That depends on whether you think your anger can change the situation. It may make a real difference to let your co-worker know how much you are upset, and the consequences of his or her action.

But more often than not, getting angry and losing your cool is ineffective and counterproductive. Exploding and venting merely increases

Key Point

your angry feelings, puts a strain on your relationships, and potentially damages your health.

If your anger leads to effective action and assertive communication, great. But if there is little you can do to affect the provoking situation, then redirect your attention and emotions elsewhere with distraction techniques (📖 see box page 175).

℞ Defusing Anger in Relationships

In situations where relationships are involved, it's usually most effective to make yourself as clear as possible in a very direct and assertive way. Here's how to do it:

▶ **State your observations about the problem.** Try to express your perceptions in an objective, non-judgmental way. You might, for example, say, *"The roof has been leaking for a month. You agreed to fix it two weeks ago, but nothing's been done."*

▶ **Say what you think.** This is your opportunity to express your opinions, beliefs, and/or interpretation of your observations. *"It seems to me that the longer the roof goes without repair, the greater the potential damage."*

▶ **State your feelings.** Say what the impact of the situation is on you. Use "I statements" to describe your own reaction rather than blaming the other person. Instead of saying, *"You never do anything you promise to do,"* say *"I'm really bothered by this leaky roof, and frustrated that it still isn't fixed."*

▶ **Say what you want.** Make a clear, specific request. Suggest consequences if that's appropriate. *"I want you to fix the roof this weekend. If you don't have time, I'll call a roofer on Monday and pay to have it done."*

For more suggestions on healthy communication see Chapter 9: *Communicate Well*, (📖 see page 121), and the box, *Deflecting Others' Anger* (see page 176).

℞ Cool Off

Anger depends on tension and arousal. Any technique that relaxes or distracts you —like meditating or taking a long walk— can help you put out the fire within. Here are some things to try:

Breathe. Slow, deep breathing is one of the quickest and simplest ways to cool off (📖 see page 90). You can combine this technique with the old standby, "count to ten." When you notice anger building, take ten slow, relaxed breaths before responding. This focused breathing gives you time to think, and it reduces the physical arousal that fuels anger. Make a deliberate effort to speak slowly and softly.

Withdraw. Sometimes temporary isolation can be healing. Many people report that spending a little time alone removes the stimulus to anger, and helps them calm down. If you have a high-stress job, give yourself a few minutes of private time to relax when you first get home. You'll probably find family interactions less anger-provoking.

Exercise. Vigorous exercise provides a good natural outlet for stress and anger. Exercise may also release endorphins, the chemicals in the brain that act as natural tranquilizers. Exercise is especially helpful for "hot reactors"—people whose distrustful, hostile attitudes pump an excess of powerful stress hormones into their bloodstream (📖 see page 112).

Laugh at Yourself. It's hard to be angry when you're laughing. Turn arguments

DISTRACT YOURSELF

Angry feelings and hostile actions thrive on angry thoughts. The more you mull over anger-provoking incidents, the greater your anger becomes, and the longer it lasts. But it can be difficult to put angry thoughts out of your mind. In fact, research shows that when you try to suppress a thought, you're likely to end up obsessing about it even more.

Imagine a situation that makes you really angry—like someone grabbing the parking place you've been waiting for. Now try not to think about how mad it makes you. Whatever you do, don't let the thought of that inconsiderate driver enter your mind. You'll probably find it nearly impossible not to think of it. You need a way to redirect your attention elsewhere. Now think about that person grabbing your spot again. Suddenly, slam your hand on the steering wheel and shout, "STOP!"

What happened to your thought about the stolen parking space? Gone, at least for the moment. You can practice this technique any time you find yourself endlessly going over an angry thought. With practice, you won't even have to shout out loud. Just whisper "STOP!" Or tighten your vocal cords and move your tongue as if you were saying "STOP!" Or picture a large stop sign.

Another technique is to put a rubber band around your wrist and snap it hard whenever you want to break a chain of angry thoughts. Some people pinch themselves. Do whatever will get your attention off the angry thought. Or use a more pleasant distracter:

▶ Seek out any positive, absorbing stimulation that is unrelated to whatever triggered your anger

▶ Read, watch television, or engage in a hobby

▶ Go over a happy moment in your imagination

▶ Concentrate on something you're looking forward to

into jokes. One couple drew water pistols when their fights went on too long. Picture the person you're angry with wearing a clown costume. Exaggeration is an excellent humor generator. Carry your irrational beliefs, fears, and resentments to ridiculous extremes (see page 54).

℞ Stay in the Present

Feelings of anger often trigger memories of other anger-provoking experiences. This can lead to a whole cascade of angry feelings. *The best clue that anger may be coming from old resentments is when just a "ten-cent" provocation triggers a "ten-dollar" response.* For example, a friend grins at you during a disagreement, and suddenly you're filled with rage and fury. The friend's expression may be triggering painful memories of a ridiculing parent.

Work to stay focused on the specific incident that's upsetting you now. Avoid making generalizations: "always" or

Key Point

13 Anger

DEFLECTING OTHERS' ANGER

If you are the target of someone's anger, the most effective way for you to deflect it is to *genuinely listen*. This isn't very easy when you are feeling attacked—the natural tendency is to defend yourself. But force yourself to listen.

Often we attribute meaning to someone's displeasure that isn't really intended. For example, your roommate says, "It makes me angry when you leave your dirty dishes on the counter." You might say to yourself, "She thinks I'm a terrible person." In reality, she is probably only saying that she doesn't like dirty dishes on the counter.

Active listening helps you to avoid misinterpreting anger (📖 see page 122). To listen well, repeat in your own words what you think the person said. "You're angry because I didn't tell the boss you helped with that report," or "I understand. You think at age thirteen you should have more freedom." This helps assure accurate communication. It also helps the other person to feel understood, and reduces the level of hostility.

If the other person still doesn't feel heard, ask for an example to clarify the grievance. Remember that saying "I understand" doesn't mean you agree. The goal is to de-escalate the anger so that you can try to resolve the problem together. Agree only to a solution if you feel it is fair, and you can live with it. Then do your best to keep to it. Monitor progress together, so you can keep the issue from building up again.

While you are working on a mutually satisfying solution, practice positive self-talk: "I refuse to let this get the best of me." "When we are both calm, we'll find a solution." Sometimes it helps to imagine yourself in a protective cocoon so the hostile comments just bounce off you.

After an argument, you may find yourself continuing to think of things you wish you'd said. This train of thought can be enough to get you angry all over again. Try some constructive coping thoughts instead, such as:

▶ *This is difficult; it takes time*

▶ *I'll get better as I get more practice*

▶ *Thinking about this just upsets me; I have better things to do with my time*

Problem resolved? Congratulate yourself:

▶ *I actually got through this fight without being sarcastic*

▶ *I'm glad I didn't get more upset over this than it was worth*

▶ *I handled that one pretty well*

Do not try to defuse anger by telling someone to relax or to calm down. This sounds condescending, and it is more likely to infuriate than calm. If you feel someone's anger is getting out of hand, say you need some "time out." Get a glass of water or take a walk around the block. Do not put up with either psychological or physical abuse. Get professional help if necessary.

"never" statements such as, "You're always telling me what to do," or "You never think about my feelings." Instead, make specific, assertive requests.

℞ Practice Empathy

Reframe an anger-provoking situation by trying to see it from the other person's point of view. There may be a perfectly understandable explanation for the other person's behavior, but you misinterpret it, or don't take the time to find out what it is.

Making up a story to explain, excuse, and forgive can help to neutralize your anger. Imagine that you're driving down the highway and someone suddenly cuts you off. If you assume that this was a malicious act, you are likely to get angry. But if you consider that the other driver might be racing to the hospital with a very ill child in the back seat, you'll be more likely to relax and wish him luck. *Even if this "explanation" is not true, your body will react as though it is.*

Maybe the slow sales clerk is at the end of a double shift or is worrying about her out-of-work brother. Imagine how you'd feel in her situation. Empathy helps you dismiss irritating incidents. Give others the benefit of the doubt. Assume their intentions are good unless you have evidence to the contrary.

℞ Help Others

Anger and hostility cuts you off from the people around you. It makes you feel apart from—rather than a part of—the larger human community. Look for ways of being connected by making a contribution to your community. Volunteering helps fight the isolation that fosters anger. It also expands your capacity for empathy.

And volunteering has an added bonus: volunteers are healthier and live longer than non-volunteers (📖 see page 136).

℞ Let it Go

There will be times when you may have been genuinely wronged, but expressing yourself assertively is impossible. Or it is inappropriate, or it will not lead to the resolution you seek. In order to be free of the anger, pain, and the ill health it causes, you may need to forgive, and let it go.

Forgiveness doesn't mean approving of hurtful behavior, or pretending something never happened. It doesn't mean you have to trust the person who wronged you. It *does* mean choosing to move on, unencumbered by the past.

Forgiveness may come more easily to you when you consider this: A person's mistreatment of someone else is often an expression of their fear. Many times that fear is based on a deeper need for help, respect, and love.

The following questions can help you evaluate whether a particular resentment is worth keeping. Ask yourself:

▶ Do I use anger as a way of feeling more powerful, or being in control?

▶ Does my anger help me to avoid communicating?

▶ Do I use anger to punish, or to make others feel guilty?

▶ Do I use anger to cover feelings I am trying to avoid?

▶ Does my anger give me an excuse for not taking responsibility for my role in what's happening?

▶ What do I gain by staying angry?

▶ What do I gain by giving up my anger?

℞ Get Professional Help

Sometimes all your efforts to curb your own or a loved one's anger fail. If you try the strategies suggested here but remain unable to control your anger (or to cope effectively with someone else's anger), seek professional help. Ask your doctor or a clergyman for a referral to a counselor or support group.

Key Point *Do not, under any circumstances, tolerate abusive anger.* You must say to yourself, "I deserve better than this." For immediate help, look in the telephone book under *Crisis Intervention Services* or *Social Service Agencies,* or call the *National Family Violence Hotline* at 1(800) 222-2000.

Remember, neutralizing your hostility and developing healthy alternatives takes considerable practice, but it can be done. You may have spent a lifetime practicing those ingrained, anger-producing, automatic thoughts and behaviors, so don't expect yourself to change overnight. With patience and persistence, you can become freed of the chronic anger and hostility that is so harmful to your health and happiness.

📖 *For more information, see page 276*

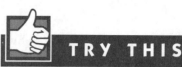

TRY THIS

OVERCOME PAST HURTS

This exercise can help you overcome the common tendency to relive old hurts. It may make you feel temporarily anxious or sad, but that's normal. It's well worth the effort to be freed of the hurt.

▶ Start by acknowledging the painful feelings you didn't fully express at the time. Remember the situations that provoked them. Then try completing this sentence: "I felt hurt when _____, and I am still hurt."

▶ You may need to share what you've learned with the person who provoked the pain, either face to face or in a letter. Even if you don't send the letter, writing out your feelings often reduces your anger and hurt (📖 see page 207).

14 Time Pressure

How to Manage Time and Deal with Procrastination

Mahatma Gandhi was once asked, "You have been working at least fifteen hours a day, every day, for fifty years. Don't you think it's about time you took a vacation?" To which Gandhi replied, "I am always on vacation."

We all have 24 hours in a day. Some of us feel like we have no time at all. Others manage to get their work done and still have lots of time to relax and enjoy themselves. They are people who have learned to structure their lives so that they focus most of their time and energy on what is most important to them, and minimize time spent on things they don't really value. The key is to discover what's really important for you to do and do those things well.

Kathleen is always running late, which stresses her and inconveniences others. From the moment she realizes that she has slept through the alarm to the moment she collapses into bed at night, she is in a constant struggle with time. Each day begins the same: "Where's the blouse that goes with this suit?" "There's no milk for cereal. Where did I put my keys?"

On the way to work she thinks, "Whew! I just made the bus. Oh, god,
poor Steve, he needs my report for his project and I haven't finished it yet. I hope he doesn't hold it against me. I hope the supervisor doesn't find out."

At work, Kathleen's desk is a disorganized mess. She can't find a letter she needs to respond to immediately. She's nervous and ill-prepared for a meeting, and a million little distractions prevent her from finishing the report for Steve. "I'll have to take it home with me."

She sees it's time to pick up her daughter at day care. She's relieved to hear that the fund-raising committee isn't meeting this week, but annoyed that she'll miss out on another evening with her family because she has to finish her work.

After finishing the report at midnight, Kathleen has just enough energy to look around her house. It's in dire need of cleaning. She wonders, "Where does the time go?"

Kathleen is not sick in the traditional sense, but she suffers from time stress. It undermines her well-being.

The world seems to be spinning faster and faster, and our newest "time-saving" devices—computers, faxes, pagers, car phones, and automated tellers—just seem to add pressure and pile on even more. We suffer from "time-poverty"; we all have too much to do, and not enough time to get it done. As the Queen said to Alice, "We're running as fast as we can to stay in place."

No wonder we're exhausted. According to a Harris survey, the average American had 37% less leisure time in 1990 than in 1973. This harrowing pace often leaves us with no time to savor or contemplate our experience before we rush on to the next task.

Life doesn't have to be so hurried. The way we break up time into units is arbitrary. In some cultures there is no word for minute or even hour. The shortest unit of time may be the time it takes for a certain food to cook.

We often make ourselves frantic. Most of the time we are too busy because we choose to be so. For some people,

> **Key Point**

being busy is a sign of importance and self-worth. For others, it gives their life a sense of meaning and purpose. Our "leisure" time is often crammed full of activities, commitments, and responsibilities. Even our children feel the pressure of a chock-full day: school, music lessons, soccer practice, and homework.

What Time Pressure Does to You

If you're reading this chapter, you're probably troubled in one way or another with time stress (📖 see box this page). This may be taking a toll on your health, and on the quality of your life. When you feel you're not accomplishing what you should be, your self-esteem plummets. If

you feel exhausted and overwhelmed all the time, you rob yourself of the satisfaction of a job well done.

There's no breather and no time to pat yourself on the back because the next task is right there in front of you. You can't fully enjoy anything because you're thinking about the end product—getting it done and over with—so you don't enjoy the process. Or you're thinking about something else you should be doing. Your personal relationships may suffer since you don't have time for real conversations and intimacy. As relationships help buffer you from stress and increase your resistance to disease, this is a serious loss.

The Toll of Time Stress

Because of the added tension and worry about getting things done, you can lose sleep, and sleep loss itself is related to many health problems (see page 192). When there's no time to relax and have fun, you can slip into bad habits—eating too much or too little, or relying on junk food or fast food for energy or comfort, or to save time. And a jam-packed schedule provides the perfect excuse to avoid healthy exercise, light up a cigarette, or turn to alcohol, caffeine, or pills to rev you up or calm you down. The most common excuse for not doing most of the simple, health-promoting things described in this book is "I don't have time."

Key Point *It sometimes takes a serious illness to awaken us to the fact that time is our most valuable asset.* Many of those who face a life-threatening illness say that they dramatically reorder their priorities. Fortunately, there are less drastic ways to change how we think about time, and how we spend our most precious resource.

The Experience of Time

"If you are sitting on a hot stove, a minute seems like an hour, but if you are doing something pleasurable, an hour can seem like a minute."
—*Albert Einstein*

Our sense of time is different from our other senses. As we don't have sensory receptors for time like we do for sight and sound, we can't experience time directly. Instead, our sense of time comes from how we interpret what happens to us. It can be relative, as Einstein observed.

Because our experience of time is largely created in our brains, it's not surprising that the way we think about time determines the way we experience it. We all know that sometimes time drags, and other times it moves swiftly. Whether time seems to drag or move swiftly reflects how we are dealing with the world. Time drags when there is too much or too little to do. On one hand, we sit around bored; on the other, we're overwhelmed with stuff to respond to. For many of us, our lives are a combination of boredom and blitz: it's always, "hurry up and wait."

But when the amount we have to do fits the time we have to do it, time glides by. During moments when we're truly connecting with others or driving on a twisty road or listening to favorite music, time seems to expand, and, in a sense, becomes almost timeless. When we have the right amount to do—so we don't feel overloaded or underloaded—time *flows* right along. The trick is to be, as Gandhi said, "on vacation" where nothing hurries us, but a lot happens.

Getting in Sync

It's not just the Gandhis of the world who can escape time pressure. Even in our speeded-up culture we can all think of someone who is relatively unbothered and unhurried. This person faces similar demands as we do, and may be as productive as others, but he or she appears unhassled and is somehow in sync with the flow of time.

So how can you get more in sync with the flow of time? There are a couple of ways. One is to listen to what efficiency experts on time management have to say. There are many around and that's where most people turn. Their techniques—better planning, making lists, using

Time pressure can cause great stress to the body. Rushing puts our bodies on perpetual combat alert. Our brain regards clocks, deadlines, and interrupted schedules as threats, and calls up the "fight or flight" stress response inappropriately. In tax accountants, for example, cholesterol levels skyrocket the weeks before the April 15th tax deadline.

Hurry Sickness and Hostility

This "hurry sickness"—along with hostility—were originally found to be components of Type A behavior among people prone to heart disease. But more recent evidence suggests that it is *the hostility alone*, not the time stress, that is related to a higher risk of heart disease.

Even if time stress does not increase the risk of heart disease directly, it has its own toxicity. It can easily erode the quality of people's lives and threaten their sense of well-being. The unending struggle to do more and more in less and less time increases our likelihood to respond with toxic anger to anyone or anything that slows us down.

Rushaholics

For some, time pressure is like an addiction. Rushaholics are dependent on hectic activity from the moment they wake up in much the same way that others need nicotine or caffeine to get them jump-started in the morning.

Stress stimulates hormones and neurochemicals such as adrenaline that keeps the body on full alert. When rushaholics try to relax, uncomfortable feelings and emotions surface, so they get busy again and stuff the feelings back down.

The 20% That Counts

An Italian economist, Vilfredo Pareto, described the "80-20 Principle: 20% of what we do yields 80% of the results." The key is to find out which 20% pays off, and let go of as much as possible of the rest. Doing so can make you both happier and healthier.

---

calendars and other tools—aim at maximizing productivity during every minute of the day. Time management techniques have been refined over the years, and have helped many people. The most effective suggestions are included later in this chapter, and we encourage you to try them.

Know What You Value

But we also want to encourage you to start thinking about time itself, and how you feel about it. This attitude is different from the cram-as-much-in-as-possible approach; it leads to feeling more relaxed. This second approach to time management emphasizes "The Big Picture": staying focused on what really matters to you. Rather than squeezing more activities into your day, you'll probably end up cutting things out.

This approach encourages you to continually evaluate what you're doing, and to ask the essential question: *Am I doing what I really need to be doing to have a satisfying and productive life?* If it isn't, it's likely to be a

Key Point

poor use of your time, no matter how well or efficiently you are getting it done.

Relaxing the Grip on Time

Trying to control time by strict scheduling is like trying to control what we eat by strict dieting. We become so obsessed with it that it becomes more—not less— important in our lives. If we relax our grip on time and not see it as the enemy that must be beaten into submission, it relaxes its grip on us. Still, there are situations in which time management tricks can help, and for most people, combining both approaches helps them lead less time-pressured lives.

How to Manage Your Time Effectively

The advice offered below begins with discovering what's really important in your life: your "Big Picture." We'll then go to strategies to help you manage the details so that you can accomplish your Big Picture goals in a more rewarding way.

THE BIG PICTURE

Recognize Your Top Priorities

We all have to do certain things, such as fulfilling our responsibilities to others. But if our time is to have meaning, it's *our own personal vision* that must take overall priority. Every few months—or at least once a year—it is essential to step back and consider what is most important to you (see box page 184).

Seek a Better Balance

Working long hours at a particularly stressful job may be necessary to pay the bills. But in many cases the motivation to overwork comes from a desire to achieve a better lifestyle or to prove one's self-worth. This may be the time to ask yourself if it's worth it.

Take a look at your life and see whether you'd lose or gain by buying and consuming less. Cutting back on work reduces income, but it can improve your standard of living in other ways. Two salaries rarely double the family income. The average two-paycheck family gains only 40% more than one with a single wage earner. And there are many other expenses when two people work, such as child care, eating out, commute expenses, home maintenance, and the like.

When people are surveyed about what is most important to them, they typically rank family life and a better society above having a nice home, car, or other belongings. They also say they wish they had more time to socialize with family and friends. Few say they want more time for work or watching TV. Almost no one on his or her death bed ever says, "I wish I had spent more time at work."

℞ Voluntary Simplicity

You can't do everything, be everything, or have everything. It's a myth that we get more out of life living it fast and cramming it full. Just the opposite seems to be true. Slowing down, streamlining, and uncluttering allows us to savor the moment, enjoy life more, and get more done. In the modern world, no one's life is going to be simple. But we can voluntarily choose to limit the things which unnecessarily complicate our lives.

The more things you want to buy, the more time you'll spend choosing, shopping, maintaining, mastering, using and earning money to pay for them. Even such "time savers" as answering machines, computers, and fax machines save less time than we think they do. They sometimes add to the complexity of our lives instead of simplifying them. How many people do you know who record a program on their VCR and then don't have time to watch it?

It may be difficult to say "no" to some things because life now presents us with so many possibilities. We have multiple options, roles, and identities. We want to be a good parent, hold down a full-time job, participate in neighborhood and community activities, take classes, go on trips, learn new skills, build new relationships, look for a better house, and cultivate sixteen hobbies. But what's the cost? In the end, it's not how much you've done or how many experiences you've collected that counts, but how well you have lived.

℞ Live in the Moment

We spend much of our time either thinking about the past or worrying about the future. In fact, there is no other moment in time other than the one that is happening *right now*. Time slips by when

CHECK YOURSELF

WAYS TO SET YOUR PRIORITIES

Imagine that you are at the end of your life. Reflect back over its course. As you look back, ask yourself:

❑ What did I enjoy doing most?

❑ What did I appreciate having most?

❑ What did I most value accomplishing?

❑ What do I wish I had done?

Or pretend that you have just learned that you have a rare, fatal disease that has no symptoms, but will kill you in six months.

Given only half a year to live, what do you want to accomplish? Experience? Have? What if you have five years to live—what are your priorities?

our minds are not paying attention to our present experience. When we are totally absorbed in what we are doing in the present, we fully appreciate that moment. It is an exhilarating experience, one that makes us feel truly alive, positive, and productive. It creates the "timeless" moments during which our tensions, fears, and pressures about time evaporate. This experience is sometimes called "flow state," or a state of "mindfulness."

To get to this state, you must break the rushing habit. Here are some things that might help:

- Try driving 5-10 mph slower
- Select the longest grocery checkout line (but not when everyone is waiting for dinner!), smile, and practice waiting patiently
- Try not wearing a watch
- Don't look at the clock for a day
- Allow yourself some time for transitions—to shift gears between activities: sit in the car for a few minutes before getting out; take a moment of silence before eating a meal; let the telephone ring several times before answering it
- Schedule some protected, free time
- Immerse yourself in a pleasurable sensory experience (see page 57), or practice some of the mindfulness relaxation techniques (page 94)
- Focus your full attention on whatever task is in front of you, whether it's washing dishes, commuting, talking with someone, or attending a meeting

℞ Establish Your Own Rhythm

Much of our time is spent according to society's schedule, which tells us when it's time to work, eat, sleep, and play. It is difficult to overcome these external pressures which preprogram and over-schedule our lives.

But occasionally, throughout the day, pay attention to your natural rhythms—your peaks and valleys of energy, alertness, concentration, and creativity. Some people prefer morning; others are night owls. Researchers have observed a tendency for us to get sleepy in the afternoon. They believe our body clocks are set to take a nap—or at least a rest—at midday.

Remember, not all days are created equal. Some days you marvel at how productive you are; others are more like swimming in molasses. Respect these differences. Don't blame yourself for not performing like a machine.

Vary the tempo of your life. Most people are not comfortable either when they are extremely busy or when they have too much time on their hands. Balance fast-paced intense activities with more relaxed ones. Until recently, human life consisted of alternating periods of harder and easier work, which usually depended on the season. It followed a natural, organic pattern. Now we work year round, except for a few paltry vacation weeks and days off throughout the year.

Take time out for fun, relaxation, daydreaming, contemplation, family, friends, and hobbies. Many "busy" people find this is not a waste of their time. It refreshes them and enables them to be more productive. Many of their best solutions and ideas come during these times off.

Some people benefit by taking a longer breather every once in a while—a month or a year to step back, get perspective, and take stock. With considerable planning and initiative, it may be possible to clear such valuable time.

MANAGING THE DETAILS

℞ Keep a Time Log

For many of us the days and weeks seem to be rushing by so fast that we don't really have a sense of how we are spending our time. One helpful exercise is to keep a time log for one day or more. Each hour of the day while you're awake, take a few seconds to record the activities you do and how much time you spent on each. It helps to have an alarm watch to remind you to

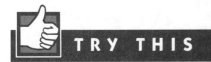
SET YOUR GOALS

Write down some short, medium, and long-term goals.

▶ Which of them are you willing to commit a lot of time and effort to?

▶ Which ones are realistic and achievable if you plan them carefully, and give them the right amount of effort?

Setting these goals will help you to determine how you spend your time. They should influence your daily decisions on how to invest your time and energy. Reassess and revise these goals periodically.

make an entry in the log each hour.

Then review each entry and add up the amount of time you spent in various categories of activities. Include things like work (including paperwork), telephone calls, meetings, and socializing along with non-work activities such as eating, cooking, personal hygiene, shopping, commuting, running errands, watching television, hobbies, exercise, reading, and managing child care. Create a list of categories that make sense to you.

Now review your list and time estimates. Any surprises? Do the investments of your time reflect your highest priorities and goals? What's missing? What things are taking up too much time for their yield? What items can be eliminated or reduced without compromising your priorities and goals?

℞ Set Your Priorities

Keep a notebook with a running list of things that require action (things to do, errands, etc.) without regard for deadlines or importance. Then evaluate the importance of the items listed in terms of your overall goals. Sometimes you'll have to set priorities not only for your own individual goals, but also for goals shared by your family or work group.

Some time management systems suggest you use numbers: #1 for the highest level priority, #2 for middle, and #3 for low. Others assign letters such as A, B, and C, or use colors to distinguish priorities. As you look at each entry, ask such questions as:

▶ *What would happen if I didn't do this?*

▶ *Is this task worth the investment of my time?*

▶ *Do I need to do this, or could someone else do it?*

℞ Divide and Conquer

Break complex tasks into smaller, more manageable steps, and then organize the steps into the best order to do them in. Set a realistic target date or time span for the completion of each task, and for its intermediary steps. Add about 25% to your first time estimate to give yourself a buffer for success. Sometimes it's easiest to determine the last step first and establish its deadline; then work backward, step by step, to the present. This way tasks seem less formidable, and you can work on them a little at a time, according to a plan. The most achievable goals are those that are moderately demanding, realistic, measurable, flexible, *and written down*.

℞ Make a "To Do" List

Translate individual steps and actions from your list of priorities to a daily, weekly, or monthly organizer. This way you can do them on a planned schedule. Cross them off as you complete them. Most of these activities should relate to your highest priority goals and projects.

Don't forget to build in some time for interruptions, unscheduled events, and unforeseen problems. Without some slack you're likely to get frustrated by not achieving your goal on time. In the movie, "Broadcast News," the Holly Hunter character was so super-organized that she scheduled a specific time slot to express her emotions and have a good cry. Few time management experts would recommend you go this far. "Make every minute count, but don't count every minute" is a good rule to live by.

No matter how organized you are or how well you've planned your day, sometimes things just don't go right. Or they don't go as expected. Be flexible. This enables you to respond to the moment, and take advantage of a spontaneous turn of events. Being flexible also allows you to use your intuitive sense for when to charge ahead and when to back off. Don't let schedules, clocks, and pre-arranged plans overrun your inner sensibilities.

Key Point

℞ Evaluate Your Progress

After about one month of priority setting and making "to do" lists, ask yourself:

❏ *Am I accomplishing more?*

❏ *Am I more effective?*

❏ *Do I feel more in control?*

❏ *Am I making progress towards the really important things in my life?*

❏ *Am I happier?*

Check to make sure you're spending most of your time on high-priority items. If you're doing too many low priority ones, you are wasting your time. Ask yourself why you are doing these low priority tasks. If things are taking longer than you expected, you need to come up with a more realistic schedule.

Remember, the goal of time management is not the elimination of relaxation time. It is to get rid of the real time wasters in your life, and reduce your struggle with time.

Key Point

℞ Combine Tasks

Instead of running a million little errands throughout the day, consolidate them. Here are some possibilities:

▶ When you go grocery shopping, drop off the camera at the repair shop on the same trip, or do other errands at the same end of town

▶ Instead of taking the car, get some fresh air and exercise by walking or biking if the distance is not too great (often you'll get there just as fast and you'll save time at the gym)

▶ Combine activities such as talking with someone while going for a walk or peeling apples while watching the news

▶ Keep a list of short, five-minute tasks to do while you are waiting or "between things"—sew on a button, polish your shoes, empty the dishwasher, or water a plant

▶ Think of waiting as a gift of time: to relax, read, write letters, or make notes

"Never do today what you can put off till tomorrow."

— **Mo Lasses**

Unless it has an adverse effect on you or someone else, there's nothing intrinsically wrong with procrastination (putting something off until later). In fact, sometimes you're better off doing some things later rather than sooner. By delaying, low-priority items may fall completely by the wayside, and no one notices or cares.

But other times you may procrastinate about important things which do need to be taken care of. Then the "undone" takes on mountainous proportions, contributes to your stress level, frustration, and embarrassment. It stands in the way of your success.

Procrastination can also undermine your health if you put off doing things to promote or protect it—like quitting smoking, starting to exercise, buying a fire extinguisher, fixing an unsafe staircase, getting marriage counseling, completing a living will, or getting medical durable power of attorney. Procrastination can also rob you of well-deserved, guilt-free vacation or valuable relaxation time.

Procrastination itself is a time and energy-waster. So why, if we are so short of time and energy, do we procrastinate? One reason is that we set impossibly high standards for ourselves. Thinking we must decorate a room perfectly, write a flawless book, or thoroughly master a new software program, we never begin for fear of failure.

Another reason we procrastinate is because the task is unpleasant. No one enjoys firing or reprimanding an employee, and so it gets put off as long as possible. Or a task may seem too overwhelming (your current filing system may not be working, for example, but it seems like too big a task to take on).

Procrastination is one method of coping. It may temporarily lessen the tension of facing a challenging or unpleasant project, or the risk of failing. But there are often more effective ways of coping and facing life's challenges.

Ultimately, when you're dealing with procrastination, the only thing that really works is to take the bull by the horns. Fortunately, we provide ways to tame the "mañana" monster. Don't put off trying some of these suggestions!

℞ Organize Your Space

Overwhelmed by clutter? Here are ways to clear some space:

❑ Purge your surroundings of unnecessary paper

❑ Get rid of things you "might need someday," "should read," or are hanging on to for no good reason

❑ Arrange the things you keep in a more orderly fashion to help you find them faster

❑ Establish a workable filing system so you know where papers go

❑ Handle each piece of paper as few times as possible

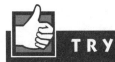

COST-BENEFIT ANALYSIS

Think of some task that you have been putting off. Make a quick list of the pros and cons of postponing this specific task. Add up the advantages and disadvantages, and decide whether to do it now, postpone it, or never do it.

Even though doing the task now may be unpleasant, consider the cost in anxiety of putting it off. Some tasks are just plain not very important. Procrastination—or not doing something at all—may make the most sense.

Think about what you'll get out of procrastination. For example, finishing your education might mean facing the difficulties of finding a job. Or leaving your current job may mean dealing with fears of inadequacy. Try to be aware of any underlying issues so the choices you make can be made consciously.

❏ Scan all your mail once and throw away as much as you can

❏ Re-evaluate your magazine subscriptions

There are many good books and professional services to help you do a "get-organized makeover" (see page 276).

℞ Let It Ring

Try to arrange your environment to minimize interruptions. If you are involved in a task, ask yourself whether you need to answer the telephone every time it rings. Make clear requests to co-workers, family members, and friends to respect your time, and thank them when they do.

℞ Change Your Negative Thoughts

If you find yourself criticizing and worrying yourself with such thoughts as "I'm never getting anything done," or "I'm wasting all of my time," or "There's never enough time," challenge these thoughts (see page 42). You can substitute kinder, gentler ones such as, "At any given moment I am doing as much as I can," or "I accomplish the most when I fully concentrate on what I am doing," or "In truth, I've accomplished a lot."

Don't let negative thinking undermine you. Observe your thought pattern as you approach (or avoid) a task. For example, if you catch yourself thinking things like:

▶ *I do not feel like doing this*

▶ *I'll never get that project done*

▶ *I'm not capable of doing so complex a job*

▶ *I always miss deadlines anyway*

▶ *I don't have the energy to do this*

Try substituting more enabling thoughts:

▶ *I don't have to be in the mood to get started*

▶ *Once I get started I'll probably feel more like doing it*

▶ *I will only work on this for 10 minutes*

▶ *If I do a little each day, I'll be able to finish the job*

▶ *I don't need to feel fully capable; I'll learn more about the project as I do it*

▶ *I will feel much better when it is done*

14 Time Pressure

189

℞ Encourage Yourself

Key Point

Usually, doing a "good enough" job is all that's required. Doing something is better than not doing anything at all. If fear of failure has you paralyzed, be compassionate toward your imperfections by using positive self-talk. For example, tell yourself:

- ▶ *Even if I fail, I'll survive*
- ▶ *If I don't do a perfect job, that doesn't make me a bad person*
- ▶ *No one is perfect*
- ▶ *I'll do the best I can*

℞ Ask for Help

Because procrastinators tend to be perfectionists, they feel they must do every aspect of a task themselves. Don't fall into this trap. It is not a sign of failure or incompetence to ask for help; it's a sign of intelligence and good management. Assign tasks you don't have to do to others. It will free you up to concentrate on the more important ones, and gets the job done better. Just be careful not to sabotage yourself. Choose the right people to help.

℞ Take a Break

When you run into an obstacle while working on a task, it's tempting to get frustrated and abandon hope. Avoid this scenario by taking some time out. Tell yourself it's just a temporary setback, and that you are not stupid, incompetent, or bound to fail. Set a specific time to come back to the snag with a fresh eye. Perhaps

you can work on another part of the task in the meantime.

℞ Create Small Steps for Success

Reduce the weight of an overwhelming task by breaking it up into smaller pieces, and focus on completing one step at a time. Reward yourself when you have completed each part.

This may be more difficult than it sounds. Procrastinators are usually better at berating themselves for failures than patting themselves on the back for succeeding.

℞ Use Your Imagination

Before you begin working on something, visualize yourself going through the steps, making progress, and completing the task. Using this kind of mental imagery prepares you for the actual activity, and helps you make the transition from thinking about it to doing it (📖 see page 99).

℞ Just Do It

Sometimes the best cure for procrastination is to just do the task. Don't think about it. Don't wait until you feel like it. Break the cycle of anxiety. Things are often not as unpleasant as you anticipate, and once you get started, the momentum gets you through.

📖 *For more information, see page 276*

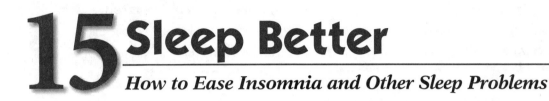

15 Sleep Better

How to Ease Insomnia and Other Sleep Problems

"Sleep...it is meat for the hungry, drink for the thirsty, heat for the cold, and cold for the hot...."

Don Quixote —*Cervantes*

Do you have trouble falling asleep? Do you lie awake tossing and turning for hours, shifting restlessly from one position to another, desperately trying to sleep? Do you wake up frequently during the night and lie restlessly for hours hoping that you'll fall back to sleep? And in the morning do you feel exhausted, irritable, and bleary-eyed?

If all this sounds familiar, you're not alone. Almost everyone has occasional sleepless nights. These restless nights often come during times of stress, illness, or along with a traumatic life experience. But about one-third of adults report chronic sleep trouble. For over 40 million Americans, the nightly ritual of drifting off to sleep is a nightmare.

Insomnia, sleep deprivation, and daytime sleepiness are so common that many of us accept them as part of normal life. We gulp down the coffee and cola during the day to stay awake.

As a population, we've reduced our average sleep time over the past century by more than 20%—that's nearly two hours less sleep each night. These days students stay up cramming; women work all day and do housework into the night; night-shift workers take part-time day jobs. None of these activities fit into the natural work cycle from sunrise to sunset, and there's little evidence that we require any less sleep than our ancestors did. Ironically, the pursuit of "The American Dream" leaves many of us without enough time for real dreaming.

How Much Sleep Do You Need?

This varies from person to person. Most people do best with seven and a half hours. Some feel refreshed with just six, but others need eight to ten to function well. Some of us conk out when we hit the pillow and are oblivious until the alarm goes off. Others take half an hour to fall asleep and wake up several times during the night. *What counts is how you feel, not how many hours of sleep you've had. If you are alert, feel rested, and function well during the day, chances are you're getting enough sleep.*

Key Point

Healthy Sleep

Sleep is a basic human need, like food and water. Getting less sleep one night is not a big problem. Most of us can adapt quite well to an occasional shortened night of sleep. Aside from feeling sleepy and perhaps a little irritable, our ability to function is usually not significantly impaired. But if you get less sleep than you require night after night, your quality of life and mood may suffer considerably.

Chronic Sleep Problems

There are three kinds of sleep problems:

1. **Sleep-onset insomnia**. Difficulty falling asleep within thirty minutes

2. **Sleep-maintenance insomnia.** Difficulty staying asleep

3. **Poor quality of sleep.** Loss of the deeper, more restful sleep

Any of these sleep problems can result in:

▶ Daytime sleepiness

▶ Impaired memory

▶ Difficulty in concentrating

▶ Depression

▶ Slow thinking

▶ Irritability or erratic behavior

▶ Poor health

When healthy sleep is restored, these symptoms may lessen dramatically.

With chronic insomnia, family and social life can suffer. Problem sleepers have twice the number of auto accidents. Sleep-deprived people are more likely to report poor health and diminished work performance. Night shift workers (some 40% to 80% of whom have difficulty sleeping) suffer more gastrointestinal and heart disorders, and have more marital problems.

Continued on next page

℞ How to Sleep Better

The self-help techniques we offer here are clinically proven with a 75% to 80% success rate. They are not "quick fixes" like sleep medications, but they'll give you more effective (and safer) results in the long run. In trying these methods, it's really important not to give up after just one or two nights. Allow yourself at least two to four weeks to see some positive results, and ten to twelve weeks for significant, long-term improvement. Each morning after awakening, record your progress on the One-Minute Sleep Log (see page 200).

One study showed that people who slept fewer than six hours each night had a 30% higher death rate (from cancer, heart disease, stroke, and all other causes) than those sleeping seven or eight hours a night. Whether the increased risk is due to sleep deprivation or other causes isn't clear.

Sleep is also connected to immune function. The same chemicals that trigger sleep also stimulate the cells of our immune system—the body's defense against infections. Even partial sleep deprivation can drop immune function. However, whether such changes in immune function increase our risk of illness is not known.

Sleep Apnea

One sleep disorder clearly associated with health problems is *sleep apnea*. It is characterized by:

▶ Stopped breathing during sleep for periods of up to several minutes

▶ Snoring

▶ Frequent awakenings and fragmented sleep

▶ Daytime sleepiness

People with sleep apnea have an increased risk of high blood pressure, coronary heart disease, stroke, and impaired mental and emotional functioning.

Just reading about the hazards of sleep loss is enough to keep anyone awake. However, sleep loss often gets blamed for many problems and symptoms that are due to other causes. *But there is good news: most people tolerate occasional sleep loss and disruption with surprisingly few ill health effects. And most can learn to sleep better without medications by using the proven, effective methods described in this chapter.*

Key Point

℞ Think Well about Sleep

The first step to getting a good night's sleep is to correct any misconceptions you might have about sleep. Here are some common myths, followed by the truth:

MYTH: *"If at first you don't succeed, try, try again."*
Not true when it comes to sleep. In fact, the harder you try to fall asleep, the more likely you'll stay awake.

MYTH: *"I didn't sleep a wink last night."*
It's unlikely you got no sleep at all. Even during the roughest nights, most people with insomnia manage to get several hours of sleep. We tend to *overestimate* the time it takes us to fall asleep and *underestimate* how much sleep we've gotten.

MYTH: *"If I don't get to sleep right now, I'll be a total wreck tomorrow."*
For most tasks, one sleepless night will not affect your performance very much unless your job is crucial or dangerous. Don't worry. When you sleep poorly, the best thing to do is go about your business the next day without focusing on last night's sleep loss. You will be able to function the next day, even though it may seem hard to believe that as you toss and turn at 3:00 a.m. the night before.

GETTING OFF SLEEPING PILLS

If you are regularly using sleeping medications, you may need to slowly reduce their use under the supervision of a physician. Here are some tips:

▶ Start by reducing the dose of the sleep medicine by half of your usual dose. For the first week, do this on *only one night* of the week.

▶ The second week, reduce the dose by half on a second night of the week. Space these nights apart.

▶ Continue to reduce your dosage by half for *one additional night* a week until you are taking half your original dose every night.

▶ Next, for one night of the week, reduce the dose of the medicine to one-quarter of your beginning dose. Continue to reduce the dose gradually until you are down to one-quarter every night of the week.

▶ Finally, choose *one night* to go without the sleep medication. Gradually extend the "no-meds" nights until you stop the medication completely, or until you use the reduced dose only twice a week or less.

▶ During your tapering-off period, use some of the other self-help advice in this chapter for restoring natural sleep.

Remember, even if you don't sleep well on medication-reduction nights, you will still be able to function the next day.

Compare, for example, your attitude toward *voluntary* sleep loss due to late-night socializing or travel with sleep loss due to a night of not being able to sleep. Both experiences result in lost sleep, but the night of insomnia is accompanied by both anxiety and frustration. *It's the frustration more than the actual sleep loss that accounts for the irritable mood the next day. Remember, sleep on any particular night is not really that important. Don't let the fear of insomnia keep you awake.*

> **Key Point**

℞ Let Sleeping Pills Lie

Sleeping pills may be good for short-term, temporary treatment. They are not the solution for chronic sleep problems. In fact, most sleep medications lose their effectiveness after several weeks or months of use. Ultimately, sleeping pills may have a reverse effect, causing "rebound insomnia." Then when you stop taking them, your problem is worse. In addition, sleeping pills may interfere with the deepest, most restorative stages of sleep. And they may give you a hangover, so you actually feel worse the next day. If you are dependent on these medications now to fall asleep, you may need professional help to stop them (📖 see box this page).

℞ Skip the Stimulants

Caffeine. Problem sleepers should avoid caffeine for six to eight hours before bedtime, especially if you are particularly sensitive to it. Watch your intake of coffee, tea, chocolate, soft drinks, and caffeine-containing medications. Look for caffeine on the labels.

Medications. Some mediations can be the cause of restlessness and sleeplessness.

These include certain decongestants, anti-depressants, asthma medications, beta blockers, steroids, thyroid medications, diet pills, and amphetamines. Learn to read labels. Review all medications with your physician or pharmacist, or look them up yourself in a drug handbook.

Alcohol. While a nightcap may make you drowsy, alcohol can also disrupt the soundness of your sleep. You may wake up frequently, especially if you drink within several hours of bedtime.

Nicotine. Smokers often find it more difficult to fall asleep, and they wake up more during the night than nonsmokers. This may be because they are experiencing nicotine withdrawal. So there's another good reason to quit.

Food and Drink. Avoid heavy meals right before bedtime, but a light carbohydrate snack such as cookies, pasta, toast or bread may actually help you sleep. Carbo-hydrates increase brain serotonin, a chemical that helps trigger sleep. Also try to decrease the amount of fluid you drink in the hours before bedtime. This will reduce your chances of waking up to the "full bladder alarm."

℞ Go for Timely Exercise

A good, well-timed workout can help you feel and sleep better. Physically fit people usually fall asleep easily and sleep soundly. Exercise may help change brain chemistry and relieve the depression and anxiety that interferes with good sleep (📖 see page 112).

People with insomnia tend to be less active during the day. This may disrupt the normal rhythmic changes in body temperature that trigger sleep. Your body temperature normally peaks in the mid-afternoon, and bottoms out around 4 to 5 a.m. If your

TRY THIS

HEAT HELPS SLEEP

To sleep better, try exercising in the late afternoon or early evening five to six hours before bedtime. This will give your body temperature time to cool down by bedtime. If, for example, you want to go to bed at 11 p.m., try to exercise between five and six in the evening.

You don't need to exercise to exhaustion, but the activity has to be vigorous enough to raise your body temperature. And it should make you sweat a little.

Relaxing for 20 minutes in a hot bath or a sauna will also stimulate a later cool-down. Enjoying one of these activities several hours before bedtime will also help you sleep better.

nighttime temperature doesn't drop, you could get disrupted, fragmented sleep. Exercise causes a rise in body temperature, followed by a sleep-inducing drop hours later (📖 see box this page).

℞ Set the Stage: Cool and Quiet

A comfortable bed and a dark, quiet room that's cool (one that's between 65 and 70 degrees) also aids sleep. The quiet hum of a fan, the soothing sound of a "nature" tape (like waves lapping the shore), or earplugs can do wonders to block out distracting sounds. And get rid of anxiety-creating clocks! If you need to set an alarm, put the clock under the bed or face it away from you. Then forget the clock until the alarm rings.

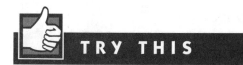
SET A "WORRY TIME"

Does a racing mind keep you awake? If it does:

▶ Designate a "worry time"

▶ Do so well before bedtime

▶ During your "worry time" write down your problems and concerns

▶ Make a to-do list to get them off your mind

Then you can relax and sleep well at night, knowing you can worry again at tomorrow's "worry time" (📖 see page 150).

℞ Get Ready for Bed

Research shows that after a stimulating day (shopping, seeing a movie, visiting a new place) people fall asleep faster and sleep more soundly than after a boring, uneventful day. On the other hand, you can't run around all day and expect to fall fast asleep within minutes of hitting the pillow. Most of us need to wind down and ease into sleep.

Many successful sleepers have established relaxing bedtime routines. They may watch television, read, write in a diary or do some soothing needlework before slipping off to sleep.

Find some quiet, relaxing activity that prepares you for sleep. You might, for example, start by practicing a relaxation exercise. Try muscle relaxation (📖 see page 92), or meditation (page 96), or imagery (page 99) as a way to calm down and prepare yourself for sleep.

If a racing mind is what keeps you

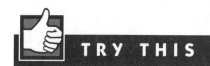
TAKE A NAP

What did Winston Churchill, John F. Kennedy, and Lyndon Johnson have in common?

Answer: They all thoroughly enjoyed (and benefited from) frequent naps.

Unfortunately, napping is becoming a lost art in the modern workday, even though our biological rhythms are programmed for a midday rest. An afternoon snooze consists mostly of the deepest, most restful stage of sleep. Studies show that a brief nap can restore energy levels, calm irritable moods, and leave you clear-headed and productive.

And naps may decrease certain health risks. A Greek study compared hospitalized patients who regularly took a siesta with those who went napless. Those who took naps had a 30% to 50% decrease in their risk of heart attack.

So if you can arrange a nap to coincide with your afternoon slump, you'll likely be healthier and happier. Try to limit your snooze to less than an hour. Longer sleep moves you into a state from which it's harder to wake up. But caution: if you are having problems sleeping at night, you may wish to skip daytime naps.

awake, designate a "worry time" well before bedtime. Write down your problems, worries, and a to-do list to get them off your mind (📖 see box this page).

YOUR BEST SLEEP SCHEDULE

To find the amount of sleep that's right for you, follow these steps:

▶ Use your Sleep Log (📖 see page 200) to calculate your average amount of nighttime sleep (the time you're really asleep, *not* the hours you lie in bed).

▶ Plan to stay in bed only the length of your average sleep time.

▶ Choose a regular wake-up time. No matter what time you go to bed, get up at the *same* time each morning, even on weekends or vacations. This regularity is crucial to establishing a natural sleep rhythm.

▶ Choose a regular bedtime based on your estimate of your average sleep time. For example, if your regular wake-up time is 6:00 a.m. and you estimate you average six hours of actual sleep, then go to bed at midnight. Do not go to bed any earlier.

▶ Stay up until your calculated bedtime, even if you're tired. You may need to distract yourself with stimulating activities—anything to keep you active and ward off sleep. Think of it as extra free time, not lost sleep.

▶ At first, your body may complain because you are not used to spending less time in bed. But stick to your new schedule for several weeks. Don't be discouraged if you are sleepy during the day. This sleepiness will help you sleep better at night.

▶ If you are still not falling asleep sooner and sleeping more soundly, then reduce your time in bed by an additional 30 minutes. Go to bed 30 minutes later but get up at your regular wake-up time. You may need even less sleep than you thought. This may sound crazy, but it works!

▶ After several weeks you may find that you are falling asleep more easily and sleeping more soundly, but you're still tired during the day. Now's the time to experiment by going to sleep 15 to 30 minutes earlier, until you find the amount of sleep that's right for you. But cut back again if you are not sleeping well.

Remember, the more you cut down on your time in bed, the more soundly you'll sleep. And you can enjoy the extra time being awake and productive.

Key Point

℞ Spend Less Time in Bed

Key Point

It may sound paradoxical, but if you spend less time in bed, your sleep may improve. You will fall asleep more easily, sleep more deeply, and experience fewer nighttime wakings. Many insomnia sufferers believe that they need to spend extra time in bed to make up for poor sleep. But going to bed earlier or sleeping in late results in less deep, restorative sleep.

For example, if you really need seven hours of sleep but try to spread it out over eight or nine, you'll spend several hours of stressful, frustrating awake time as you struggle to get sleep you don't need. In addition, your sleep becomes shallower and less refreshing.

The next day you feel tired and think you need even more sleep to "catch-up." But you really don't. Restricting your time

Use Your Bed Only for Sleep

Some people can sleep anywhere except their own bedroom—on the couch, in a hotel, or even a sleep laboratory! Perhaps you associate your bed or bedroom with just about everything but restful sleep and relaxation.

For many, the bedroom has become an activity center: a place for paying bills, talking on the phone, completing work assignments, planning tomorrow's activities, family arguments, worrying, and other activities incompatible with sleepiness. The very thought of your own bed may trigger frustration or anxious memories of sleepless nights.

Relearning How to Sleep

One effective strategy for reversing this attitude toward your bed is called "stimulus control." The idea is simple: over

time, *you learn to associate your bed solely with relaxation and restful sleep.* Here is how to use this technique:

Key Point

▶ Use your bedroom only for relaxing, pleasurable activities, and sleep.

▶ Make anything stressful off limits.

▶ Do not use your bedroom for arguments, eating, worrying, talking on the phone, or other rousing activities (with the exception of enjoyable, relaxing sex).

▶ Relax in bed for 10 to 15 minutes with a calming activity like reading, listening to music, watching television, doing needlework, or a relaxation exercise.

▶ Avoid stimulating TV programs or reading material. This is not the time for an engaging mystery or an exciting page-turner novel.

Continued on next page

in bed results in a deeper, more restful sleep. You also get extra free time (📖 see box page 197).

℞ Reset Your Internal Clock

Each of us has an internal clock. It controls our natural body rhythms, including when we sleep and when we wake. Some people are more alert at night than others (the so-called "owls"), while some naturally wake up early (the "larks").

Many people find that their daily schedule is out of sync with their natural rhythms. If you have trouble falling asleep and getting up on time, try to reset your in-

ternal clock with *phototherapy*. Here's how:

Every morning for a week, expose yourself to an hour of morning sunlight. Or strong artificial light (at least 2,500 lux—that's four shop lights with two 4-foot fluorescent tubes each, or a commercially available light box with eight fluorescent tubes). Sit about 3 feet away from the light source. After about a week of morning phototherapy, you should find it easier to fall asleep at night, and wake up more easily in the morning. Consult a professional experienced in phototherapy (📖 see page 277).

▶ Turn off the lights only when you feel very drowsy. If you are not asleep within 15 to 20 minutes (estimate the time, don't watch the clock), go back to a relaxing activity until you are drowsy again.

Caution: Don't force yourself to sleep (the harder you try to sleep, the longer you'll stay awake). Don't frustrate yourself by trying to sleep when you're not ready. Instead, do a relaxing activity. If you have to repeat it more than three or four times, you're going to bed too early.

▶ If you're wide awake and your mind is very active, leave your bedroom. Go do something relaxing until you feel drowsy. Leave as often as necessary.

▶ If you wake up in the middle of the night, use the same suggestions that are described above.

Important: No matter how much you sleep or how often you get up during the night, get up each morning at the same time. A consistent get-up time helps your body develop a regular sleep rhythm. Resist the temptation to sleep in late on weekends.

Even if you feel more tired and worse at first, follow the above advice faithfully for at least three weeks. Remember, even if you don't sleep, just relaxing, reading, or watching television is more restful than tossing and turning. Keep this basic strategy in mind:

▶ Don't go to bed until you are really drowsy.

▶ Don't try to force yourself to sleep.

▶ Distract yourself with relaxing activities until you are drowsy and ready to sleep.

Key Point

℞ Get Professional Help

The majority of sleep problems can be solved with the techniques mentioned above. But there are times when you need professional assistance. Get help:

▶ If your insomnia persists for six months or is seriously affecting your daytime functioning (your job or your social relationships), despite faithfully following the self-help program described here

▶ If you have great difficulty staying awake during the day, especially if your daytime sleepiness causes or comes close to causing an accident

▶ If your sleep is disturbed by breathing difficulties including loud snoring with long pauses, chest pain, heartburn, leg twitching, excessive pain, or other physical conditions

▶ If your difficulty sleeping is accompanied by depression, problems with alcohol, sleeping medications, or addictive drugs

If you have any of these problems, consult a physician who can help you or refer you to a sleep specialist or clinic. Don't put it off. Most sleep problems can be solved. Without them you'll enjoy a better night's sleep and better health.

ONE-MINUTE SLEEP LOG

▶ Date _____

▶ What time did you first turn out the lights to sleep? _____

▶ About how long did it take you to fall asleep? _____

▶ About how many times, if any, did you awaken during the night? _____

▶ Overall, how many hours did you actually sleep last night? _____

▶ What time did you wake up for the last time this morning? _____

▶ How well did you sleep last night? (circle)

    Terrible night   1   2   3   4   5   *Great night*

▶ How rested did you feel this morning? (circle)

    Not at all rested   1   2   3   4   5   *Very well rested*

▶ How would you rate your overall mood and functioning during the day? (circle)

    Poor   1   2   3   4   5   *Very good*

Other comments:

▶ Naps _____

▶ Sleeping medications _____

▶ Caffeine _____

▶ Alcohol _____

▶ Exercise _____

▶ Stress _____

📖 *For more information, see page 277*

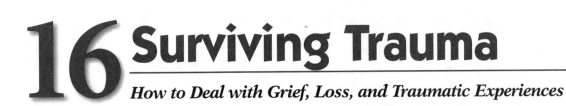

16 Surviving Trauma

How to Deal with Grief, Loss, and Traumatic Experiences

Every life has its ups and downs—ordinary stresses woven almost unnoticeably into our daily lives. But a major trauma—death, divorce, violent crime, life-threatening illness, natural disaster, job loss, infertility, or major betrayal—can tear a hole in our world. The emotional fallout can jolt our mental and physical health for years.

Traumas usually follow from loss. And any loss—even the loss of an object—can disrupt our sense of self, identity, and permanence. We easily recognize some losses like that of a loved one, of health, of possessions, or of affection. Some losses are more subtle, such as loss of an ideal, or one's sense of purpose, goals, hopes, or plans.

A natural disaster like an earthquake can shake our basic belief that life is predictable, controllable, and fair. A burglary can rob us of more than possessions. It takes away our view of the world as a safe place. A serious illness can undermine the illusion of our own immortality. The most common reaction among victims of rape, illness, or other tragedies is a disturbing feeling of loss of control. This can lead to depression and loss of self-esteem. Victims may also feel that the world is a dangerous place, and that they are likely to be victims again.

Even positive experiences can be traumatic. Although a promotion can bring prestige and a bigger paycheck, it may also mean the pain and separation from old friends and the stresses of moving to a new city. Having a new baby brings joy and fulfillment, and it can also mean good-bye to sleep, freedom, and sometimes, even marital harmony.

Rebounding from Trauma

Why do some people rebound quickly from the most serious traumas, while others have ongoing difficulties after even relatively minor losses? *How the event is experienced and how a person comes to terms with it is more important than the event itself.* Many factors can shape your response to trauma:

Key Point

▶ How well you have coped in the past

▶ Your sense of control and self-esteem

▶ The strength of your social support

▶ The nature of the loss (whether it was sudden or expected, common or extraordinary)

▶ Personal, cultural, and religious beliefs

Even how society views the trauma can affect your ability to cope with it. For example, people dealing with suicides, AIDS,

Many researchers note the relationship between traumatic events and health risk. After bereavement there's an increase in deaths from all causes— especially heart disease and suicide. And there are also higher rates of cancer, colitis, rheumatoid arthritis, asthma, anxiety, and depression. Several studies of traumatic losses have also found a decrease in immune function.

Physical and emotional symptoms may also be present:

- Heart palpitations
- Chest pain
- Headaches
- Dizziness
- Ringing in the ears
- Loss of appetite
- Indigestion
- Nausea
- Difficulty swallowing
- Tightness in the throat
- Muscular pain
- Damp hands
- Dry mouth
- Insomnia
- Inability to concentrate
- Irritability
- Fear of intimacy

Bereaved persons may also change their behavior. They may drink more, exercise less, and eat less healthfully. All of these can undermine health.

The ill health effects are reduced for those who maintain close supportive relationships. One study examined the health of the surviving spouse after the other had committed suicide or died in a car accident. These three important findings emerged:

1. The more people talked about the death, the fewer health problems they had during the year following.

2. The more time they spent talking, the less time they spent thinking about it.

3. The less time they spent thinking about it, the fewer health problems they had.

abortion, and rape often get less support from others than they would for more "acceptable" traumatic experiences.

People who withstand stress more successfully do so, in part, because they believe they have some control. They view change as a challenge, not just as a threat. Even when a traumatic event shatters their illusion of control, they work to regain it. They think about how much worse the situation could have been. They com-pare their case with others who are even less fortunate. They make changes in their lives that confirm they have control over some things.

People who focus all their energies on one relationship, one role, one identity, or one set of skills become more vulnerable when trauma strikes. People who lose their only friend or close confidant are more susceptible to problems than people who have cultivated several and varied

POST-TRAUMATIC STRESS DISORDER

Many people rebound fairly quickly from trauma. They seek new relationships, a new job, go to a new country, or find a new reason for living. For others, trauma leads to ongoing disturbing symptoms called *post-traumatic stress disorder.* They include:

▶ Reliving or re-experiencing the traumatic event in flashbacks, nightmares, or daydreams

▶ Avoidance or numbness. This may include detachment and distancing from others, avoidance of anything associated with the trauma, and loss of interest in the future

▶ Increased anxiety with difficulty concentrating, outbursts of anger, sleep problems, and an exaggerated stress response

close personal relationships. People who invest their entire identity in their work, for example, are at greater risk if they lose their job or become disabled.

Perhaps one of the best hedges against a devastating loss is to have "multiple investments"—in work, hobbies, and relationships. We have a great range of abilities and talents within us. The more we use them, the hardier we are.

The Value of Separate Identities

Most of us like to think of ourselves as one unified person: we're the same when we are at work, meeting with our children's teachers, talking with friends or taking a class. But in fact, we are a collection of multiple selves. And the more developed and distinct each of these selves is, the less vulnerable we are to stress.

Each of our selves acts to absorb the hard times in life. They help us laugh when work isn't going well, and to maintain some good feelings, even for a moment's relief, when a loved one dies. It's healthier not to put all our eggs in one basket.

Marcia is an attorney going through a divorce. Her personal and professional worlds are closely linked. She met her husband at law school, and they share the same circle of acquaintances in their private and work lives.

When the divorce hit, it shattered Marcia's world. It eroded her sense of confidence. Her self-doubt, anger, and sadness spilled over to cloud both her personal and professional life. There was nowhere for her to retreat for solace. She'd put everything in one basket.

In contrast, Cecilia has developed separate identities as wife, teacher, mother, and friend. When she faced a divorce her sense of confidence was not completely devastated, and she could enjoy other parts of her life. She could still enjoy conversations with friends, and relish intimate moments nurturing her baby.

People who are complex, diverse, and have many sides that reach out in different directions suffer fewer signs of life stresses. They report less depression, bad moods, colds, coughs, stomach pains, headaches, and muscle aches than less complex and diversified people.

The more you develop different aspects of your selves, the more resilient you are. Nurturing variety in

Key Point

GRIEF

yourself makes you healthier, less vulnerable, and more likely to find solace within during trying times.

Myths about Loss and Grief

Our beliefs play a role in how well we cope. But there are a number of prevailing myths about loss and grief that can hurt as much as help us.

MYTH: *Everyone goes through the same fixed stages of grieving.*

Grief is a natural process. And though some common stages of grief can be identified (see box this page), they do not necessarily follow a fixed, sequential pattern. Some people go through only a few of the stages; others proceed from one directly to the next. Most people move back and forth among them, or experience several stages simultaneously.

MYTH: *If you don't feel intense distress or depression right away, you'll suffer problems later.*

While sadness and depression are common, a large minority of people come through traumatic experience without ever having any intense distress. One team of researchers interviewed widows within 30 days of losing their spouses. They found that only a third of the widows could be classified as depressed. Another study found that less than a quarter of people with spinal cord injuries were clinically depressed. In fact some losses, such as a divorce from an embittered spouse, may even be relief.

MYTH: *The lack of intense distress after a trauma means trouble later (delayed grief).*

Studies showed that the widows who were most upset shortly after the death of their spouse were those who also had difficulty coping two years later. In spinal cord injury patients, absence of depression predicts more successful long-term adjustment. In a study of parents who lost a child to Sudden Infant Death Syndrome (SIDS), those who spent a lot of time and energy working through the loss, trying to make sense of the death, and being preoccupied with it were still distressed a year and a half later.

MYTH: *Denial is bad for you.*

Denial—the mental operation by which thoughts, feelings, acts or threats are reduced—has received too much bad press. We often assume that it's unhealthy to linger in denial; that it's always better to face reality, get in touch with our feelings, and be honest with ourselves.

However, denial is a valuable part of the brain's complex pain-relief system. That system evolved to aid surviving dangers, like the attack of a wild animal, when we must decide to flee or fight. Denial blocks overwhelming anxiety allowing other, more useful thoughts and actions.

Whether denial is healthy or unhealthy depends on the circumstances, and on the outcome. It's generally healthier to minimize, ignore, or deny minor traumas than to get upset about them. In major traumas, denial can create some time and space for healthy hope. This is better than a mind flooded with anxious thoughts about something that can't be changed. For example, denial might help burn victims buy time until they can face the facts, and mobilize other means of coping.

But denial can interfere with necessary action and undermine health. The diabetic who needs to regulate insulin dosages or the woman who discovers a breast lump must take action to preserve their health. Ignoring insulin regulation can lead to life-threatening complications. Denying a breast lump can lead to delays in treatment for breast cancer.

MYMTH: *You should expect to recover quickly and completely from a loss.*

The expectation of a swift, full recovery ignores the findings that some people are still distressed and sad four to seven years after a trauma. Sometimes they feel that way forever. Some losses just never "make sense." Anniversaries, subsequent losses, or watching someone else go through a similar experience can evoke distressing feelings months or years later. This is neither unusual nor abnormal unless it seriously disrupts your life.

℞ How to Survive Traumatic Experiences

Some severe traumatic experiences require professional assistance. The self-help advice that follows, however, may be sufficient for others, or can supplement professional help.

℞ Feel Your Feelings

Allow yourself to grieve. When you're suddenly confronted with a traumatic experience, you may feel numb and emotionally limited. It may not be so easy if you have spent years controlling your emotions to suddenly let yourself freely express sorrow or anger. Or you may be afraid that you will be perceived as weak, or vulnerable, foolish, crazy, or "you've got to be the strong one."

On the other hand, don't feel bad if you don't feel bad. Those around you are likely to send subtle (or not so subtle) messages about how you "'should" feel. Some may pressure you to explore sadness or anger. They may even react negatively if you don't feel what they expect you to feel. Others may avoid you or prematurely encourage you to "put the event in the

205

past." The most important thing is to *allow yourself to feel whatever you feel.*

℞ Expect Ups and Downs

Many reactions to trauma are normal and natural healing responses; they're not signs of failure, weakness, or "going crazy." For example, nightmares and flashbacks may have a value. They can be a signal that you are working through the events, or they may be a sign that you are searching for some new meanings. Or your mind may be pacing itself with numbing denial and avoidance to allow you to deal with manageable doses of the stressful experience.

Even distress itself can help you mobilize ways of coping and healing. In one study of patients with malignant melanoma, a deadly skin cancer, patients who felt *higher* levels of emotional distress at the time of diagnosis had *lower* rates of recurrence and death years later. Those at the highest risk were those who minimized or expressed little distress. *When faced with a serious, threatening situation, it is appropriate to feel distressed—especially if such feelings motivate you to take constructive action.*

Key Point

However, emotions can sometimes feel overwhelming. In other chapters we give specific advice for defusing anger (📖 see page 169), lightening depression (page 159), and calming anxiety (page 147) as well as suggestions for how to communicate your feelings (page 123).

℞ Don't Do It Alone

A traumatic experience can disrupt your ties with others, leaving you feeling isolated. Talk about your feelings with other people. Seek out people who have gone through similar events. There are self-help groups for nearly every major trauma including rape; unemployment; loss of a child, spouse, pet; child abuse; domestic violence; divorce or separation; and missing children.

If the thought of participating in a support group is not appealing to you, a one-on-one relationship with a friend or counselor is a good alternative. Several computer services also offer health and community forums with information and on-line dialogue.

The need for help and support is normal, so don't be afraid to ask others to help you. People usually care about each other and want to be useful.

℞ Talk About It

There is mounting evidence that it's healthy to confess and confide. One survey showed that adults who experienced trauma as children and never talked about it were more likely to develop cancer, hypertension, ulcers, and serious cases of the flu than those who talked about their experiences with others, or never experienced the trauma. Another study of widows and widowers showed that those who spoke with others about their personal tragedies were healthier one year following the death.

℞ Writing Really Helps

It's hard work to keep our deep negative feelings hidden. Over time, this cumulative stress undermines our physiological defenses and seems to weaken our immunity. Confiding our feelings in others or writing them down puts them into words, and helps us sort them out. Words help us understand and absorb the traumatic event, and eventually put it behind us. It gives us a sense of release and control.

THE WRITE THING

WRITING AS A WAY OF DEALING WITH TRAUMATIC EXPERIENCE

Try the "write thing" when something is bothering you: when you find yourself thinking (or dreaming) too much about an experience; when you avoid thinking about something because it is too upsetting; when there's something you would like to tell others, but don't for fear of embarrassment or punishment.

Here are some guidelines for writing as a way to help you deal with any traumatic experience:

▶ Set a specific schedule for writing. For example, you might write 15 minutes a day for four consecutive days, or one day a week for four weeks.

▶ Write in a place where you won't be interrupted or distracted.

▶ Don't plan to share your writing—that could inhibit your honest expression. Save what you write or destroy it, as you wish.

▶ Explore your *very deepest thoughts and feelings,* and why you feel the way you do. Write about your negative feelings such as sadness, hurt, hate, anger, fear, guilt, or resentment.

▶ Write continuously. Don't worry about grammar, spelling, or making sense. If clarity and coherence come as you continue to write, so much the better. If you run out of things to say, just repeat what you have already written.

Even if you find the writing awkward at first, keep going. It gets easier. If you just cannot write, try talking into a tape recorder for 15 minutes about your deepest thoughts and feelings.

If you are coping with death, divorce, rape, or other major trauma, don't expect to feel better immediately. But you are much more likely to gain a deeper understanding of your thoughts and feelings, and get a better perspective on your life.

You may feel sad or depressed when your deepest feelings begin to surface. This usually fades within an hour or two, or a day or two at most. *The overwhelming majority of people report feelings of relief, happiness, and contentment soon after writing for several consecutive days.*

Key Point

Writing may help you to clarify what actions you need to take. But don't use writing as a substitute for taking action or as a way of avoiding things.

Adapted from James Pennebaker, author of Opening Up: The Healing Power of Confiding in Others

A series of studies investigated the healing effects of confiding or writing. One group was asked to write about their deepest thoughts and feelings about a traumatic event they experienced. Another group wrote about ordinary matters such as their plans for the day. Both groups wrote for 15 to 20 minutes a day for three to five consecutive days (📖 see box this page).

The results were surprisingly powerful. When compared with the people who wrote about ordinary events, the ones who wrote about their traumatic experiences reported fewer symptoms, fewer visits to the doctor, fewer days off work, improved mood, and a more positive outlook. Their immune function was enhanced for at least six weeks after writing. This was especially true for those who expressed previously undisclosed, painful feelings.

Another study involved recently unemployed people. Some wrote their deepest thoughts and feelings about losing their job. Eight months later, they had twice the success in finding a new job than those who just wrote about their job seeking plans.

℞ Look for the Positive

After a natural disaster, we often hear victims comment on the remarkable help they received from complete strangers, or how the community seemed closer. Crisis can bring families closer together, or serve as a turning point for personal growth.

Many victims of trauma find they reorder their life's priorities, and appreciate life more. Some even work to change the conditions that led to their misfortune. For example, a woman whose 16-year-old daughter was killed by a drunk driver founded MADD (Mothers Against Drunk Driving). The father of a child who was kidnapped and killed developed a national network to help find missing children.

Many people participate in self-help support groups. Sometimes helping others is the best way to help heal yourself (📖 see page 134).

Traumatic experiences can lead some people to renewed or deeper religious and spiritual involvement. Religious beliefs can make stressful events more bearable by providing a meaningful, coherent explanation. They can also offer hope, comfort, and community support.

Try to consider the trauma from a larger perspective. Challenge the negative thoughts and self-talk that lead to bad moods (📖 see page 42). Ask yourself:

▶ *Has anything positive come out of this experience?*

▶ *Am I in a better or worse situation compared to others?*

▶ *Could the situation have been worse?*

▶ *Is there anything about this that makes me feel lucky or fortunate?*

Finally, give yourself some credit for coping with all you've been through. And devote some time and attention to pleasurable activities (📖 see page 57). They can help boost your mood as well as counterbalance the trauma.

Some trauma comes to every life. But keep in mind there are some ways of coping with it that are better than others. They lessen the negative impact on your health, and help your sense of well-being. If you have a major traumatic experience, try the advice here. But don't hesitate to ask for additional support from family, friends, clergy, physicians, or mental health specialists.

📖 *For more information, see page 277*

17 Addiction

How to Control Addiction and Bad Habits

▶ *"If I drink too much a couple of times a month am I an alcoholic? If my father was an alcoholic will I be one too?"*

▶ *"My son smokes marijuana. Should I put him in an expensive residential treatment program?"*

▶ *"I slipped up once and smoked crack cocaine at a party. Now I feel doomed to becoming an addict for the rest of my life."*

▶ *"I've been smoking for years. I've tried to quit and failed. What can I do?"*

Ask ten people what they think about addiction, and you're likely to get ten different answers. The same is true of most "experts" in the field. There is a wide range of opinions and beliefs:

▶ Addiction is the sign of moral or spiritual weakness, or perhaps a sin or a crime

▶ It stems from poverty, social deprivation, or lack of a meaningful job

▶ Personality traits, character, and upbringing sow the seeds of the "addictive personality"

▶ It's a defect in the genes or brain

▶ Addiction is an irreversible, incurable "disease"

Characteristics of Addiction

One reason there are a wide range of beliefs is that "addiction" covers a wide range of problems: abuse of drugs like alcohol, cocaine, and nicotine, and uncontrollable behaviors like gambling, shopping, and overwork. So addiction is neither simple nor well understood, but experts agree the following are some of the most common characteristics of addiction:

▶ The substance or activity first produces pleasure or other desirable changes in mood

▶ The body usually develops a tolerance to the substance or activity which then requires larger doses to produce similar effects

▶ Stopping usually causes painful or uncomfortable withdrawal symptoms

▶ Addiction usually involves psychological dependence that reinforces cravings and the addictive behavior

▶ Addictions are typically associated with an increasing obsession with the drug or activity and involve increasing amounts of a person's time, attention, and resources

Addiction is sometimes accompanied by a range of problems from bad livers to lost livelihood, and the consequences on mental, physical, and financial health can be profound. By some estimates, addiction and bad habits account for nearly three-quarters of all disease, illness, and injuries. None of us are untouched by the social impacts of alcohol and drug abuse, smoking, and physical violence.

Addiction and Bad Habits

Attitudes about addiction shape what actions people take to help themselves or treat others. It's unfortunate that there are so many myths, misconceptions, and partial truths surrounding the problem. We need to ask:

▶ How well are the different beliefs supported by the current scientific evidence?

▶ How useful are they in helping people overcome addiction and control bad habits?

Sometimes these beliefs are unsubstantiated. Sometimes they are untrue, but may still help people seek care. In some cases, the beliefs may *prevent* individuals from overcoming their addiction (📖 see box page 213).

Very few people exposed to an addictive substance or activity become addicted. *It is probably most helpful and accurate to think of addiction as a bad habit. It is a behavior that is learned and can be unlearned, not a disease that always requires intensive, ongoing treatment.*

If addictions are viewed largely as "bad habits," even when they're very disabling, a different approach becomes possible. Though some people with addictive habits may benefit from self-help groups or professional treatment, the vast majority of people successfully control the habit by making behavior change strategies such as those described in this chapter.

Just Do It

The writer Russell Baker said: *"To give up smoking, you quit smoking." The first way to try beating a destructive habit is to simply stop—without a lot of planning, techniques, or a group support.* This advice may seem too simple. But this is the way most people quit or control their bad habits. They decide that it is unacceptable to continue the habit. After a firm decision, the rest is often surprisingly easy. *Just do it. You can quit.*

When addiction counseling professionals are asked which is the most difficult habit to change, they often rank cigarette smoking above cocaine, heroin, and alcohol. Yet most of these professionals have successfully quit smoking on their own, without any help.

In a large survey of people who were able to successfully stop substance abuse, only 3% were helped by doctors, and less than 1% were helped by psychologists, psychiatrists, or self-help groups. So where did rest of the help come from? The largest number of people (30%) did it entirely on their own! The rest got help from friends or family, especially spouses. The most successful people were those who quit on their own; those who used programs were only half as successful.

In a series of studies of treatment for alcoholism, patients who received printed self-help materials did just as well as those who got counseling and Antabuse, a drug that produces nausea when combined with alcohol. The self-help materials reinforced the belief that the patients were

ARE YOU ADDICTED?

The *consequences* of the behavior (rather than the behavior itself) usually help you determine if your habit is harmful. Here are some questions that may alert you to a potential problem:

❑ Is more and more of your life revolving around the habit?

❑ Do you find yourself thinking about it or planning when and where you'll next engage in it?

❑ Do you find yourself denying it's a problem, or acting secretively about it?

❑ Do you ever feel guilty about the habit?

❑ Do other people annoy you when they suggest that you should stop or cut down?

❑ Do you feel that you are not able to stop or control the behavior?

❑ Have you ever tried to stop the habit, even for a few days, and found yourself making excuses for not stopping?

❑ Has your habit ever created problems between you and your family or friends?

❑ Have you ever gotten into trouble at work or school because of your habit?

❑ Do you have any medical problems (diseases, symptoms, abnormal laboratory tests) due to your habit?

❑ Have you ever endangered yourself or others by your behaviors (for example, driving under the influence, or caused physical or mental abuse to someone)?

❑ Has your habit put serious financial pressures on you and your family?

❑ Is the habit illegal and likely to lead to significant problems if you are caught?

If you checked one or more of these boxes, your habit is causing problems or potential difficulties. Fortunately, habits are not fixed in stone. You can choose to change them.

not helpless "victims of a disease," but were capable of making the change.

How Successful is AA and Other Support Groups?

For some, self-help, recovery, and support groups are the answer, *especially after failing to quit on their own.* But others find the principles and methods of groups like Alcoholics Anonymous difficult to accept. These groups encourage participants to "confess" their weaknesses, surrender themselves to a higher power, and to associate with other people who have the same dependency.

We don't know how well AA or other treatment programs work. There have been few controlled, long-term studies. The little

Is Addiction a Disease?

The disease model, popularized by Alcoholics Anonymous, holds that an addiction is:

An incurable, abnormal condition like diabetes or asthma which you either have been afflicted with or you're free of. It is treated only with complete abstinence, vigilance, and lifelong therapy.

This view is a great advance over calling addiction a "sin." The disease model relieves the moral stigma and guilt of addiction because it considers "addicts" victims of disease who need treatment. It is also reassuring to the general public who view themselves as "well" because they don't have "the disease." But this model doesn't fit the facts about addiction. It is not a condition fixed in the brain that compels you to use a substance or engage in a destructive behavior for life. It doesn't necessarily require total abstinence and lifelong treatment.

It is helpful and accurate to think of addiction as a bad habit or an attempt to cope with stress, anxiety, and difficult situations. Rather than speaking of "addiction," it's more useful to focus on "addictive behaviors." From this perspective, addiction has more in common with other bad habits than with

Key Point

a disease fixed in your body and mind. You can change a bad habit. You are not put in an all-or-nothing (diseased-or-well) situation.

Is There a Gene for Addiction?

Genetics does influence some addictions: if you have alcoholic relatives, your risk of becoming alcoholic is greater. But genes are not destiny. More than 80% of people with alcoholic parents do not become alcoholics. In fact, there is still no way to accurately predict who will become addicted.

An "Addictive Personality"?

Some researchers claim the following predisposes a person to addiction:

▶ Low self-esteem

▶ Criminal and antisocial behavior

▶ Excessive dependency

▶ An inability to control strong feelings

▶ An inability to turn to others for comfort

But which comes first: the personality and social problems, or the addictions? Many people have these personality characteristics without becoming addicted. Research has failed to find any consistent link between personality traits and addiction. In fact, such character-

Continued on next page

evidence available suggests that the treatment programs may help some people in the short-run, but it is uncertain in the long-run.

If these programs don't suit you, there are other support groups which operate on different principles. For example, there are programs that help problem drinkers learn to moderate their habit.

Research continues on ways to help people with addictive behaviors. New medi-

istics as emotional insecurity, depression, dependency, and criminality seem to be the *result* of alcohol, drug abuse and addiction, not the cause. Fortunately once the abuse or addiction is under control, the undesirable traits tend to go away. In many cases criminal behavior, aggressiveness, selfishness, pessimism, and so on fades along with the addiction.

Is it Easy to Become Addicted?

Addiction is a bad habit that is repeated frequently. Yet many people fear that one drink, one cigarette, or one encounter with a narcotic will sentence them to a life of addiction. Almost no one who drinks, sniffs cocaine, or even smokes crack or a cigarette once becomes addicted. Most people with an alcoholic parent do not become an alcoholic. And hospitalized patients who are treated for weeks with morphine do not tend to become addicted.

Key Point

You may be surprised to learn that cigarettes may be even more addictive than cocaine. About 36% of the people who begin smoking cigarettes become addicted; the percentage of those who have used cocaine and are now regular users is less than 1%. Each exposure requires a choice and a decision.

Do Our Beliefs Affect Addiction?

Addiction is determined as much by our culture's beliefs as by physical dependencies, or the substances themselves. It takes more than repeated exposure to produce addictive behavior. *Much of addiction has to do with what we believe rather than being physically dependent.* For example, consider this experiment: Male drinkers who had relapsed after an alcohol treatment program were asked to sample some drinks. Some were told they were drinking three brands of vodka; the others were told they were drinking three brands of tonic water.

Key Point

In reality, however, each group received the *opposite* of what they were told they were drinking. Those expecting alcohol drank more than those expecting tonic water. They thought they were drinking alcohol even when they were not!

Other experiments show that people who were led to believe they were given alcohol, even when they were not, acted and felt intoxicated just as though they had really been given alcohol. What we believe and expect changes our behavior. The good news is that you can learn to change and control your behavior by changing what you believe.

cations, new skills training programs, and different types of support groups are being tried and evaluated. Until some proven ways are developed, it's useful to remember that many people change bad habits on their own. If you're not successful on your own, then consider self-help groups or professional help.

How to Control Addiction and Bad Habits

If you regularly use too much of some substance or engage in a destructive activity, take heart. We can help you take steps to stop. And don't be discouraged if you don't succeed the first time. The evidence shows that the more times you try giving up, the better your chances are of being successful the next time.

In one study, nearly two-thirds of the people who tried repeatedly to give up smoking and overeating eventually succeeded. So put past efforts down to experience. You have learned valuable lessons from past attempts, whether you realize it or not. Think of yourself as being successful in the long run.

The strategies you can use for changing bad habits are described in Chapter 1: The Power to Change (see page 17). To quit, first try just quitting, second, try the other self-help suggestions in Chapter 1, and third, if you are still not successful, try a recovery group or professional program.

Key Point

For more information, see page 277

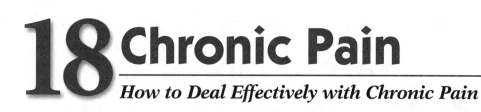

18 Chronic Pain

How to Deal Effectively with Chronic Pain

"I hate my pain. It's ruining my life. I'm frustrated by doctors who can't find what's wrong and fix it. I really resent them saying 'it's all in my head.' My family doesn't understand. No one believes my pain is real. I feel so helpless."

If you have chronic pain, these feelings may be all too familiar. In the face of unremitting or recurrent pain, it may be difficult to believe that pain is essential for our survival. But put your hand on a hot stove and you'll be thankful for the painful reminder to remove it immediately. While acute pain—sharp and immediate—may be excruciating, it serves as a warning, and protects you from further damage. Acute pain also tends to go away.

But when pain persists, it ceases to be a useful warning, and the pain itself becomes the problem. Chronic pain—the kind that is almost always with you or recurs frequently—is unfortunately common. Ten to thirty percent of Americans suffer from chronic or recurrent pain that serves no apparent purpose. Chronic pain takes a heavy toll on health, the ability to work, and a sense of well-being.

Vicious Cycles of Pain

Chronic pain can lock you in a vicious cycle. Here are four scenarios:

1. Inactivity: Because of the pain, you tend to avoid physical activity, which, in turn, causes you to lose strength and flexibility. The weaker and more out of condition you become, the more frustrated and depressed you feel. These negative emotions can open the "pain gates," and cause pain levels to rise.

2. Overdoing. You may be determined to prove that you can still be active, so you overexert. This increases the pain and leads to more inactivity, more depression, and more pain.

3. Misunderstanding. Your friends, family, boss, and co-workers may not understand that you are suffering, and dismiss your pain as "not real." This evokes more anger or depression.

4. Overprotection. Friends, family, and co-workers coddle you and make excuses for you. This can lead you to feel and act more dependent and disabled.

Fortunately, this downward spiral can be interrupted. Being told you have to learn to live with pain doesn't have to be the end of the road. It can be a new beginning.

KEEP A PAIN DIARY

Get a clear understanding of how your moods, activities, and conditions affect your pain. Begin by recording your activities and pain levels three times a day, at regular intervals (see the *Pain Diary* below).

At first you may resist keeping these records since focusing on your pain may make it seem worse. But a pain diary will allow you to identify important patterns.

▶ Is the pain worse after sitting for long?

▶ Less when you are engaged in a favorite hobby?

Notice how your awareness of pain varies according to your mood, fatigue, muscle tension, and degree of focus on it. This record enables you to track the effectiveness of your pain management.

It's important to distinguish between *physical pain sensations* (the physical stabbing, burning, aching sensations) and your *emotional pain distress* (the accompanying anger, anxiety, frustration or sadness). This is useful because while your physical pain may not be reduced, you may feel better about the pain, and experience less distress, anxiety, helplessness, and despair.

Pain Diary

1. Record date and time

2. Describe situation or activity (watching TV, housework, arguing, etc.)

3. Rate Physical Pain Sensation on a scale of 0 to 10 from 0 (no pain) to 10 (worst pain)

4. Describe pain sensation ("deep aching pain in left lower back," etc.)

5. Rate emotional pain distress scale of 0 to 10 from 0 (no distress) to 10 (terribly distressed)

6. Describe type of emotional distress (felt very angry, depressed, etc.)

7. Describe if you did anything for the discomfort (medications, massage, relaxation exercise, took a walk, etc.), and its effect

Date	Describe Situation	Physical Pain Sensation (0 - 10)	Describe Sensation	Emotional Distress (0 - 10)	Describe Distress	Actions or Medications Taken (and effect)
Time 1						
Time 2						
Time 3						

You can learn to:

▶ Redirect your attention to control pain

▶ Challenge negative thoughts that support pain

▶ Cultivate more positive emotions

▶ Slowly increase your activity and recondition yourself

It is important to become an active partner in your pain treatment. Using behavioral techniques to gain more control may not make your pain go away, but emotional suffering and distress can be lessened enabling you to become more active in your life again.

Key Point

℞ How to Manage Chronic Pain

The following "prescriptions" are in addition to your doctor's recommendations, not a substitute for it. If these self-help techniques are not working for you alone, consider a group program. In addition to reinforcing the techniques, interacting with other sufferers helps reduce your feelings of isolation. Group members can learn a lot from each other about practical ways of coping with pain.

℞ Take Control

Chronic pain tends to take over and become the focus of your life. It tells you how much you can do and when you can do it; it keeps you from living life to its fullest. Though life may never be the same as before the pain began, you can get it back in control.

If your physical condition has been thoroughly evaluated and nothing further can be done medically, your first step may be to accept the pain, and make the best of it. Resist the tendency to blame others and don't put your life on hold, waiting for someone—physicians, members of your family, or society—to fix your problem. Take charge. Identify some steps toward more independence. Reading and trying some of the exercises in this chapter is a good beginning.

℞ Recognize Costs and Benefits

It's helpful to understand what pain means to you, and its impact on your life. What is the cost to your family activities? Your work? Your play? Most people find chronic pain very disruptive to themselves and the people around them.

Surprisingly, chronic pain can also yield some hidden "benefits." Here are some examples:

▶ People who can get attention and support only when they have pain often have higher levels of pain, and are more disabled.

▶ Pain can also be used as an excuse for avoiding something else, such as problems in a relationship: a woman may experience pain during sex, for instance, as an expression of unhappiness with her relationship, a

Controlling the "Pain Gates"

Recent research suggests that we are not helpless in the face of pain. The brain does not just passively receive pain signals from the body. It can regulate the flow of these pain messages by sending electrical and chemical signals that open and close "pain gates" along nerve pathways.

For example, the brain can release powerful opiate-like chemicals—endorphins—which can effectively block pain. When people are very seriously injured, they sometimes experience little pain while they are focused on survival. How you focus your attention, your mood, and the way you view your situation can open or close the "pain gates."

Many factors can contribute to chronic pain. Most experts now believe that almost all unexplained chronic pain is rooted in some type of physical problem: damaged or hypersensitive nerves, blood vessels, muscles, or other tissues. These underlying physical problems simply can't be pinpointed. It's not "all in your head."

Both physical and psychological responses to chronic pain play important roles in determining the degree of the pain and distress that's experienced. The body quickly attempts to limit the movement of the damaged area. This causes muscle tension, which, in itself, can cause more pain. Since chronic pain often leads to inactivity, muscles often become weakened and hurt with the slightest use.

Feelings of anxiety, anger, frustration, and loss of control also amplify the experience of pain. This doesn't mean that the pain is not "real," it just means that emotions can make a painful situation worse.

Managing Chronic Pain

There are several ways to manage chronic pain. Following are some alternatives:

Physical Treatments

▶ Acute pain usually responds to painkilling drugs, from mild over-the-counter analgesics for headaches to

Continued on next page

fear of sex, or a fear of getting pregnant; a man who is threatened by his wife's career may use his pain to control her and undermine her independence; a parent may unconsciously use pain to get a grown-up son or daughter to visit regularly.

Key Point · *To begin to manage your pain, be honest with yourself about both the costs and the "benefits" if any.* Then you can begin to find other, less painful ways to get those needs met.

℞ Express Your Feelings

George developed chronic lower back pain which aroused many fears. Would he be crippled? Lose his job? Would his wife leave him? Was he dying? He kept these worries to himself, and that made his pain worse.

Keeping fears and anxieties to yourself can increase pain. In talking about your fears, you often discover they are unfounded, or not so serious. And the relief you feel in not shouldering burdens

powerful narcotic medications for post-operative and cancer pain.

▶ Some types of chronic pain respond well to anti-inflammatory medications or antidepressants.

▶ Narcotic (opiod) medications can sometimes be used to relieve chronic pain and improve functioning. While such medications can have side effects, such as disturbance in mental functioning, addiction is rare (📖 see page 211). Narcotic medications need to be monitored carefully as part of a treatment plan to avoid misuse. Medications are more effective when used at a regular time-interval, not just when the pain gets severe.

▶ Sometimes injections of a local anesthetic or a surgical procedure can block pain signals from a painful area. This provides temporary or sometimes lasting relief from chronic pain. Ice, heat, massage, and physical therapy also can be helpful.

▶ Early, aggressive treatment of acute pain may prevent hypersensitization of nerves and development of chronic pain.

Self-Management

Mind/body techniques such as relaxation, distraction, and changing negative thought patterns have been used in clinically tested programs to help patients cope better with chronic pain. In one such program, participants with chronic pain saw the doctor 36% fewer times within a two-year period after practicing these behavioral self-management techniques. They said they felt more in control, and had less depression, anxiety, and pain severity. The degree to which pain interfered with daily activities was also decreased.

In treatment of low back pain and headache, relaxation techniques have been used successfully. Several studies have shown that relaxation alone can produce a 38% reduction in the intensity, frequency, and duration of migraine headaches, and a 45% improvement for those with tension headaches.

Biofeedback training, in which sensors give feedback about muscle tension or skin temperature, is also helpful for some people to learn to relax and control their bodies.

alone can help lessen pain.

Suppressed anger can also heighten pain. Often the anger is related to loss: of the ability to work, of friends or family members, or of cherished activities. The anger may also be triggered by an inability to say no, or an inability to ask for help. Learning how to communicate assertively (📖 see page 127), writing about your deepest thoughts and feelings (page 207), and learning ways to defuse automatic anger responses can all be helpful (page 169).

℞ Challenge Your Thoughts

Thoughts can profoundly influence moods and pain. Constantly telling yourself things like, "I'm always in pain," "I don't know how much longer I can take this," or "I don't see how this can ever get better," can cause you to tense up and open the "pain gates" in your nervous system. Such negative thoughts also undermine your sense of control and keep you from taking positive action.

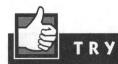

TRY THIS

SOME WAYS TO RELAX

Abdominal (belly) breathing: Place your hands just below your belly button. Move your belly rather than your chest. Take a deep breath. Imagine a balloon inside your belly filling with air. As you slowly exhale, feel it deflate (📖 see page 90).

Progressive muscle relaxation: Start with your feet, then your legs, and progress up to the top of your head. Systematically tense—and then relax—each muscle group. Gradually build up the tension, and then release it. Pay attention to the way your muscles feel when they are tense, and, by contrast, when they are relaxed (📖 see page 92).

"Mini relaxation" exercise: Take a deep breath. As you exhale, let the word "relax" fill your thoughts. Allow all tension to flow downward, from the muscles of your face and neck, through your arms and legs, and out of your hands and feet. Hold that feeling of relaxation for 10 to 15 seconds before you return to your activity. Repeat each time you feel pain or tension. Or do it at other regular times, such as each time the phone rings.

Massage: This is another pleasant and helpful way to relax and reduce pain. You don't need a professional. Get a self-help massage book and practice with a partner or friend.

Learn how to monitor and challenge this negative self-talk (📖 see page 42). Write down your thoughts and feelings as part of a "pain diary" (see box page 216). If you find yourself waking up in pain and saying, "I'm going to be miserable all day; I won't get anything done," say to yourself, "I've got some pain this morning, so I'll start with some relaxation and stretching exercises. Then I'll do some of the less demanding things I want to get done today."

℞ Refocus Your Mind, and Relax

Pain is a stressor. It triggers the "fight-or-flight response." Chronic pain can lead to chronic stress. These things include:

▶ Sleep disturbance

▶ Fatigue

▶ Poor concentration

▶ Increased muscle tension

▶ Anxiety

▶ Depression

▶ Loss of sense of control

All of these responses can amplify pain.

When you feel pain, it's natural to tense up and tighten muscles all over your body. In response to lower back pain, for example, you may change your posture. This can create tension and pain in your neck.

Consider learning a variety of relaxation exercises to reduce muscle spasm and tension, and help correct abnormal muscle patterns (📖 see page 92). Focusing on the breath is a good start. It is difficult to maintain tension (pain, stress, anger, anxiety) while concentrating on the breath. Self-hypnosis and imagery can also help (📖 see page 99).

℞ Distract Yourself

Our minds have trouble focusing on more than one thing at a time. You can use this to lessen the intensity of pain by refocusing your attention. This is something we do unconsciously all the time. Many athletes often don't realize they have injured themselves, for example, until after the competition is over.

Distraction techniques can be especially helpful to get through a brief painful procedure or activity. Distract yourself with something neutral or try swapping pain for pleasure. Experiment with these distraction techniques:

▶ **Focus on something in the environment.** Listen to music, stare at some object in the room, or watch TV.

▶ **Do a rhythmic activity.** Sing a favorite song to yourself, or drum some rhythm with your fingers.

▶ **Challenge yourself.** Name all 50 states, or go through the alphabet listing names (A: Alice, B: Bruce, ...).

▶ **Think of the future or past.** Concentrate on plans for tomorrow, or recall a movie you have seen.

▶ **Create a dramatic image.** Imagine rescuing a child from an accident, and feel your pain as part of the heroic act.

▶ **Conjure up a pleasant scene.** See yourself relaxing on a beach or sitting by a brook. Immerse yourself in vivid, detailed images, and use all your senses (📖 see page 104).

▶ **Imagine healing.** Find your specific pain sensations, and imagine soothing them. If your pain is hot and throbbing, envision cool fingers lightly stroking the area. If it feels like a tight band, see a warm liquid dissolving it (📖 see page 106).

TRY THIS

RENAME THE PAIN

Try relabeling your sensations of pain.

1. Get into a comfortable position. Allow your breathing to become slow and regular. Scan your body for areas of discomfort. When you find one, focus all your attention on that area.

2. What is the exact location of the pain? Simply "my leg" won't do; zero in: "an inch below the center of my knee."

3. Now describe the quality of the sensation. Is it burning? Cold? Stabbing? Aching? Tight?

4. Be precise. The sensation may change, increasing or decreasing, or perhaps going from "sharp" to "dull aching." Just go along with it. See if you can change the way you feel about it by relabeling it.

5. By concentrating on the pure physical sensation, you may be able to disconnect the emotional distress you link to the word "pain." Pain by any other name may be less painful.

℞ Engage in Healthy Pleasures

At age 29, Jan suffered a lot of pain from rheumatoid arthritis. When she decided to get involved at her own pace in raising funds for arthritis research, her pain was diminished, and she had a much brighter outlook on life.

Chronic pain can cause us to eliminate the

TRY THIS

FOCUS ON YOUR PAIN

Gently focus your mind on the pain, and observe the accompanying stream of thoughts. You might hear something like this: "My back is killing me. If I hadn't lifted that dresser I would never have gotten into this mess. It's my own fault. I'm so stupid..."

The idea is to *simply observe*, and not react with judgments or feelings. Instead say to yourself: "Okay, I'm feeling some pain, and I'm angry about it."

Becoming aware of those judgments will help you gain a sense of control. With practice, you will be able to identify them when they first come up. You'll simply observe them, then watch them fade away (📖 see page 94).

fun from life. This is a serious mistake; we all need a daily dose of pleasure (📖 see page 57). Stay open to enjoyment. Keep a long list of things you like to do, refer to it whenever you start tuning in to your pain, and choose one of them to do.

Attention to pleasure deserves some long-range planning. You might take up a hobby and immerse yourself in it. Your pain will be helped considerably, even if at the outset you think you are in too much pain to do anything at all.

Don't feel guilty about having fun when you "should" be doing something "productive." If giving yourself pleasure relieves your pain, it is productive. Try doing something to help others. You'll distract yourself from your own problem,

feel better about yourself, which in turn will help reduce your pain (📖 see page 134).

℞ Focus on Your Pain

The opposite approach to "distraction" has also proven to be effective. In one study, participants were asked to immerse a hand in ice-cold water for four minutes. One third of the group was told to *suppress* any thoughts of the pain; another third to *distract* themselves with a vivid mental image of their bedroom; the last group was told to *focus* all their thoughts on the pain. Although none of the participants could tolerate the pain for more than a few minutes, the pain faded much more quickly for those who focused directly on it.

℞ Reclaim an Active Life

With chronic pain, you may find yourself attempting to do your usual activities until the pain gets really bad. Then you are forced to stop and rest for long periods of time. The link between increased pain and activity can lead to a pattern of fear, and that fear can lead to an avoidance of activity. This can result in greater weakness and fatigue. Maintaining a more active lifestyle in the face of chronic pain requires time and patience, but it can be very satisfying as you watch yourself very gradually take on more and more. *The key is to pace yourself carefully.*

Key Point

℞ Get Some Exercise

Gentle exercise is likely to decrease—not increase—persistent pain. It strengthens muscles that help you become more mobile and independent. It can be a pleasant distraction from the pain. It also gets you out of the house and gives you a change of scene. Exercise may release endorphins, the body's natural painkillers, which gives you an emotional lift while they reduce your pain.

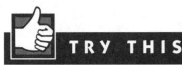
ALTERNATE ACTIVITY AND REST

Keep a log of your daily activities for three days. Record how many minutes of activity and how many minutes of rest. You may notice a pattern of overactivity, extreme pain, followed by prolonged rest.

To break that vicious pain/inactivity cycle, set an initial goal of so many minutes of moderate activity that doesn't increase your pain to very high levels (note: this may initially be less activity than you usually do!). For some people moderate activity may be spending 30 minutes up and out of bed, for others it may involve 30 minutes of walking.

If you find your pain level rising, *stay active* but slow down or switch to less demanding activity. *Time,* not pain, should be the measure of your activity.

Follow each scheduled activity period with a limited rest period (sitting or lying down) that gives you some pain relief. But the total amount of rest time should be *less* than you recorded in your baseline log. Repeat the cycle of moderate activity followed by limited rest frequently throughout the day.

Keep a written record each day and gradually increase the time of moderate activity and decrease rest periods.

Get professional advice on the best exercise for your particular condition. Once you begin, keep at it on a regular schedule, and increase your efforts very gradually (📖 see page 114).

℞ Modify Your Environment

By changing your environment and/or the way you use your body, you can avoid pain from everyday activities. Learning how to bend, lift, reach, and sit can make a critical difference in pain flare-ups. Use helpful devices such as adjustable desk chairs and wrist supports. Carts for carrying heavy objects can also prevent further injury.

℞ Plan Ahead for Flare-ups

It may be more difficult to respond effectively when you are in the throes of an acute flare-up of pain. It's a good idea to prepare ahead of time a list of the specific pain relievers that work best for you. Here are some examples of things you might include:

1. Do a relaxation exercise
2. Use heat or ice
3. Take a bath
4. Do something distracting
5. Focus on the pain as though you were an outside observer
6. Remind yourself of the things you do have control over
7. Find a book or television show that will make you laugh or completely engage you
8. Use visualization to imagine yourself with less pain
9. Remind yourself that the pain is temporary; it will pass
10. Ask others close to you for support

Sometimes your pain may not respond, no matter what you do. Just accept it, and call it a bad day. Tomorrow will probably be better. Your path to improvement may follow an up-and-down course.

📖 *For more information, see page 277*

223

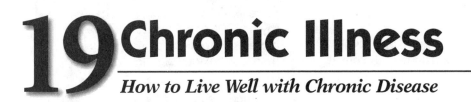

19 Chronic Illness

How to Live Well with Chronic Disease

"It is much more important to know what sort of patient has the disease than what sort of disease the patient has."
— *Sir William Osler, M.D. (1849-1919)*

Same Disease, Different Response

Arthur suffers from severe arthritis. He is in pain most of the time and can't sleep properly. He took early retirement because of his arthritis and now, only 55, he spends his day sitting at home bored. He avoids most physical activity because of the pain, weakness, and shortness of breath. He has become very irritable. Most people, including his family, don't enjoy his company anymore. It even seems too much trouble when the grandchildren he adored come to visit.

Isabel, age 66, also suffers from severe arthritis. Every day she manages to walk several blocks to the local library or the park. When the pain is severe, she practices her relaxation techniques and tries to distract herself. She works several hours a week as a volunteer at a local hospital. She also loves going to see her young grandchildren and even manages to take care of them for a while, when her daughter has to be out. Her husband is amazed by how much zest she has for life.

Arthur and Isabel both suffer from the same condition with similar amounts of physical impairment. Yet their ability to function and enjoy life is very different. Why? The difference is their attitude toward the disease and their life. Arthur has allowed his life and physical capacities to wither. Isabel has learned to take an active role in managing her chronic illness. Even though she has limitations, she controls her life instead of letting the illness control it.

Attitude cannot cure chronic illness. But a positive attitude and certain self-management skills can make it much easier to live with. Much research now shows that the experience of pain, discomfort and disability can be modified by circumstances, beliefs, mood, and the attention we pay to symptoms. For example, with arthritis of the knee, how depressed a person is better predicts how disabled, limited, and uncomfortable they will be than the evidence of physical damage to the knees on x-rays. *What goes on in a person's mind is often more important than what is going on in their body.*

Key Point

MIND MATTERS

Thousands of studies link psychological states and social conditions to the onset, course, and recovery from chronic illness. Even when the underlying physical disease cannot be made better, positive psychological states can change the way you experience your symptoms and how disabled you are. Mental factors are, of course, not the only things that determine who becomes ill (📖 see box page 46). But the accumulation of evidence adds up to a very strong case that mind *does* matter (📖 see page 14). Here are some examples:

Onset of Disease

▶ Inadequate social support is as dangerous to your health as lack of exercise, high blood pressure, obesity, smoking, and an elevated cholesterol level. *Social isolation is associated with twice the overall rate of premature death.*

Key Point

▶ An analysis of over 100 studies suggests people who experience chronic anxiety, depression, pessimism, incessant hostility, and cynicism tend to have double the risk of many kinds of diseases such as asthma, arthritis, ulcers, and heart disease. Chronically nervous, tense, and anxious people, for example, are more likely to have abnormal heart rhythms. They are two to six times more likely to die of a heart attack than less anxious people.

▶ Women younger than 45 who are divorced, separated, or widowed have significantly higher levels of total cholesterol and "bad" LDL cholesterol than married women.

▶ Men with a lot of hostility are seven times more likely to die within 25 years (from any cause) than less hostile men. Reducing anger and hostility appears to reduce the risk of recurrent heart attack, and may even prevent heart disease.

▶ If you are wealthy, well-educated, and hold a high-status job, you are less likely to have nearly all chronic illnesses or die from them.

▶ Older people who believed that they were in "poor" health were nearly three times more likely to die than those who rated their health as "excellent" over a seven-year period. These self-ratings more accurately predicted who would die than their doctors' objective reports.

Health pessimists who thought they were in poor health (despite a clean bill of health from their doctors) had a slightly greater risk of dying than the health optimists. These optimists,

Continued on next page

who viewed themselves as well even though their doctor's reports suggested their health was poor, had a slightly less risk of dying.

▶ A long-term study of college graduates found that optimistic men were physically healthier and had less chronic illness in later life than the more pessimistic alumni.

▶ Women with a history of depression have bone density that is 15% lower than nondepressed women of the same age. Bone loss is the critical factor in osteoporosis. It is a disease marked by thinning of the bones. This thinning often leads to crippling fractures.

Course of the Illness

▶ How depressed a person is better predicts how disabled, limited, and uncomfortable they will be with arthritis of the knee than physical damage shown on x-rays.

▶ Group education sessions for patients with arthritis led by other patients reduced pain levels by 20%. They also decreased visits to the doctor by 43%, saving an average of $400 per patient over four years.

▶ Women with advanced metastatic breast cancer who received group psychotherapy and support in addition to standard medical care survived (on average) more than twice as long as those who received only standard care.

Recovery from Disease

▶ In addition to standard surgical treatment, one group of patients with a deadly skin cancer (malignant melanoma) received a group support and education program for six weeks. They learned about their condition, stress management, relaxation, and coping skills. The group who received this training had a 60% reduction in death rate six years later.

▶ Depressed patients with coronary heart disease are more likely to have heart attacks, undergo bypass surgery, and suffer other heart-related problems than heart disease patients who aren't depressed. In a study of patients who had a heart attack, depression related more closely to future heart problems than the severity of artery damage, high cholesterol levels, or cigarette smoking. In heart attack survivors, depression triples the risk of dying within six months.

So managing your moods and learning how to cope effectively with chronic illness can be an important addition to your regular medical treatments.

How to Cope with Chronic Illness

The more confident and determined you feel, the more you will be able to maximize your health. Whether you have arthritis or diabetes, heart disease or cancer, lung disease or multiple sclerosis, or a combination of chronic conditions, you can learn to be more active, cope better, and be more in control.

To live well with chronic conditions you need to learn how to:

1. Manage your illness and symptoms
2. Manage your normal daily activities
3. Manage your emotions

1. MANAGING YOUR ILLNESS

Any illness requires that you learn new things. You may not even know that you have a pancreas gland until you're told you have diabetes. *Successful self-managers of chronic illness become experts in their own disease. This doesn't mean they become doctors, but it does mean they learn enough about the condition and how their body reacts to minimize disability and complications successfully.*

Key Point

℞ Be an Active Partner in Your Own Health Care

Learn about your medical condition. What makes it worse or better? What action plan should you take if symptoms flare? What are the warning signs that signal you should get professional medical help? What can you expect from medical care, and what must you do for yourself? There may be specific skills you need to learn: how to measure your blood sugar if you are diabetic, how to properly use an inhaler if you have asthma, how to safely exercise with a heart or lung condition, how to use assistive devices if you have arthritis.

Learn how to prepare for a medical visit (see page 240), questions to ask about medical tests (page 247), medications (page 256), and surgery (page 267). Find community resources, talk with health care providers, friends, family, and:

▶ Check out the yellow pages of the telephone book (look under "Health," "Hospitals," "Community," "Social Service Organizations," "Local Government—Information and Referral")

▶ Call the national offices or local chapters of the voluntary agencies such as the American Heart Association, American Cancer Society, or National Arthritis Foundation

▶ Visit a library and ask the reference librarian to help you find information

▶ Check out the "calendar of events" in your local newspaper

See *Resources For More Information* (see page 278)

℞ Learn to Cope with Symptoms

Most chronic disease symptoms wax and

wane. When symptoms are bad, you can take some consolation that they are likely to improve. But there are also specific skills you can learn to lessen the discomfort from symptoms:

- ▶ **For pain** (📖 see page 217)
- ▶ **For tension** (📖 see page 88 and 99)
- ▶ **For depression** (📖 see page 159)
- ▶ **For anxiety** (📖 see page 147)
- ▶ **For insomnia** (📖 see page 192)

2. MANAGING DAILY ACTIVITY

Life doesn't end if you have a chronic illness. There are still chores to do, jobs to perform, and relationships to maintain. But things you once took for granted can become much more complicated in the face of chronic illness. You can learn new skills to maintain your daily activities and continue to enjoy life.

℞ Break the Cycle

Most people with chronic disease suffer some fatigue, pain, shortness of breath, or other symptoms that discourage physical activity. They may not sleep well and their energy levels drop. The less active they are the more physically weakened and deconditioned they become. Deconditioning then leads to feelings of helplessness which in turn discourages physical activity. And so the cycle of weakness, inactivity, deconditioning, and helplessness increases the original chronic disease problem.

The solution is to break the cycle with gentle, gradual physical activity. As your physical activity increases, your strength and stamina grow, your mood improves, and you can restore or preserve your ability to carry out your normal daily activities.

℞ One Step at a Time

Chronic disease often carries with it a sense of limitations and disabilities, rather than of one's potential. We assume it is not safe to extend ourselves, but such assumptions may be too restrictive. There are safe limits within which people with chronic disease can live a vital and fulfilling life.

Identify a specific action you would like to take. Then figure out how to break it down into specific small steps to help insure your success (📖 see page 23). For example, if you want to be able to walk one mile to the park, you may need to begin with walking just one block. Successfully completing each step brings satisfaction, boosts your mood, and enhances your confidence.

3. MANAGING EMOTIONS

When diagnosed with a chronic illness, your future changes. And with it also comes changes in your regular routine, your life plans, and your emotions. The emotional shift can magnify your symptoms and disabilities. You may react with any of the following feelings:

Anger. *"Why me—it's not fair. I am frustrated that I can't do what I used to."*

Anxiety. *"I'm afraid of what might happen to me. The future is so uncertain."*

Depression. *"I can't do anything well anymore. What's the use of trying."*

Isolation. *"No one understands. No one wants to be around someone who is sick."*

Living well with chronic illness, then, also means learning new skills to manage these negative limiting emotions.

℞ Explore Your Feelings

▶ *"The blood test shows that you have diabetes"*

▶ *"You have had a heart attack"*

▶ *"The biopsy results show that you have cancer"*

Learning you have a disabling chronic disease can be a profound shock to your sense of self. It changes your perceptions of who you are, who you were, and who you will now become. Suddenly you discover that you are not invulnerable after all; that "these things" don't always happen to someone else. These traumatic feelings can hit hard and you may need time to come to terms with them. Like bereavement, chronic illness can bring with it powerful feelings of loss: loss of aspirations, plans, or physical abilities (📖 see page 201).

People often go through various stages of feelings when diagnosed:

▶ **Denial** (denying or not believing the diagnosis)

▶ **Anger** about being ill and blaming others

▶ **Bargaining or guilt** (attempts to reverse the diagnosis by offering something in exchange)

▶ **Depression** (feelings of helplessness and loss of control)

▶ **Acceptance**

These are normal responses to having a chronic disease. *Expressing your feelings is very important. Pent-up anger or unvoiced sadness can undermine actions you can take that may help you manage your illness.* There are specific "prescriptions" that can help you manage your angry feelings (📖 see page 169) and depression (page 159).

Key Point

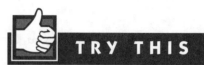

TRY THIS

When you're dealing with a chronic illness, you might find it helpful to keep a journal for a while. Write down exactly how you feel about what has happened to you (📖 see page 207):

❏ How did you feel about yourself before the diagnosis?

❏ How do you feel about yourself now?

❏ How do you feel others will react to you?

❏ What is the meaning of the illness to you?

❏ When you replay the diagnosis (heart disease, cancer, hypertension, etc.), what thoughts and feelings come to mind?

❏ Have you known others with this condition, and how does that experience shape your hopes and fears about the future?

You will probably come up with some very useful information. You'll find areas you need to work on to rebuild your self-esteem and sense of control.

℞ Watch Your Self-Talk

The explanations that you tell yourself about your symptoms and disease can strongly influence your mood and ability to function. *Many of the limitations and restrictions associated with chronic illness lie more in our beliefs than our bodies.* Your expectations can become self-fulfilling prophesies. If you think heart disease means that you'll never be able to work, have sex, or see your child graduate, then your actions and

Key Point

feelings are likely to reflect these beliefs. You can learn to eavesdrop on your internal dialogue and to challenge and rewrite restrictive, inaccurate, negative self-talk (📖 see page 42).

℞ Don't Do it Alone

Key Point *One of the side effects of chronic illness is a feeling of isolation. As supportive as friends and family members may be, they often cannot understand what you are experiencing as you struggle to cope with a chronic illness.* Chances are, however, that there are others who know firsthand what it is like to live with a chronic condition just like yours. Connecting with other people with similar conditions can:

▶ Reduce your sense of isolation

▶ Help you understand what to expect based on a fellow-patient's perspective

▶ Offer practical tips on how to manage symptoms and feelings on a day-to-day basis

▶ Give you the opportunity to help others cope with their illness

▶ Help you appreciate your assets, and realize that things could be worse

▶ Inspire you to take a more active role in managing your illness by seeing others coping successfully

Support can come from reading a book or a newsletter about how someone lives with a chronic illness. Or it can come from talking with others on the telephone, in support groups, or even linking on-line through computer and electronic support groups (📖 see page 273). However you connect with others, practice clear communication skills to express your feelings and wishes (📖 see page 123).

℞ You're More than Your Disease

When you have a chronic disease, too often the center of attention becomes your disease. But you are more than your disease—more than a "heart patient" or "lung patient." And life is more than trips to the doctor and managing symptoms.

It is essential to cultivate areas of your life which you enjoy. Small daily pleasures can help balance the other parts in which you have to manage uncomfortable symptoms or emotions. Find ways to enjoy nature by growing a plant or watching a sunset, or indulge in the pleasure of human touch or a tasty meal, or celebrate companionship with family or friends. Finding ways to introduce moments of pleasure is vital to chronic disease self-management (📖 see page 57). Focus on your abilities and assets rather than disabilities and deficits. Celebrate small improvements. If chronic illness teaches anything, it is to live each moment more fully. Within the true limits of whatever disease you have, there are ways to enhance your function, sense of control, and enjoyment of life.

℞ Illness Can Be an Opportunity

Illness, even with its pain and disability, can enrich our lives. It can make us reevaluate what is really important, **Key Point** *shift priorities, and move in exciting new directions that we might never have seen before.*

Jill has breast cancer. Since her diagnosis she lives more fully than ever:

"I was a housewife, lost and aimless after my children grew up and left home. One of the first things I did after the diagnosis was go and teach myself to swim with my head in the water. I had always kept it above, too scared to put

SOMATIZATION

Charlotte has visited her physician nine times in the past year. Her complaints vary—dizziness, joint pain, difficulty swallowing, palpitations, and shortness of breath. Her physician discussed every symptom in detail, examined her carefully, and ordered appropriate tests and x-rays. *Her test results and examinations always were completely normal. No physical cause was ever identified.*

Charlotte was not imagining or faking her symptoms. She was truly suffering, and her life was significantly disrupted. Charlotte is not alone. In 25% to 50% of all visits to a primary care physician, no physical cause can be found to explain the patient's bodily symptoms. Psychological stress appears to play the major role in prompting the visit.

Physical Symptoms and Stress

Many of these patients experience *somatization*. Somatization is the reflection of psychological distress through bodily symptoms. It is the tendency to minimize the mental and emotional aspects of distress and amplify physical symptoms. Through somatization, the body speaks its mind by expressing emotional stress in terms of physical symptoms.

Somatization is quite common; we all do it to some degree. But for some people this becomes a predominant pattern. While the symptoms are not life-threatening, they can be more disabling than a major medical condition such as diabetes or heart disease.

Somatization takes a heavy toll in health and dollars. Somatizing patients may average up to five days a month in bed while most patients with major physical problems average one day or less. Somatizing patients also spend more than twice as many days in the hospital, and visit the doctor much more frequently.

A Rising Problem

Healthy people commonly experience isolated symptoms and minor illnesses. In any two-to-four week period, over 90% of all people have at least one bodily symptom. Fatigue, rashes, stiffness, diarrhea, dizziness, headache, backache, and cold/flu symptoms are very common. These are very rarely caused by serious disease. But our tolerance for mild ailments and our ability to manage stress seems to be declining. There are four factors that can cause you to amplify bodily symptoms:

1. **Your current circumstances**

2. **Your beliefs about their cause**

3. **How much attention you pay to them**

4. **Your mood and sense of well-being**

Many patients fear that their symptoms represent a serious condition. This drives them restlessly from one physician to another. Each time tests are ordered, their belief in some elusive physical

Continued on next page

cause is reinforced. The result is often frustration for both patient and doctor, and a waste of health care resources. Most importantly, the patient continues to suffer.

When confronted with unexplained physical symptoms, physicians often say "there's nothing else that can be done." This is not actually the case. Both patient and doctor can take action to reduce suffering and unnecessary procedures, and improve health.

Unexplained Symptoms

Pain, suffering, and physical symptoms can be generated by either your mind or your body. Good health care depends on identifying the source of the symptoms, and then targeting the treatment appropriately. To help manage frequent, unexplained physical symptoms:

▶ Recognize the problem. If you frequently visit the doctor with physical complaints and all the tests and exams come up normal, consider that the source of your problem may be psychological. Physical complaints and symptoms may be signals that you're distressed and not coping well.

▶ A consultation with a mental health professional might do more for you than the pursuit of medical solutions. Although the symptoms are not "all in your head," the solutions may be. Finding new ways to express yourself or get attention other than through physical symptoms can help (📖 see

page 88). Learning how to cope and relax effectively may help you feel more at ease and in control.

▶ Stick with one physician you trust— it's usually your best hope for improvement. "Doctor hopping" is unlikely to benefit you.

▶ Schedule regular visits rather than waiting until troubling symptoms arise. While waiting for your next visit, your symptoms may subside.

▶ Don't pressure your doctor to find a physical cause (there may not be one). One of the goals is to protect you from unnecessary, costly, and sometimes risky surgical or medical procedures and tests.

▶ Reduce your stress and anxiety. They can amplify normal aches, pains and bodily sensations. Practicing some of the techniques in this book should help. Learn to think more positively (📖 see page 42), relax (page 88), use imagery (page 99), calm anxiety (page 147), ease depression (page 159), and manage pain (page 217).

▶ Shift your focus away from your symptoms. Everyone has aches and pains. Expecting a perfect, pain-free life is unrealistic and sets you up for frustration and disappointment. The vast majority of symptoms improve on their own with time. The more you focus on your symptoms, the more worrisome they become. Distract yourself with pleasurable activities (📖 see page 57), or by helping other people (page 134).

my whole self in. That had been the story of my life. Now I do whatever I want. I don't think about how much time there is, just what I want to do with mine. Surprisingly, I feel less afraid of living."

A heart attack sometimes makes people decide to slow down. They would rather have more time to deepen relationships with family and friends. A chronic disease that restricts movement may lead some to think again about unused intellectual talents. Meg learned a new language and found a pen pal from that country to write to; Fred dared write the novel he always thought he was too "stupid" to do. Though chronic illness may close some doors, you can choose to open new ones.

℞ Plan for the Future

Living well with chronic illness may also involve preparing for death. Death may be feared, welcomed, accepted, or, all too often, pushed away. A large part of the fear of death is a fear of the unknown. But facing dying can intensify living. The most useful way to come to terms with your eventual death is to take positive steps to prepare for it. Here are some suggestions:

▶ Talk openly about your feelings about death. Most family and close friends are reluctant to bring up the topic, but appreciate it if you do.

▶ Finish "business." Mend relationships. Say what needs to be said to those who need to hear it. Don't leave words of love, forgiveness, and thanks unspoken. Forgive others, and yourself.

▶ Put your affairs in order. Make a will. Get your financial records organized. Make plans for your memorial.

▶ Make your wishes known. Let others

WATCH OUT

YOU ARE NOT TO BLAME

Chronic diseases are caused by a combination of genetic, biological, environmental, and psychological factors.

For example, stress alone does not cause most chronic illnesses. Mind matters, but mind cannot always triumph over matter. If you fail to recover, it is not because of lack of right mental attitude.

There are many things you can control that will help you cope with chronic illness. *Remember, you are not responsible for causing the disease or failing to cure it, but you are responsible for taking action to manage your illness.*

Key Point

know how and where you want to be during your last days, when you want life-support procedures to be stopped.

▶ Write out a *Durable Power of Attorney for Health Care* which documents your wishes and designates someone to make decisions when you cannot. Discuss these wishes with your family and physician.

Having a chronic illness doesn't have to close down your options. You can still participate actively in life, learn new and interesting skills, make a contribution, and have a rich and satisfying life.

📖 *For more information, see page 278*

20 Doctor-Patient Partnership

How to Work Effectively with Health Professionals

Once there was a time when there weren't any doctors. No nurses. No dentists. No hospitals. No lab tests. No x-rays. People treated themselves and their families. But that's now drastically changed.

Today we have access to a wide variety of skilled health professionals, dazzling medical technology, and highly effective medications. But these advances in medical care have not been without their price. Medical costs have sky-rocketed. Dissatisfaction with medical care is rising. And we have become increasingly dependent on professional medical care. Our confidence in managing our own health has declined.

Many people think there is a medical solution for every physical problem, a test for every ailment, and a pill for every pain. We present our bodies to the doctor with the expectation that he or she will fix it. Today's health care system raises some important questions:

▶ What is our responsibility for our own health?

▶ How can we take a more active role in managing our own health care?

▶ What problems can we safely and successfully treat ourselves?

▶ When should we get professional help?

▶ How can we get information to make good decisions?

Your New Role: Active Partner

Think of the health care system. You probably envision physicians, nurses, clinics, hospitals and medical laboratories. But that leaves out one crucial person—you. Today you play a critical role in the health care system. In fact, the professional medical care system *depends* on assistance from you.

The average person has about 48 new medical symptoms each year, and yet consults a physician only four times. So that means 80% to 90% of the medical symptoms people experience are self-diagnosed and self-treated. If people were to stop practicing self-care and seek professional help for even a small percentage of their complaints—colds, backaches, stomach aches, headaches, fatigue, and so on—the professional health care system would be overwhelmed. And, if people's ability to manage their own health problems increased even by a small amount, the demand for costly professional services would decrease dramatically.

Your vital role as the *primary provider of health care* for yourself and your family has not gotten the credit it deserves. Even the term *patient* carries with it a sense of

Key Point

passivity, submissiveness, and helplessness. Confidence in managing your own health problems has been undermined. The knowledge of when to self-treat and when to seek professional care has not been widely shared. If you have a medical problem and put off seeing your doctor when you really need to, you may suffer unnecessary discomfort or harm.

On the other hand, if you go to the doctor when you don't really need to, you waste time and money, and you may subject yourself to unnecessary (and possibly harmful) medical tests, medications and procedures. This can subtly erode your confidence in your own abilities. It can also work against the natural healing capacities of your own body and mind.

But a major shift is now occurring **Key Point** *in the health care system towards much greater participation by you, the patient. People are beginning to reclaim their own healing power, transforming the doctor-patient relationship.* Many patients now ask more questions of their doctors, consider a wider range of options, and educate themselves about the issues that are important to their health.

The view of the physician as an all-knowing authority, and patient as helpless and passive is changing. A new doctor-patient partnership is emerging in which the doctor's role is more like a consultant, and the patient's responsibility is to participate more actively. But as with all major changes, the road can be bumpy.

Doctors now find the ground radically shifting under them. Trading autonomy for a partnership isn't always easy. Patients are becoming more knowledgeable. They are also making greater demands, and have higher (and sometimes unrealistic) expectations. They are more apt to sue for malpractice. Insurance companies, hospitals, and group practices are putting even more constraints and demands on today's doctors. No wonder many are becoming increasingly frustrated.

The role of the patient has also become more difficult. They are asked to take more responsibility. People who are used to doctors making all the decisions and blindly following orders find themselves confronted with decisions they don't know how to make. And, for various treatments and procedures, they find themselves presented with a disturbingly long list of what can go wrong, which the doctor now must spell out for legal reasons.

So there may be some confusion as the new roles and relationships are sorted out. Meanwhile, more patience and understanding is needed as doctors and patients alike learn to work together in new ways. *A successful doctor-patient partnership is composed of knowl-* **Key Point** *edgeable, caring physicians willing to share power, and a well-informed, prepared, and assertive patient willing to take responsibility.*

Central to this transition in the traditional doctor-patient relationship is the reality that people are becoming managers of their own health and health care. And managers, whether they're running a home or a business, don't do everything themselves. They use others to get the job done. But as managers, they are responsible for the decisions, and for seeing that the decisions are carried out.

As manager of your own health care, you need to seek information from a wide variety of sources: friends, family members, books, magazines, and self-help groups. Think of your relationship with your doctor as though you hired him or her as a consultant, or hired a team of consultants including physicians and

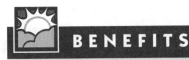

A WIN/WIN DOCTOR-PATIENT PARTNERSHIP

Patients win when they get:

▶ More respect

▶ Improved self-confidence

▶ Higher quality medical care

▶ Better health

▶ Lower medical costs

Physicians win when they get:

▶ Better information from patients to make a diagnosis and adjust treatment

▶ Better adherence to prescribed medical regimens

▶ More satisfaction from better use of their skills and knowledge

▶ More gratification when their efforts pay off in healthier patients

▶ More satisfied patients

▶ Patients who know when to seek medical care, and when and how to treat themselves

▶ Potentially greater financial reward

other health professionals. Once they have given you their best advice, it is up to you to make the decisions, and to follow through with the treatment.

Key Point *Not everyone can be an active partner all of the time. Depending on the* situation, you may wish to shift more of the responsibility for decision-making onto your physician, entrusting yourself to the best judgment and skills of your doctor. It is important for you to find a comfortable and flexible way of interacting with your doctor. It should suit both your personal preferences as well as your medical and psychological condition (☐ see box page 243).

No matter how carefully you follow the advice in this book, how well you use your mind to manage your health, or how optimistic, confident and in control you feel, it is likely that you will become a patient at some point. This chapter and the three that follow will help you summon the skills and attitudes essential for maximizing your health, whether you are sick or well.

From now on you are not only a consumer of medical care, you are also a primary health care provider. *Key Point* *Learning and using new skills will result in getting better health care.* You'll also feel increased competence about managing your own health, and this confidence itself may result in better health. Skills for better health care include:

▶ Managing common medical problems

▶ Knowing when and how to self-treat

▶ Knowing when to seek professional help

▶ Being able to communicate clearly and concisely with your physician

▶ Knowing what to ask about medical tests, medications, and surgery

▶ Knowing how to get more information on health topics (☐ see page 278)

20 Doctor-Patient

VALUE OF INVOLVEMENT

Research in mind-body health suggests that taking greater control of your medical treatment can *itself* contribute to better health. Your beliefs, attitudes, and expectations about medications or surgery have a significant effect on your body's response and recovery. And studies show that patients who interact more with their doctors and ask more questions enjoy better health outcomes.

When patients with diabetes, hypertension, and peptic ulcers were coached to be more assertive with their physicians, the result was an improvement in their health. While waiting to see their physician, trained aides reviewed the patient's medical records with them. They helped them identify important medical decisions to discuss with the doctor. They also encouraged them to ask questions, and to participate actively in the decisions. Patients were coached in how to overcome communication barriers such as embarrassment, fear of appearing foolish, or intimidation by the physician. Some patients even rehearsed their questions out loud before seeing the doctor.

These coached patients were more assertive with their doctors. They asked more questions, interrupted when necessary, and obtained a good deal more information about their medical condition. They reported better overall health and fewer limitations in their social and work life due to illness. The diabetic and hypertensive patients also demonstrated better control of blood sugar and blood pressure levels. Being actively involved in your health care pays off.

HEALTHY COMMUNICATION

"It is not enough for the doctor to stop playing God. You've got to get off your knees."

—Melvin Belsky, M.D.

The key to making the health care system work for you lies in good communication with your physician, and the other members of the health care team. But many people are intimidated by their doctors, and are afraid to communicate freely. The use of unfamiliar medical terms (jargon) is often intimidating, and it's easy to get confused. One study revealed that a quarter of college-educated people misunderstood the meaning of such common medical terms as *hypertension, virus, herpes, tumor, pap smear, strep throat,* and *uterus*—let alone more complex medical terminology.

And yet patients are often reluctant to ask their doctor what a word means because they are afraid of looking stupid. They hesitate to ask why a test or treatment is needed for fear of appearing to challenge the doctor's authority. And many times patients conceal personal concerns about such things as sexuality, drug abuse, emotional problems, and cancer or other delicate issues. This blocks vital communication with the doctor.

Physicians share the responsibility for

KNOW WHAT'S POSSIBLE

Although many doctors do not communicate well, there are inspiring examples of how some do talk and listen to their patients. Consider the wonderful communication skill of a Houston cancer specialist described by Norman Cousins:

When he gets patients with a new diagnosis of cancer, he sits down with them and tells them he's convinced they are going to make it. He tells them it's nonsense to equate the word "cancer" with death. He says he has an excellent treatment for their condition, and that they have an excellent treatment of their own—their body's own natural healing processes.

"And you can activate that healing process," he tells them, "by building up your confidence in yourself and your confidence in me. Build up your joy, your appreciation of life, and your urge to do everything you've always wanted to do." He tells them that they have one of the most magical systems the world has ever known for the treatment of disease.

"Now," he says, "Here's the partnership I propose. I'll work with you on the things you'll be doing to build up your confidence, your joy, your hope, and your faith. Beginning tomorrow, I'm going to introduce you to five other patients who had exactly the same kind of cancer you have and came through it successfully. I'm going to make sure you receive the best treatment medical science has to offer. We're going to have a lot going for us, and I'm convinced that we can whip this thing, and that you can make it." Then he holds out his hand and says, "Now how about a partnership?" They always take his hand.

Of course, every encounter with a doctor is not like that. The doctor, the patient, and the clinical situation don't always allow for such unbridled confidence. Still, you can hope for that level of encouraging communication. And there is a lot you can do to insure that you get the information you need, and, at the same time, help your doctor communicate better with you.

poor communication. Sometimes they feel too busy or important to take the time to talk with patients. And sometimes they may ignore questions, use jargon, or respond in an unsupportive way to your attempts to assert yourself.

Remember, doctors are human, too. They have bad days, they get headaches, they have family problems. And they get frustrated by paperwork. And sometimes they make mistakes, like everyone else. Or your doctor may feel discouraged—like you—when treatments don't work in spite of the best intentions.

You don't have to think of your doctor as your best friend, but you should expect this person to be attentive, caring, able to listen, and able to explain things clearly to you. You also have to do your part. As an involved patient you need to:

- Be assertive in a polite manner (not challenging, confrontational, or aggressive) (📖 see page 126)

- Be respectful of your own and your doctor's needs

- Express your feelings and concerns openly and honestly

- Ask questions

- Be persistent

If your physician is unable to communicate clearly with you in spite of your best efforts, you probably need to find a new one. Remember, your doctor is there to help and support you.

How to Communicate with Your Doctor

One of the realities of medical care today is that physicians are often pressed for time. We all wish they had more time to discuss things, explain things, and explore options. The time constraints make it even more essential that you prepare for your visit, and use your time to maximum advantage. Although the advice below is written to support your communication with your doctor, it also applies to your interaction with nurses, pharmacists, dentists, physical therapists, psychotherapists, or any other member of your health care team.

BEFORE YOUR VISIT

℞ Prepare a List

Have you ever thought to yourself after you walked out of the office, "Why didn't I ask about...?" Preparing a list of your observations, concerns, and questions *ahead of time* helps insure they get addressed. Here are some things to do:

❑ Decide what you want to get out of this visit to the doctor.

❑ Before a visit make a written list of your most important questions or concerns.

❑ Be realistic. If you have a dozen problems and questions, the doctor probably can't adequately deal with

them all in one visit. So prioritize your main concerns or problems.

❑ Prepare notes about your symptoms:

- When they started

- How long they last

- Exactly where they are located

- What makes them worse; what makes them better

- What treatments you have already tried

- What you think might be causing the problem

❑ If you have questions that you are uneasy about, practice discussing them ahead of time. Or write them down and hand the paper to your doctor.

❑ Bring a list of all the medications (both

prescription and nonprescription) that you are taking, or bring the containers and show them to your doctor.

❑ If you have previous medical records or test results which might be relevant to your condition, bring them along. Or have them sent from elsewhere.

This checklist will help you clearly state your major concerns, and answer concisely the questions your physician is likely to ask. It provides vital information to help in your diagnosis and treatment.

DURING THE VISIT

℞ Present Your Concerns First

The first few moments of the visit are the most important. Be sure to state your concerns at the very beginning of the interview because that's when the purpose of the visit is best clarified.

Key Point

A study of medical visits found that physicians allowed patients to talk an average of only 18 seconds before interrupting them with questions. Take the initiative and use this time to list briefly your concerns. They will then form the agenda for the visit. For example, you might say, "I have several things that I'd like to discuss with you today if there is time. The things that most concern me are my shoulder pain, my dizziness, and the possible side effects from one of my medications."

Be straightforward and honest. If you are concerned about a sexual problem, difficulty with bladder control, or cancer, don't disguise your concern. And don't wait until the end of the visit to bring it up. It's very frustrating for both you and the doctor when concerns are brought up

at the end of a visit ("Oh, by the way, could you look at this odd-looking growth..."), and there isn't enough time to give it the attention it deserves.

℞ Be Concise and Specific

In well over 70% of cases your description of symptoms alone leads to a correct diagnosis. You are the expert about how you feel and how you experience symptoms. By telling your story you can share your expertise with the physician, and help increase the odds of a speedy and accurate diagnosis.

Key Point

When the doctor asks a question, try to answer it as concisely and specifically as you can. If asked when the symptom started, "a while ago," is not very helpful. Was it a few minutes ago, or hours, days, years, or decades?

If you've been having numbness in your right thumb and index finger, for example, say that, rather than "my hands are numb." The more specific you can be (without overdoing it with irrelevant details), the clearer a picture the doctor will have of your problem, and the less time will be wasted for both of you.

℞ Be Open and Honest

Try to be as open as you can in sharing your thoughts, feelings, and fears with your doctor. Remember, your physician is not a mindreader. If you are worried, try to explain why: "I am worried that what I have is contagious"; "My father had similar symptoms before he died"; "I think my symptoms are caused by (a recent trip to Mexico, stress, chemicals at work, a change in weather, etc.)."

Share your hunches or guesses about what might be causing your symptoms, as they often provide vital clues to an accurate diagnosis. Even if it turns out your guesses are not correct, it gives your doctor the opportunity to reassure you or address your hidden concerns.

If, for some reason, you don't think you can (or will) follow the doctor's advice, say so. For example, "I don't think I will take the aspirin because it badly upsets my stomach," or "I don't think I can afford that medication. It isn't covered by my insurance." If your doctor knows why you are unlikely to follow advice, alternative suggestions can sometimes be made to help you overcome the barriers. If you don't talk about the barriers to following the instructions, it's hard for your doctor to help you.

℞ Ask Questions

Your most powerful tool in the doctor-patient partnership is the question. You can fill in vitally important missing pieces of information and close critical gaps in communication with your questions. And asking all your questions reflects your active participation in the process of care, a critical ingredient to restoring your health.

Key Point

To help you better understand the power of questions, we suggest ones you might ask whenever medical tests are ordered (📖 see page 247), medications are prescribed (page 256), or surgery is recommended (page 267). Don't be afraid to ask what you may consider a "stupid" question. It often indicates an important concern or misunderstanding.

℞ Share in Medical Decisions

Many decisions in medical care are not clear-cut, and often there is more than one option. The best decisions, except in life-threatening emergencies, depend on your values and preferences, and should not be left solely to your doctor. For example, if you have high blood pressure you might say, "I'm very conservative about taking medications. What's a reasonable period of time for me to try exercise, diet, and relaxation first, before I start taking the medication?"

To make an informed choice about any treatment, you need to know what the cost and risks of the proposed treatment are. This includes the likelihood of possible complications such as drug reactions, bleeding, infection, injury or death. It also includes the personal costs such as lost time from work, and financial considerations such as how much of the proposed treatments your insurance will cover.

You also need to understand how likely it is that the proposed treatments will benefit you in terms of:

▶ Prolonging your life

▶ Relieving your symptoms

▶ Improving your ability to function

Sometimes the best choice may be to delay a decision about treatment in favor of "watchful waiting."

No one can tell you which choice is right for you. But to make an informed choice, you need information about the treatment options. Informed choice, not merely informed consent, is essential to quality medical care. The best medical care for you combines your doctor's medical expertise with your own knowledge, skills, and values.

℞ Be Clear on the Instructions

When appropriate, ask your physician to write down instructions. Or ask how to get more information on a particular subject.

MAKING A MEDICAL DECISION

Suppose you're having trouble with your knees, and your doctor lays out all the alternatives, one of which is surgery. He or she also describes the benefits and risks of each. Then the doctor says, "It's completely up to you."

This can be a bewildering moment if you are unsure as to what to do. And you may take your doctor's evenhandedness as indifference, which only adds to your uncertainty. You may even long for the old days when an authoritarian physician decisively ordered surgery or prescribed specific medications—in short, made the decision for you. No one is promising that being an active partner in your own health care is always simple, easy, or comfortable. But the decisions to be made are yours. How do you handle it? Here are some suggestions:

▶ Ask the doctor, "What would *you* do if you were me?"

▶ Or ask, "If I was a member of your family, what would you recommend?"

▶ Ask if you could speak to other similar patients who have been through making this decision.

▶ Bring a tape recorder so you can listen to the conversation with your full attention after you leave the office. You can also play it for others and get their reactions.

▶ Ask for the best way to get questions answered if you have any after you leave the office.

▶ Get a second opinion from your primary care physician or another doctor (📖 see page 268).

▶ Don't rush to a decision. If it's not an emergency, tell your doctor you need more time to think it over.

Taking some of these steps may seem awkward or time-consuming. But it may take some extra effort to assure yourself. You want to be certain that the choice you make is the very best one for you. After you have made your decision, relax, trust your doctor, trust your body, and hope for the best.

If you tend to have trouble remembering instructions, take notes during the visit, or bring someone else along to act as a second listener or take notes for you. Another set of eyes and ears can help you remember the details, and you can discuss them together when you leave the office.

AT END OF VISIT

℞ Repeat Key Points

It is extremely helpful to repeat these five key points to your doctor at the end of your visit:

1. The diagnosis (the nature and cause of your symptoms, or what might be causing your symptoms)

2. The prognosis (the expected duration, course, and outcome of your condition)

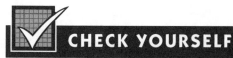

ACTIVE PARTNER CHECKLIST

Before Your Visit

❑ Prepare a list of concerns, questions, and observations

During Your Visit

❑ Present your concerns at the beginning

❑ Be specific and concise

❑ Be open and honest

❑ Ask questions

❑ Share in medical decisions

❑ Be clear on the instructions

At the End of Your Visit

❑ Repeat back key points

❑ Know the follow-up plan

❑ Give feedback to your doctor

3. The doctor's treatment recommendations and instructions

4. The follow-up plan

5. What you are going to do

This confirms that you clearly understand the most important information. Repeating also gives the doctor a chance to correct any misunderstanding. If you don't understand or remember something the physician said, admit that you need to go over it again. You might say, for example, "I'm pretty certain you told me this before, but I'm not clear on it."

℞ Know the Follow-up Plan

Before you leave the office, make sure you understand the next steps:

▶ Should you return for a visit?

▶ If so, when and why?

▶ Should you phone for test results?

▶ Are there any danger signs you should watch for and report back to your physician?

℞ Give Feedback to Your Doctor

Your doctor needs to know how satisfied you are with your care. If you don't like the way you have been treated by your doctor or someone else on the team, let him or her know. If you have been unable to follow the doctor's advice or had problems with a treatment, tell your doctor so that adjustments can be made.

Also, most physicians very much appreciate compliments and positive feedback. Doctors are human, and praise is very nourishing for a busy, hard-working professional. One of the best ways to make doctors feel good about helping you is to let them know you appreciate their efforts. Patients are often hesitant about praising their doctors, but if you are very pleased, let your physician know. You might say, "I really appreciate your taking the time to explain that so clearly to me," or drop your doctor a note to express your thanks.

📖 *For more information, see page 278*

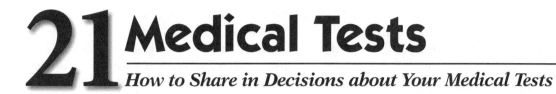

21 Medical Tests

How to Share in Decisions about Your Medical Tests

Solving a medical problem is like solving a mystery. The problem is presented, clues are discovered, confirming evidence is sought, possibilities are tracked down, and finally, a diagnosis is made.

There are three main sources of information (clues) on which to base a medical diagnosis:

1. The first—and usually most helpful—is your medical history: your own description of what has happened

2. The next is the physical examination

3. The third is the results of diagnostic tests and procedures

The information, gathered from these three sources, is evaluated to reach a diagnosis. The diagnosis names and explains your problem, and guides your treatment.

The New World of Medical Tests

Gone are the days when medical tests only meant a microscope and a drop of blood or some urine. High-tech, high-cost medical testing is now a burgeoning industry, accounting for nearly a third of our national health bill. No bodily fluid, opening, or cavity is beyond the reach of a medical probe. There are blood and urine tests, x-rays, biopsies, taps, scans, electronic monitors, and tiny viewing instruments that can peer into nearly

every part of the body.

More than 10 billion medical tests are done in the U.S. each year. That's over 40 tests per person. The cost is a staggering $140 billion, or an average of $600 for each of us every year. Patients cannot afford to take a passive role in this important phase of their medical care.

The Use and Misuse of Tests

Medical tests can save lives and improve the quality of life. Good reasons for doing a medical test are:

▶ To help your doctor diagnose symptoms accurately

▶ To monitor the progress of a known disease

▶ To screen for a hidden disease

But many unnecessary tests are performed for other reasons. Doctors sometimes order tests to protect themselves from malpractice. One survey found that at least three out of every four doctors admitted having ordered tests for the sole purpose of having a better defense, should a patient bring a suit against them. Unnecessary tests may also be ordered because they are personally profitable. Physicians can sometimes earn more by ordering tests and doing diagnostic procedures than by taking the same amount of time to question, examine, counsel or think about a patient's problem.

Data from several studies suggest that at least 25% of all medical tests contribute very little to patient care; yet they contribute a lot to patient bills. When researchers studied 2,000 patients hospitalized for surgery, for example, they found that 60% of the blood tests routinely ordered were unnecessary. Of these tests, only one in about 400 revealed an abnormality that might change pre-operative management.

Further, in those rare cases where abnormalities were detected, the results were ignored, presumably because they were either not noticed or were dismissed as not significant. The researchers concluded that if a thorough history turned up no hint of a medical problem, most routine testing at the time of hospital admission is a waste.

Patient demand, real or imagined, also affects the number of tests that are done. Many patients feel that more tests means better care. People often say, "My doctor is so thorough, he did nearly every test available." *Although tests can provide a measure of reassurance, an accurate diagnosis can be made 80% to 90% of the time with a thorough history and physical exam alone—without tests.*

Key Point

The challenge is to have the right tests done at the right time. Consider Anne, a 45-year-old woman complaining of a mild burning discomfort in her upper abdomen. It had gone on for about two weeks. Her doctor asked her several brief questions, examined her abdomen, and ordered "a few tests": a urinalysis, a 12-test blood panel, a complete blood count, and an upper GI series (x-rays that outline the esophagus and stomach).

All these studies added an extra $2000 to her bill, but they did little to change her doctor's suspected diagnosis of reflux esophagitis, an inflammation caused by back-up of stomach acid into the esophagus. Nor did the tests affect her treatment (antacids). The most likely diagnosis and treatment could have been determined from her description of her symptoms without a lot of testing. In this respect she was *overtested*. But she was also *undertested*. In the previous five years, she hadn't had a mammogram or pap smear, important cancer-screening tests generally recommended for women her age.

Shared Decisions

Patients are not helpless in the face of overtesting or undertesting. You may be surprised to learn that except for life-threatening emergencies, doctors cannot order medical tests (or surgical procedures or treatments, for that matter) without your permission. Though most doctors make sure they get written consent for tests with significant risks—those requiring general anesthesia, or the insertion of tubes or catheters—other tests are usually "ordered" without much explanation.

You can help assure that your medical tests are not "just what the doctor ordered," but what you really need. In practice, most doctors simply order tests without much explanation. And most patients go along with such "orders," never exercising their right to ask questions or make the final decisions.

When your physician recommends a test, you should ask certain questions described below. For most minor tests, you need only assure yourself that the test is necessary and safe. However, if the test is complex, expensive, uncomfortable, or potentially harmful, you would be well advised to gather more complete information. Clear communication is the key. In some cases, a second opinion may be worthwhile before agreeing to the test.

Medical tests sometimes save lives, but in other cases, they are unnecessary, anxiety-provoking, and may actually be harmful. A frank, informed discussion with your doctor is the best way to decide if tests are needed, and what the results might mean.

QUESTIONS ABOUT MEDICAL TESTS

WHAT TO TELL YOUR DOCTOR

If your doctors don't ask, volunteer this information:

Are you taking any medications?
Report to your physician the names and dosages of all the prescription and non-prescription medications that you are taking. Include birth control pills, aspirin, and ibuprofen.

Have you had any allergic or unusual reactions to medications, anesthetics, or x-ray contrast materials?
Be as specific as possible about the medication or anesthetic you had, and exactly what your reaction was to it. This information can be life-saving.

Do you have any major chronic diseases or other medical conditions?
Some diseases can complicate or interfere with a test. Tell the doctor if you have a history of bleeding problems, or if you think you might be pregnant.

WHAT TO ASK YOUR DOCTOR

Why do I need this test?
The most important question is whether the test is necessary to diagnose your problem or change your treatment. Ask the questions:

▸ What happens if the result is *abnormal*?

▸ What happens if the result is *normal*?

If the answers are the same, then you probably don't need the test.

"Because you need it" or "because we usually do it in this situation" are not satisfactory answers. Here's an example of a better explanation: "I'm recommending a scoping exam of your colon because you've been passing blood in your stool. A previous test shows the blood isn't due to hemorrhoids, so we need to find the source of the bleeding. It may be quite harmless, but it could also be a serious problem such as a bowel cancer, and that would need prompt treatment."

Ask about alternatives. For example, if you have already had the proposed test, find out if those earlier results can be used. It is wise to keep a record of all your medical tests. Record when and where the tests were done, and the results.

Also ask your physician about the risk of postponing the test. *Sometimes the best test is the test of time.* Monitoring the symptoms under a doctor's supervision may allow time for new diagnostic clues to emerge or for the symptoms to go away on their own.

Sometimes medical tests are recommended for healthy people without symptoms. Ask about these screening tests so you can decide if they are worthwhile for you (📖 see box page 248).

DO YOU NEED TESTS IF YOU FEEL HEALTHY?

Each year patients faithfully flock to their doctors for their annual physical exams and testing. But is all this testing really necessary if you are generally healthy and have no symptoms?

Doctors and patients alike tend to assume that if a few tests are good, more must be better. Unfortunately, very few screening tests have been shown to be of benefit. Here are the main issues in determining if a screening test is worthwhile:

> **Key Point**

▶ **Significant Risk.** The screening test must be used only for those people at significant risk for the particular disease or condition. For example, people over age 50 or with a family history of colon cancer are at increased risk and more likely to benefit from regular colon cancer screening tests. *There is no such thing as a standard package of screening tests for everyone.* The tests you need should be selected based on your age, sex, race, or medical or family history.

> **Key Point**

▶ **Accurate Early Detection.** The screening test must reliably detect a significant disease before symptoms develop. If a test is not sensitive enough to identify people with the disease, then many diseased people will be missed ("false negatives"). On the other hand, if the test shows that many healthy people have the disease ("false positives"), further testing, sometimes risky and expensive, may be required.

▶ **Effective Early Treatment.** The treatment must be proved to extend lives or improve the quality of life. For example, if a screening chest x-ray reveals an *incurable* lung cancer, the person would not survive any longer because of early diagnosis and treatment. The test merely informs the person of the cancer earlier. Early diagnosis and treatment does seem to make a difference for such conditions as high blood pressure, HIV disease, as well as breast, cervical, and colon cancer.

▶ **Acceptable Cost.** Since screening tests are usually performed on large numbers of people, the expense of even low-cost tests can mount rapidly. Screening tests should prove worthwhile in terms of prolonged life and decreased suffering to justify the cost.

Only a few tests currently meet these evidence-based requirements. There are many "gray zones" in which the benefits are as yet uncertain and unproved. At which age should women begin to have mammograms? Who needs to have cholesterol screening, and how often? Does screening for prostate cancer extend lives? In the absence of strong proof for benefits, most people would do well to forgo the test. Keep the above points in mind as you discuss with your doctor what screening tests might be helpful to you.

Remember that what's most important to your health often doesn't show up on medical tests at all. The truth is that a healthy lifestyle can do more for your health than all the screening tests in the world.

What are the risks?

No test is entirely risk free. Begin your evaluation by weighing the balance between potential benefits and risks. To start with, the test results may be wrong. An inaccurate result can lead to a wrong diagnosis, or delayed or inappropriate treatment. A "false positive" or an abnormal finding when you're actually healthy might label you as "sick." This could provoke needless anxiety and job or insurance difficulties.

There can also be direct physical risks. Anytime your body is penetrated by a needle, tube, or viewing instrument, there is some risk of infection, bleeding, or damage to vital structures. The hazards of radiation exposure, though minimal, must also be considered. Reactions to anesthetics, drugs, or dye-contrast materials used in certain imaging techniques may also produce complications. Physical risks vary depending upon the nature of the test, your age, past medical history, general state of health, and ability to cooperate, plus the skill and experience of your physician.

How do I prepare for the test?

For some tests, preparation is very important. Ask whether there is anything special you should do before the test, such as fast or discontinue medications. Some tests cannot be done or interpreted correctly if you don't prepare properly. For example, eating breakfast may interfere with a "fasting" blood-sugar test for diabetes, or if your bowel isn't cleaned out thoroughly, a barium enema may have to be repeated. Also find out if there may be a long wait. If so, bring along something to read or do. Finally, check whether you'll need help getting home after the test.

What will the test be like?

For many tests, knowing how it's done and how it will feel can decrease your anxiety and discomfort before and during a test. You may want to know:

▶ *Will it hurt?*

▶ *How long will it take?*

▶ *How will I feel afterward?*

▶ *How is the test done?*

▶ *Who will perform the test?*

Health professionals tend to significantly *underestimate* the physical and mental discomfort of tests. The physician may see the patient only briefly, and may not fully appreciate the inconvenience or discomfort before and after the procedure.

Patients, on the other hand, tend to *overestimate* the discomfort before a test. They prepare for the worst. Afterwards, they often say, "It wasn't nearly as bad as I expected."

The amount of discomfort can vary considerably according to the skill, gentleness, and sensitivity level of the professional doing the test. With certain tests such as a pelvic exam, sigmoidoscopy (to check the rectum) or a barium enema, discomfort may be due more to embarrassment than pain. It helps to remember that the physician and staff understand how you feel. If you are particularly anxious, try talking about it beforehand.

During and after the test, it is important to let the doctor or assistants know what you are feeling. If you're uncomfortable, something can usually be done. But if you don't speak up, there's no way to help you. Besides, your sensations may provide the first clue to stopping a developing complication.

What do the results mean?

No test is 100% accurate. When faced with an abnormal result, the natural tendency is to assume that you have a disease. But the test may be a "false positive," a test result that is wrong. It incorrectly indicates *ill health* when the patient is actually well. A false positive can be caused by:

▶ A mistake in measurement

▶ A mistake in recording (you may be given the results of another person's test)

▶ A statistical error based on the way "normal" is defined

How normal values are set. The "normal," or reference values for many blood and urine tests are often established by testing young, white, healthy volunteers—often lab technicians or medical students. The "normal range" is then set to include only 95% of those healthy people. *So approximately 5% of healthy patients will have abnormal or borderline values on any given lab test. Statistically, if you have 12 separate tests done, you run nearly a 50% chance of having one "abnormal" result, even though you are healthy.* If you are older, overweight, non-white, or otherwise differ significantly from the reference group, the "normal" range may not be appropriate for you.

Key Point

"Normal" usually only means "average." Your tests results are compared with averages that are typical of our general population. But "normal" in this sense does not necessarily mean healthy, optimal, or desirable. For example, although your blood pressure or cholesterol levels may be "normal" (average), that doesn't necessarily mean they're fine; lower levels may actually be healthier.

False negatives. *On the other hand, normal test results do not necessarily indicate health.* A certain percentage of tests are "false negatives"— *normal* results even though the person is

Key Point

actually *sick.* Many smokers, for example, are falsely reassured by a "negative" (normal) chest x-ray. Yet a chest x-ray is not necessarily a sensitive test for early detection of lung cancer or emphysema.

Other causes of test inaccuracies. Medications, exercise, stress, eating, or time of day can influence certain test results. And even in the best laboratories, a small percentage of results may be wrong because of variation in test reagents, or errors in handling or labeling test specimens.

Interpretations of medical tests are often subjective, although they give the impression of being objective and precise. Some tests, such as x-rays, electrocardiograms, and scoping procedures require human interpretation, and can miss important abnormalities. A study of chest x-ray interpretation, for example, found that more than 70% of the reports contained disagreements among experienced radiologists. In 25% of the reports, doctors missed important findings. So getting an experienced second opinion on a diagnosis may be important, particularly when serious symptoms are present, or when risky therapies or procedures are prescribed on the basis of one abnormal test.

Above all, remember that medical tests contribute only one piece of the diagnostic puzzle. To get the full picture, this piece must always be seen in combination with the other information about you: your medical history, age, family, habits, medications, symptoms, and the physical examination. Good medical care treats patients—not test results.

📖 *For more information, see page 279*

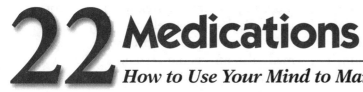

22 Medications

How to Use Your Mind to Manage Your Medicines

When something feels wrong with our body, we reach for the pills. Americans take nearly 40 billion doses of medication a year. Over a lifetime, that amounts to nearly 76,000 pills per person, almost a thousand a year, birth to death!

Thousands of lives are saved or improved with medications such as antibiotics, heart drugs, bronchodilators, and insulin. But we pay a price: all medications have undesirable side effects. Some are predictable and minor; others are unexpected and life-threatening. From 5% to 10% of all hospital admissions—and many deaths during hospitalization—are due primarily to bad reactions to drugs. And most medications are not curative. Instead, they relieve symptoms, improve functioning, prevent future disease, or make the unbearable bearable.

So reaching for a pill may not always be the best solution. When given time to work, your body is often its own best healer. The "prescriptions" filled in your body's internal pharmacy are usually safer and more effective than any drug. Non-drug treatments such as relaxation, effective communication, healthy thinking, and the use of humor support your internal healing system, without the undesirable side effects. So consider every option before choosing pills. There simply isn't "a pill for every ill."

If you do take medications, call on your internal healing system to get the most benefit from them. How you think about your medications can often determine whether you use them safely, and, most importantly, how your body responds to the medication. Your attitude plays a critical role in reducing the risks and maximizing the benefits of the pills you take.

The Placebo Effect in Your Brain

Any medication sets off two reactions in your body. The first is determined by the chemical nature of the medication. The second is triggered by your beliefs and expectations for the medication. *Any time you take medications, your beliefs and confidence can change your body chemistry and your symptoms. This reaction is called the "placebo effect."*

Thousands of scientific studies have now demonstrated the power of the placebo—the power of our mind. When people take a plain sugar pill, about one-third of them improve. Placebos relieve headaches, ulcers, asthma, arthritis, hay fever, colds, warts, constipation, angina, insomnia, and pain after surgery. Cholesterol levels, blood pressure, blood counts, gastric acidity, and even immune function have been altered by taking a placebo.

No system in the body is immune to the placebo effect. For example, a woman with unremitting nausea and vomiting is given a "new" medication by her doctors. They assure her that within minutes her symptoms will be relieved. Sure enough, within 20 minutes she reports less nausea, the vomiting stops, and her stomach contractions return to normal. The drug she was given was *ipecac*, a medication that *induces* vomiting. Her belief in the "new" medication was so strong that it counteracted the specific pharmacological action of the drug.

Our beliefs and expectations can also work against us. In one classic experiment, medical students were given a sugar pill they believed to be either a stimulant or an antidepressant. About half of them reported side effects such as dizziness, watery eyes, or abdominal pain, and had measurable changes in their blood pressure and heart rates.

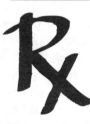 *Your internal pharmacy has its own personal interpretation of the medication you take.* Injections and capsules are interpreted as more powerful than pills. Small yellow placebo pills seem to work well for depression; while large blue placebo pills work better as sedatives. And the more bitter tasting the medicine or the more unpleasant the treatment, the more likely it is that the placebo will "work."

The way the doctor prescribes a treatment also affects our response. When it is with an enthusiastic endorsement, patients get more relief compared with the same treatment offered in a skeptical manner. When some patients are told to expect immediate improvement and others are told that their improvement will be delayed, the patients expecting an immediate effect get it; the others' improvement is delayed.

How beliefs translate into physiological changes is not known. In studies of pain relief following extraction of wisdom teeth, the placebo appears to relieve pain by releasing endorphins, powerful opiate-like pain-relieving chemicals. Endorphins are produced by the body's pain regulation system. However it works, the placebo effect clearly demonstrates that our positive beliefs and expectations turn on our self-healing mechanisms. You can learn to take advantage of your powerful internal pharmacy.

℞ How to Use Your Mind to Manage Your Medicines

Every time you take a medication, you are swallowing your expectations and beliefs as well as the pill.

℞ Expect the Best

The key to taking advantage of your internal pharmacy is to develop positive expectations. Here's how:

Examine the beliefs you have about the treatment. If you tell yourself, "I'm not a pill taker," or, "Medications always give me bad side effects," how do you think your body is likely to respond? If you don't think the prescribed treatment is likely to help your symptoms or condition, your negative beliefs will undermine the therapeutic effect. You can challenge those negative stories and change them to more positive ones (📖 see page 42).

Many people find it easier to associate healthful images with vitamins than with medications. Each vitamin pill affirms that the person taking it is doing something positive to prevent disease and promote health. If you regard all medications as health-restoring and health-promoting, like vitamins, more powerful mental benefits might be realized.

Imagine how the medicine is helping you. Develop a mental image of how the medication is helping your body. For example, if you are taking thyroid hormone replacement medication, tell yourself it is filling a missing link in your body's chemical chains, and helping to balance and regulate your metabolism.

For some, forming a vivid mental image is helpful. An antibiotic, for example, might be seen as a strong broom sweeping germs out of the body (📖 see page 106).

Don't worry if your image of what's happening chemically inside of you is not 100% physiologically correct. It's your belief in a clear, positive image that counts.

Keep in mind why you are taking the medication. "Because my doctor told me to" is not nearly as effective as understanding how the medication is helping you. Suppose you are given chemotherapy for cancer. You've been told that it is highly toxic and that it's likely to cause your hair to fall out and nauseate you. How do you think you will feel?

You could revise the expectation. Think of chemotherapy as a very powerful medication designed to kill rapidly producing cells like cancer cells. Other rapidly growing cells in your body may also be affected, such as the cells that line your hair follicles and your stomach. But fortunately, your healthy cells can recover and reproduce themselves, while the weak, poorly formed cancer cells are killed off. So if you have nausea or hair loss, remember it's temporary, and that the primary effect of chemotherapy is to destroy the cancer cells.

℞ Don't Miss Your Medicine

Joe is taking a medication to lower his high blood pressure. He often forgets to take his pills, and he's not even aware of how often he misses them. When his doctor asks him, Joe says he probably forgets his pills once or twice a month. His doctor is baffled. Joe's blood pressure just isn't responding to the medication the way it should. The doctor is about to prescribe an additional blood pressure medication.

No matter what medicine is prescribed, it won't do you any good if you don't take it. Just the act of *remembering* to take your medications may itself have a powerful benefit. Several studies suggest that patients who faithfully take their medications, *even if the medication is a placebo*, do better than those who don't.

People tend to overestimate their pill taking. When patients are asked about taking their medicine, only 7% report that they don't take them regularly. Yet when their medication-taking is monitored, nearly 50% actually miss doses more than one or two days a week. There are many reasons people don't regularly take their medications (📖 see box page 254).

Whatever reason you have for not taking your medicine, talk about it to your doctor or someone else you trust. Often an adjustment or some information can make it easier. For example, if you are

MISSING YOUR MEDICINES?

❑ Do you tend to be forgetful?

❑ Are you confused about the instructions for how and when to use the medications?

❑ Is the schedule for taking your medications too complicated?

❑ Do your medications have bothersome side effects?

❑ Is your medicine too expensive for you to be able to afford?

❑ Do you feel your disease is not serious or bothersome enough to need regular medications (some diseases such as high blood pressure, high cholesterol, or early diabetes may not have any symptoms)?

❑ Do you feel that the treatment is unlikely to help?

❑ Are you denying that you have a disease that needs treatment?

❑ Have you had a bad experience with the medicine you are supposed to be taking, or another medication?

❑ Do you know someone who had a bad experience with the medication, and you're afraid that something similar will happen with you?

❑ Are you afraid of becoming addicted to the medication?

❑ Are you embarrassed about taking the medication, view it as a sign of weakness or failure, or fear you'll be judged negatively if people know about it?

currently taking five different medications, sometimes one (or more) can be eliminated. Or if you take one medication three times a day and another four times a day, your doctor may be able to simplify the regimen, so you only need to take them once or twice a day. If the cost of the medication is a significant barrier, let your doctor know. Often an equally effective but less expensive medication can be substituted. If psychological barriers stand in your way, be frank with your doctor. Your fears and beliefs may be keeping you from getting a medication your body needs. If you don't understand how your medication can help you, ask. Understanding more about your medications will help motivate you to take them regularly.

℞ Communicate, Communicate

The goal of your medication treatment is to maximize the benefits and minimize the risks. This usually means taking the fewest medications in the lowest effective doses for the shortest period of time. *In a good doctor-patient partnership, you actively participate in determining your need for a medication, and its appropriate use.*

Key Point

How does a doctor know whether or not to prescribe a medication in the first place? In most cases, your doctor depends on the information you provide about your symptoms. This is critical.

How does your doctor know how well the medication is working? In most cases, again, your report is critical. You must

TRACKING YOUR MEDICATIONS

If you want to know how often you really forget your medications, keep a written record. Write out your medication calendar, and check off each time you take the medicine (see example below). You can also count out a week's supply, and see how many pills are left at the end of the week.

	Time	Drug Name and Strength	Amt	1 M	2 T	3 W	4 Th	5 F	6 Sa	7 Su
Morning	8 am	Micronase 5 mg	2	✓	✓	✓		✓	✓	✓
	8 am	Lisinopril 5 mg	1	✓	✓	✓		✓	✓	✓
	8 am	Azmacort inhaler	3	✓	✓	✓		✓	✓	✓
	8 am	Motrin 600 mg with food	1	✓		✓		✓		✓
Afternoon	1 pm	Azmacort inhaler	3	✓	✓	✓		✓	✓	✓
	1 pm	Motrin 600 mg with food	1	✓	✓	✓		✓	✓	✓
Evening	6 pm	Micronase 5 mg	2	✓		✓		✓	✓	✓
	6 pm	Lisinopril 5 mg	1	✓		✓		✓	✓	✓
	6 pm	Azmacort inhaler	3	✓		✓		✓	✓	✓

MEDICATION CALENDAR Month: April

Notice that some medications are missed in this example. Keeping a calendar like this allows you to see which medications are missed and when.

communicate any change in your symptoms, or any side effects.

Unfortunately, this vital interchange too often doesn't happen. Fewer than 5% of all patients receiving new prescriptions ask any questions, and doctors tend to interpret silence as understanding. Mishaps occur because patients don't receive adequate information about medications. They often don't understand how to take them, or fail to follow the instructions. You must ask questions about any medications you are prescribed (see next pages).

Many patients are reluctant to ask their doctor questions. They are often afraid of appearing ignorant, or they're concerned about challenging the doctor's authority. But asking questions is a necessary part of a healthy doctor-patient relationship. Whether the medications you take are helpful or harmful might depend on how much you know about your medications, and how well you communicate with your doctor. Don't be shy.

QUESTIONS ABOUT MEDICATIONS

WHAT TO TELL YOUR DOCTOR

If your doctors don't ask, be sure to volunteer this information:

Are you taking medications now?

Report the names and dosages of all the prescription and nonprescription medications that you are currently taking. Include birth control pills, vitamins, aspirin, antacids, and laxatives. This is especially important if you are seeing more than one physician. One may not know what the others have prescribed.

Knowing all the medications is often essential to correct diagnosis and to avoid problems from drug interactions. Be sure to carry with you an up-to-date list of all medications you are taking.

Telling the doctor that you are taking "little green pills" usually doesn't help identify the medication. Sometimes it is very beneficial to "brown bag it." Bring in all your medications (including over-the-counter medications) in a bag so that your doctor can review them. He or she can advise you as to which ones you should continue, which ones to stop, and which ones to discard.

Have you had allergic or unusual reactions to any medications?

Be specific. Say which medications, and exactly what type of reaction. A rash, fever, or wheezing that develops after taking a medication is often an allergic reaction. Nausea, ringing in the ears, lightheadedness, and agitation are likely to be side effects rather than true drug allergies.

Do you have any major chronic diseases or other medical condition?

Some diseases can interfere with the action of a particular drug or increase the risk of using certain medications. Diseases involving the kidneys or liver are especially important to mention since these diseases can slow the metabolism of many drugs and increase toxic effects.

Let your doctor know if you are breastfeeding, possibly pregnant, or planning to get pregnant. Many drugs cannot be used safely in these situations. Also tell the doctor what medications were tried in the past to treat your disease.

If you have a chronic disease, keep your own written record of the effect of any treatments tried in the past. This could help you avoid ineffective repetition.

What do you think might make it difficult to take the medication?

Try to anticipate any barriers to taking medications such as cost, complexity of the regimen, fear of side effects, or conflict with your usual lifestyle. If you are not confident about being able to take the medication, chances are you won't.

WHAT TO ASK YOUR DOCTOR

Do I really need this medication?

Many physicians often feel pressure to do *something* for the patient, so they reach for the prescription pad. If your doctor doesn't prescribe a medication, consider that good news rather than a sign of rejection or

REMEMBER YOUR MEDICINE

If you have trouble remembering to take your medications, here are some tips to help you:

▶ **Reminders.** Place the medication (or a reminder) in a conspicuous place: next to your toothbrush, on the meal table, or in your lunch box. Or put a reminder note on the bathroom mirror, the refrigerator door, the coffee maker, or your television set. Be careful where you put the medication if children are around.

▶ **Establish a Routine.** Link taking the medication with some well-established habit: meal times if it's okay to take the medicine with food, or brushing your teeth, getting dressed, or watching your favorite television program. If you have problems remembering on certain days, look for a pattern. If you forget on weekends, for example, try to connect your medication-taking with some regular weekend activity.

▶ **Use a Medication Calendar.** Make your own medication chart. For each of your medicines, note when you are to take them (see box, *Tracking Your*

Medications page 255). Check each off on the calendar when you take it.

▶ **Use a Medication Organizer.** You can buy a "medication organizer" at the drugstore, or use an empty egg container. Separate pills in the container according to when they should be taken. Fill your organizer once a week so that all of your pills will be ready to take at the proper time. This system prevents double doses and it lets you know at a glance if you missed any.

▶ **Use a Timer.** Set your watch to beep at pill-taking time. Or get one of the medication containers that beeps at a pre-programmed time. You might also get help from others. Ask household members to help by reminding you to take your pills.

▶ **Plan Ahead.** Don't run out. Don't wait until the last pill to get a refill. Stay at least a week ahead. If you travel, plan ahead. Put a note on your luggage reminding you to pack your pills, and a note inside reminding you to take them. Ask your doctor for an extra prescription and keep it in your carry-on luggage in case your pills or your luggage get lost.

disinterest. Ask the doctor about non-drug alternatives. *In some cases, lifestyle changes such as exercise, diet, and stress management should be considered.* Also ask what consequences are likely if you postpone treatment. Sometimes the best medicine is none at all.

Key Point

What is the name of the medication?
If a medication is prescribed, it is important that you know its name. You should

write down both the brand name and the generic (or chemical) name. If the medication you get from the pharmacy doesn't have the same name as the one your doctor prescribed, ask the pharmacist to explain the difference.

What's the medication supposed to do?
Your physician should tell you why the medication is being prescribed, how it is expected to help you, and how soon you

should expect results. Is the medication intended to cure the disease, prevent complications, or just make you more comfortable? Is it fast acting, or does it take days or even weeks to notice an effect?

How and when do I take the medication, and for how long?

Understanding how much to take and how often to take the medicine is critical to its safe, effective use. Ask questions such as:

▶ *Does "every six hours" mean "every six hours while awake?"*

▶ *Should the medication be taken before meals, with meals, or between meals?*

▶ *What should I do if I accidentally miss a dose? Should I skip it, take a double dose next time, or take it as soon as I remember?*

▶ *Should I continue taking the medication until the symptoms subside, or until the medication is finished?*

▶ *What food, drink, other medicines, or activities should I avoid while taking this medication?*

What are the most common side effects, and what should I do if they occur?

All medications have side effects. Some may be minor annoyances; others may signal a life-threatening allergic reaction. Some disappear over days or weeks as your body gets used to them. You need to know what symptoms to watch for and what action to take, should they develop. You also need to know when to seek immediate medical care, discontinue the medication, or call your doctor.

While the doctor cannot be expected to tell you every possible adverse reaction, the more common and important ones should be discussed. In a recent survey, 70% of patients starting a new medication did not recall being told by their physicians or pharmacists about precautions and possible side effects. So it may be up to you to ask, and you may want to write down the answers.

Are there any tests necessary to monitor the use of this medication?

The effects of some drugs can be detected only by lab tests. Levels of some drugs need to be measured periodically in the blood to make sure you aren't getting too much or too little. Find out if yours is one.

Can a less expensive alternative or generic medication be prescribed?

Generic medications are generally considered as safe and effective as the original brand name drug, but they often cost half as much. If cost is a significant concern of yours, ask your doctor if there is a lower cost (but equally effective) alternative. In some cases, your doctor may have a good reason for preferring a particular brand.

How can I get more information about the medication?

Realistically, your doctor may not have time to answer all of your questions in sufficient detail. Even if he or she does, it is difficult for anyone to remember all this information. Fortunately, there are many additional sources of information available. Pharmacists, nurses, videos, computer programs, and printed material can all be valuable resources. Several particularly useful reference books to consult are included at the end of this book (see page 279).

___

📖 *For more information, see page 279*

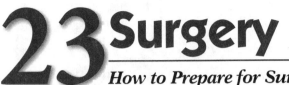

23 Surgery

How to Prepare for Surgery and Other Medical Adventures

Preparing for surgery is somewhat like preparing for a big athletic event, only more important. You've got to understand the rules of the game and devise a good game plan—it helps insure success. Having confidence in yourself and your teammates prepares you for the event.

Imagine running a race without knowing what the course is, or without having successful strategies in mind. No wonder so many surgical patients feel helpless. This feeling can also significantly inhibit their physical recovery.

Preparation Pays Off

As a patient facing an operation or other invasive medical procedure, you may feel that your fate is entirely in the hands of the surgeon and the medical staff. But this is just partly true. You can do a lot to minimize your own discomfort and speed recovery. If you know what to do and what to expect before, during, and after the procedure, it's likely to go better.

The better you are prepared mentally for your operation, the better your body also responds. In an analysis of over 190 studies of psychological preparation for surgery, 80% of the patients showed significant benefits: quicker recovery, fewer complications, less post-surgical pain, less need for pain medication, less

anxiety and depression, fewer complications, and an average of 1.5 days less in the hospital. For example, one group of patients who received educational sessions before their surgery returned to work sooner than patients who got none.

Take advantage of these findings. By preparing yourself for surgery before you go into the hospital for your stay, you can do a lot to minimize trauma and discomfort of your surgery. Doctors are often fond of saying, "the way a patient goes into anesthesia is the way a patient will come out of it." It certainly seems true that those patients who go in feeling relaxed, optimistic, and in control are likely to feel better and recover faster than those who feel highly anxious and vulnerable.

WHAT'S YOUR COPING STYLE?

People generally use one of two major coping styles to manage stressful situations like surgery. Some are "avoidant copers"; others are "vigilant copers." Which are you?

Avoidant Copers

If you like to avoid things, you don't want to be overwhelmed with information or asked to make too many decisions. Avoidant copers deal with stressful situations by distracting themselves, concentrating on pleasant thoughts, and not asking many questions. If this is your coping style, then immersing yourself in details of the operation may *raise* your anxiety.

Of course, there is some information about the procedure you'll need to know. But you'll probably feel better if you don't know every detail. There are better ways for you to feel confident and in control. They include trusting that the surgical team knows what they're doing; believing that all will work out for the best; using relaxation techniques before

and after the procedure, and listening to soothing music during the operation.

Vigilant Copers

If you are a vigilant coper, you're likely to feel more comfortable and in control by asking a lot of questions and getting detailed information about the operation. If there are choices to be made, you'll want to be the one to make them, and base your decision on carefully weighed information. You will definitely want to look at the questions to ask about surgery (📖 see page 267).

Both ways of coping can be useful. But either one, when taken to extremes, can be harmful. *Excessive avoidance may prevent you from taking appropriate action in preparing for surgery. And excessive vigilance can lead to an insatiable thirst for information, raise your anxiety, and alienate the medical staff.*

Whatever style of coping you use, measure its success by the degree to which it helps you feel more relaxed, confident and in control.

Key Point

How to Prepare for Surgery and Other Medical Adventures

The best way to make surgery less stressful depends somewhat on how much information and involvement you prefer (📖 see box above). Below is a wide range of advice on how to prepare for surgery. Go with the suggestions that seem right to you.

℞ Be Convinced You Really Need It

Americans are the most operated-on people in the world. Each year over 50 million operations are performed. About 20% of these are in response to an emergency such as a severe injury; 80% are "elective," meaning that the patient can choose when and where to have the operation, if at all.

The numbers of operations performed vary widely from country to country, state to state, city to city, and even from surgeon to surgeon. The best way to estimate of the amount of surgery in a given community is the number of surgeons in the community, not the prevalence of disease! The more surgeons, the more surgery.

Even the rates of surgery for a given condition can vary widely within a community. One study showed that the rates of hysterectomy (removal of the uterus) were four times higher in one town than the one next to it.

When surgery is recommended for you or a family member, ask a lot of questions to help insure that the operation is really necessary (🕮 see box page 243). You may want to consider getting a second opinion (🕮 see page 268).

℞ This is *Your* Operation

A hospital can often be a confusing and insensitive environment. You may need to assert yourself by asking directly and repeatedly for what you need, whether it is a blanket, a pain medication, or some information.

Remember, this is *your* life; it's *your* operation. You are renting the operating room, and paying for the nurses, the surgeon, and the anesthesiologist. That doesn't mean that you turn the hospital

schedule and practice upside down for your personal needs. But it does mean making your needs known to increase your comfort and peace of mind.

For instance, it may mean a lot to you if someone holds your hand while you're waiting for the medical procedure to start, or in the recovery room. Ask someone to do it if it's not done automatically. You might also want to ask to sign your informed consent form for the anesthesia a few days prior to your surgery rather than immediately before it. Reading a list of possible complications (however rare) could unnecessarily alarm you at a very vulnerable moment.

℞ Learn To Relax

Being able to relax as much as possible during your hospital stay is important for two reasons. First, it will reduce your anxiety. Second, it will also reduce your experience of pain. Anxiety causes tension, and tension increases pain. There are many relaxation exercises you can practice before and after your procedure (🕮 see page 88). Mini-relaxation exercises—like focusing on your breath or counting backwards—may be particularly helpful during brief procedures such as having blood drawn or an IV set up.

℞ Give Your Body Instructions

The research shows that giving specific instructions to your body encourages quicker physical recovery. *By focusing your attention on positive therapeutic suggestions, you can influence pain perception, bowel contractions, blood flow, and perhaps even immune functioning.* These functions which are controlled by the autonomic nervous system, were once thought to be

Key Point

INSTRUCT YOUR BODY

Below are some specific suggestions that can help you prepare for surgery. You can record them on an audio tape, place them on note cards and have someone read them to you, or repeat them to yourself. Use these suggestions frequently in the days before your surgery, during surgery (if they are recorded), and after the operation.

Pain Control

Relaxing the muscles around the area of the incision can help reduce discomfort after surgery. This usually results in less need for post-operative pain medications, and may speed recovery and discharge from the hospital.

Say to yourself: "All of my muscles in my _____ (area of surgery) will be completely relaxed as I come out of the operation. It is very important that all of these muscles remain completely relaxed, as limp as a rag doll, so that the blood will flow easily into that area and heal me, and so that the pain medicine will work more easily and better. With relaxed muscles I will recover more quickly and more comfortably. So all of the muscles in my _____ (area of surgery) will be completely relaxed after surgery, and will stay relaxed."

Bowel Activity

After abdominal or pelvic surgery, the stomach and intestines usually go on strike. Gut movement and digestion are halted. Nothing can be eaten or drunk for several days, until the bowel gets back to work. The first reliable sign that the gut is working is the passing of gas. This indicates that the bowel is beginning to function, food can be eaten, and you are getting ready to go home. An early discharge from the gut usually means an early discharge from the hospital!

In one study, patients undergoing abdominal surgery were given specific pre-operative instructions about restoring their bowel function (see the script below). They recovered faster, passed gas sooner, began eating earlier, and were discharged from the hospital an average of a day and a half sooner than patients who just received a general reassurance.

Jump-Start Your Gastrointestinal System

Tell yourself: "Because I need to eat food to bring nutrients to my body, it is important that my stomach and intestines begin to move and function as soon as possible after my operation. An abdominal operation causes my stomach and intestines to stop moving for a short time. This will be kept to a minimum in my case, because I will be very relaxed and comfortable. My stomach will pump and gurgle, and I will become very hungry soon after the operation. My stomach and intestines will begin to move and churn so that I can eat_____ (my favorite food) soon after the operation."

Continued on next page

Blood Loss

How much blood you will lose during surgery is difficult to predict. A large amount of bleeding can be dangerous. It can block the surgeon's view of the surgical site, and make the operation more difficult. But research has demonstrated that when people are given appropriate verbal instructions, they can learn to redirect blood flow in their bodies, and, to some degree, control blood loss.

We know that words alone can influence blood flow. When people blush in response to another's words, blood flow reddens the face. In one study, patients undergoing extensive spinal surgery received specific instructions on how to control blood flow. They lost *half* the amount of blood as those who received either general relaxation instructions or no pre-operative preparation.

Control Your Blood Flow

Say to yourself: *"Blood vessels contain smooth muscle; they contract or relax to alter blood flow to specific areas. So that I'll have very little blood loss during my surgery, it is important that the blood moves away from _____ (area of surgery) to other parts of my body during the operation. Afterwards, it will return to that area and bring nutrients to heal my body quickly and completely."*

Immune Function

After surgery, the immune system can be depressed. This can lead to a longer recovery time. Surgery often generates high levels of the stress hormone cortisol, which is associated with fewer antibodies and infection-fighting white blood cells. But patients can learn to enhance their immune function. A review of 22 studies suggests that the use of relaxation, imagery (with or without music), self-hypnosis, meditation, and/or biofeedback can help improve immune function.

In one study, subjects were taught how to induce a relaxed, hypnotic state in themselves. They were instructed to create an image of *neutrophils,* a type of white blood cell that is an important defense against infection. One subject imagined her neutrophils as ping pong balls with honey oozing out, causing them to stick to everything they touched. In tests of the subjects' blood samples, this relaxation/imagery exercise increased the stickiness of their neutrophils, while no other measures of immune function were changed.

Boost Your Immune System

Tell yourself: *"My immune system helps my wounds heal and protects me against infections. It will become active before, during, and after surgery. My antibodies and white blood cells will carry away any bacteria that have gotten into the wound, and will prevent infections. My tissues will heal quickly and smoothly. My recovery will be speedy and complete."*

Scripts adapted from the research of Henry L. Bennett, Ph.D. and Elizabeth A. Disbrow, M.A. of the University of California, Davis, Medical Center.

completely beyond voluntary control. New research has demonstrated that both humans and animals can learn to alter them to some degree. Your body already has these built-in healing systems. They can be activated by:

▶ Positive thoughts

▶ Words and suggestions

▶ Images

You can make your own audio tape of positive suggestions based on the scripts given here (📖 see box page 262), or use one of the prepared surgical tapes (page 280). Preparing and listening to such positive messages can help you feel more relaxed and in control.

℞ Choose What You Hear

Contrary to popular belief, general anesthesia does not completely "shut off" your brain during an operation. Studies demonstrate that patients are sometimes aware of speech or sounds around them even when they are anesthetized, and even though they do not usually remember them afterwards.

Your body may respond to what you hear. Surgeons sometimes say something during an operation that, if overheard, could unnecessarily alarm you. *Protect yourself by wearing earplugs, or preferably, by listening to audio tapes. This will both block out disturbing sounds and provide you with relaxing music or positive suggestions.*

Key Point

Listening to music you like can be advantageous. Studies show that people who heard soothing music before, during, and after surgery needed less sedative. One investigator calculated that music in the operating room equals roughly two and a half milligrams of Valium. Another study found that listening to music both before and during surgery reduced stress hormones in the blood.

Verbal suggestions can be heard subconsciously. In one well-controlled study, women underwent abdominal surgery while listening to taped suggestions such as, "Everything is going very well"; "We're very pleased with your progress"; "You feel warm, comfortable, calm, and relaxed"; and "Any pain that you feel after your operation will not concern you."

The women who heard these "positive therapeutic suggestions" needed 24% less pain medications the day after surgery than patients who were given a blank tape. The women did not consciously recall hearing the suggestions, but their recovery reflected the positive subconscious effects.

In a similar study, women who were undergoing hysterectomies listened to positive suggestions during surgery. They left the hospital one and a half days earlier, and had fewer complications than those who were given blank tapes.

So you may want to arrange ahead of time for some earplugs or an autoreverse cassette tape player with headphones (don't forget fresh batteries). Bring a tape of soothing music or positive therapeutic suggestions. Tell your surgical team that you plan to listen to tapes during the procedure.

℞ A Little Fear is Okay

There is good reason to worry about the prospect of being operated on. In fact, it would be unusual not to be concerned. While overwhelming anxiety can delay your recovery, you don't need to deny your fear completely, or put on a happy face for everyone around you.

It may be helpful to talk with others

about your concerns, especially other patients who have experienced the same surgical procedure. Your surgeon or the hospital staff may be able to put you into contact with other patients who have gone through the same thing.

Key Point *Channel your fear and anxiety into your own program for preparing for the operation. Not all fear is bad anyway.* Studies have indicated that we may actually need a certain level of fear and arousal to prepare us for the stress of surgery. So don't be afraid of being a little afraid.

℞ Think Positively

However frightened you might be about the prospect of surgery, keep in touch with the fact that you are doing this to help yourself. You're electing to have surgery to improve your health, and to maximize your chances of living a full life again. So think of your surgery as a positive event that will have positive outcomes. The way you think about the whole experience is important. You can make it positive if you think, for instance, about the good care you will receive at the hospital, the chance you will have to relax, read books, catch up on sleep, meet new people, and, of course, get well.

Research shows that people who take control of their own thoughts and feelings when they get upset about the prospect of surgery suffer less pre- and post-operative stress. If you find yourself thinking things like: "I feel so helpless, there's nothing I can do" or "I can't stand it, this is too difficult," try substituting more positive thoughts such as:

▶ *I can get through this*

▶ *The discomfort will pass*

▶ *Everyone is doing everything they can to*

insure a safe operation and a speedy recovery, including me

▶ *I will feel better and be healthier as a result of the surgery*

▶ *I know how to relax, distract myself, and feel better*

Reshape your negative thoughts and feelings into more positive, encouraging ones (see page 149

see page 149.

℞ Develop a Pain Control Plan

People used to think that severe pain after surgery was something they just had to put up with. But that's no longer true with current treatments. You can work out a plan with your doctors and nurses both before and after surgery to prevent or relieve pain. *Putting up with pain is neither heroic nor wise. In fact,* **Key Point** *good pain control can help you recover more quickly. With less pain you can start walking, do your deep breathing exercises, cough, and get your strength back more quickly.* You'll also be less likely to develop complications like pneumonia or blood clots. You may even be able to go home from the hospital sooner. Although complete elimination of post surgical pain is neither practical nor desirable, you should expect to be reasonably comfortable. Here are some tips:

▶ **Know what to expect.** Before surgery, find out what will happen. Will there be much pain after surgery? How long is it likely to last?

▶ **Develop a plan to prevent pain.** Work out a pain control plan with your doctors and nurses. Some people get pain medicines in the hospital only when they call the nurse to ask for them. Sometimes there are delays, and the pain gets worse while they wait. There are better, more effective ways to

23 Surgery

265

control pain. *Pain prevention and comfort rather than complete pain relief should be the goal. The pain pills or shots can be given at set times every few hours instead of waiting until the pain breaks through.*

Key Point

Some hospitals now offer "patient controlled analgesia" (PCA). This allows you to control when you get the pain medicine. When you begin to feel pain, you press a button, and a small amount of pain medication is released through an intravenous (IV) tube in your vein. PCA pumps are designed with safety features so that you cannot overdose. Studies show that patients are often more comfortable and use *less* pain medication when they can control their own doses.

▶ **Don't wait for the pain to get bad.** Take (or ask for) pain relief medicines when your pain first begins. It is critical to take action as soon as the pain starts. Severe pain is much more difficult to control.

▶ **Don't be afraid of pain medications.** Short-term use of narcotic pain medications is not addicting, so you don't have to be afraid to take them when you need them.

▶ **Measure your pain.** Everyone reacts to pain differently. Only you know how you really feel. Help your doctors and nurses "measure" your pain. Reporting your level of pain helps them know how well your treatment is working, and if any adjustments are needed. The best way to measure your pain is to answer the question, "On a scale of 0 to 10 (0 is no pain and 10 is the worst possible), how would you rate the pain?" Repeated measurements are helpful to track your progress.

▶ **Speak up.** Don't be shy about reporting your pain. If it won't go away despite the medication, say something. You may be afraid of being a nuisance, but unrelieved pain could be a sign of a complication that needs prompt attention.

▶ **Try non-drug approaches as well.** For greater relief, combine non-drug strategies with medications. Breathing exercises (see page 90), relaxation exercises (page 88), imagery (page 99), music (page 63), distraction (page 221), and massage, heat, and ice can all be very effective for reducing pain and anxiety.

℞ Get Up!

Rest is great, but too much of it is not. You can help yourself by getting some gentle exercise and movement as soon as possible after your operation. Inactivity increases the risk of blood clots forming in leg veins. So walk around wherever you can. Do whatever exercises your condition allows, or ones that the staff recommends.

℞ Choose a Room with a View

This may seem like odd advice, but at least one study has shown the healing effects of looking at nature. Patients who had a room with a view of a wooded scene after surgery suffered less post-operative distress, required less strong pain medications, and were discharged from the hospital one day sooner than those who looked out on a brick wall. Unfortunately, few hospitals have windows with beautiful views. If this is the case, you can bring in your own pictures or photographs of nature scenes. Or you might want to watch nature programs on television.

QUESTIONS ABOUT SURGERY

WHAT TO TELL YOUR DOCTOR

If your doctors don't ask, volunteer this information.

Are you taking any medications?
Tell your physician the names and dosages of all prescription and nonprescription medications you are taking. Include everything: birth control pills, vitamins, aspirin, antacids, anti-inflammatory medications, pain medicines, and narcotics.

Do you smoke?
Smoking greatly increases the risk of anesthesia. Quitting at least two weeks before surgery is extremely important. Your scheduled operation may provide just the added incentive to get you to quit (📖 see page 21).

Key Point

Have you had surgery in the past?
Let your surgeon and anesthesiologist know what operations you have had. Also tell them if you have had any problems or complications either during or after any previous surgeries.

Have you had allergic or unusual reactions to any medications or anesthetics?
Try to be specific. Say which medication or anesthetic, and exactly what type of reaction you had. This information could save your life.

Do you have medical conditions?
Some diseases can make the operation, anesthesia, and your recovery more complicated. Let your doctor know if you have a cold, flu, rash, or fever before the scheduled operation. Also be sure to mention any history of bleeding problems, or if there is a possibility that you are pregnant.

Do you have concerns or fears about surgery?
Express both your concerns and your hopes for what the operation will do for you. This will alert the surgeon to your needs, and enables him or her to talk realistically about the expected outcome.

WHAT TO ASK YOUR DOCTOR

Why do I need this surgery now?
Many experts estimate that one in five operations aren't necessary, and that many more could be prevented if we changed our lifestyles. So ask your surgeon:

▸ *Why do I need this operation now?*

▸ *Are there any suitable and equally effective alternatives?*

▸ *Can something less invasive be tried first?*

▸ *What is likely to happen if I don't have surgery at this time?*

▸ *How is this surgery supposed to help me?*

▸ *What is the success rate for this surgery?*

▸ *Is the hoped-for gain worth the risks and costs?*

Then consider a second opinion (📖 see box page 268), and ask the second doctor the same set of questions.

How often have you performed this operation?
Key Point

In general, the more often a surgeon performs an operation in a particular hospital, the lower the rates of death and complications for that surgeon and that hospital. Some surgeons may have low complication rates and excellent recovery rates for a particular operation they do frequently, but less impressive results with surgery they do not perform that often. Whatever surgeon you decide on, it is

GETTING A SECOND OPINION

Many health insurance plans now require a second opinion before elective surgery, so you won't be offending the first surgeon by getting a second one. Some studies show that the second surgeon disagrees with the first about the need for surgery in over a quarter of the cases. This is particularly true for operations of the womb (hysterectomy), coronary arteries, tonsils, gallbladder, varicose veins, back, knee, nose, and prostate gland.

Your second opinion should be independent from the first and preferably from someone not associated with or recommended by the first surgeon. Think about getting a second opinion from a non-surgeon to see if there are realistic alternatives to surgery. Also consider a second opinion for any medical treatment or diagnostic procedure that carries significant risk or cost. For example, for some patients, changes in their diet, exercise, stress management, and cholesterol lowering medications may offer an alternative to coronary artery bypass surgery.

Key Point

If the second opinion you get agrees with the first recommendation you get for surgery, then you can feel more confident in proceeding. If the second opinion conflicts with the first, you may want to have the doctors talk to each other to clarify their recommendations. Or get a third opinion.

Disagreements between doctors are usually honest differences of opinion; there are gray areas of medical knowledge where agreement has not yet been reached. In all cases, you must weigh the opinions yourself, and make the final decision about your own treatment.

important to feel comfortable with him or her, and confident in this person's abilities. This will make a difference as to how you will approach your surgery on the day.

What are the risks and complications?
Every surgical procedure carries some risk. Be very suspicious of any surgeon who tells you there are none. You should ask about the risk of death (mortality rate), as well as the risk of complications (morbidity rate). Risk will vary depending upon your general state of health, the type of operation to be performed, the type of anesthetic to be used, and the skill of the surgeon. Hospitals keep records and may be willing to share them with you.

Several governmental agencies and consumer groups now also publish ratings of hospitals based on the mortality and complication rates. Most are appropriately adjusted for the estimated severity of the disease, so that you can more fairly compare them.

If your problem is very rare, you may want to see an expert in a university medical center or a specialty hospital—one experienced in the condition. Ask your doctor where to start your search for specialists. Bear in mind, however, that it is not always advantageous to go far from home. Consider how the distance will affect the ability of your family and friends to visit and support you.

Blood transfusions may be needed in some operations. Blood banks now carefully screen all blood products to reduce the risk of transmitting infection or transfusion reactions. If your operation is scheduled a few months ahead, however, you can often donate and store your own blood before your operation. Using your own blood reduces the already low risk of contracting a blood-borne infection such as HIV/AIDS or hepatitis.

What are my options for anesthesia?
Modern anesthesia is generally highly effective in eliminating pain, and it is very safe. Depending upon the kind of operation, you may have several choices in the type of anesthesia that can be used.

Local anesthesia. This involves injecting an anesthetic in the area around the site of the surgical incision. This temporarily numbs the immediate area but leaves the rest of the body unaffected. Local anesthesia is the safest type. It can be used instead of general anesthetic in some cases.

Regional anesthesia. An injected medication temporarily blocks pain in an entire region of the body. For example, in a spinal block or epidural anesthesia, the medication is injected in the area around the spinal cord. It produces numbness from the chest down to your feet. With regional anesthesia you remain conscious, so you can let the medical team know if anything feels uncomfortable.

General anesthesia. This involves administering medications to create unconsciousness, eliminate pain, and produce amnesia (memory loss) of the surgical experience. Unconsciousness is usually brought on by injecting a medication into an IV placed in a vein in your arm. To stay unconscious, you are given a mixture of anesthetic gases to breath. Sometimes people have some reactions to the anesthetic after the operation. They may feel a little dizzy or nauseous for awhile. Although modern general anesthesia is quite safe, the risk of death from it is estimated somewhere between one in 3,000 to one in 10,000.

Find out what kinds of anesthetics are available and appropriate for you, and go with your preference. Some people prefer a local anesthetic; others would rather be asleep during an operation, even though it carries greater risk. As a general rule, it's best to select the least invasive and risky type of anesthesia that produces the desired results.

Can this be out-patient surgery?
With out-patient surgery, you are admitted in the morning and are observed for a period of time after the procedure. Then you're released to go home. Out-patient surgery has many advantages:

▶ Stress is reduced

▶ Cost is usually half as much

▶ The risk of hospital-acquired infection is less

▶ The disruption to your family is minimized

Of course, out-patient surgery is only possible for less complex operations, but 30 percent of all surgery now falls into this category. It includes breast biopsies, cataract surgery, dilatation and curettage, sterilization for both males and females, some plastic surgery, some orthopedic procedures, and some hernia repairs.

What should I expect?
Ask your surgeon to help you prepare for your surgery, and help you get useful information. You might ask:

- *How should I prepare for the operation?*

- *Should I continue taking my usual medications before or after surgery?*

- *How long before surgery should I not eat or drink?*

- *Are any tests required before the operation?*

- *Who else will be involved on the surgical team?*

- *What the surgery will be like?*

- *How long will recovery take?*

- *What can I do to speed it?*

- *When will I be able to return to work and normal activities?*

- *When will you or other members of the surgical team visit me in the hospital?*

- *What will the operation cost? You don't need any more shocks after the operation. If this doctor doesn't know, find out who can tell you.*

- What should I watch for in terms of complications, and which ones need to be reported to a doctor?

How can I get more information?

Realistically, your doctor may not have time to answer all of your questions in sufficient detail. Even if he or she does carefully answer your questions, it is difficult for anyone to remember all the information. You might want to review one or more books which describe the surgical experience in more detail (📖 see page 279). There may also be videotapes you can watch, classes you can take, support groups you can join, or experienced patients with whom you can talk.

By taking advantage of the advice in this chapter, you can prepare yourself mentally for surgery, significantly reduce your discomfort, and speed your recovery.

📖 *For more information, see page 279*

Resources for More Information

GENERAL SELF-HELP RESOURCES

Benson, Herbert and Stuart, Eileen M.: *The Wellness Book: The Comprehensive Guide to Maintaining Health and Treating Stress-Related Illness.* New York: Birch Lane Press, 1992.

Butler, Gillian and Hope, Tony: *Managing Your Mind: The Mental Fitness Guide.* New York: Oxford, 1995.

Davis, Martha; Eshelman, Elizabeth; and McKay, Matthew: *The Relaxation & Stress Reduction Workbook.* Oakland, CA: New Harbinger Publications, 1995.

Eliot, Robert S.: *From Stress to Strength: How to Lighten Your Load and Save Your Life.* New York: Bantam, 1994.

Goleman, Daniel and Gurin, Joel (Editors): *Mind/Body Medicine: How To Use Your Mind for Better Health.* New York: Consumer Reports Books, 1993.

Miller, Lyle H.; Smith, Alma Dell; and Rothstein, Larry: *The Stress Solution: An Action Plan to Manage the Stress in Your Life.* New York: Pocket Books, 1993.

GENERAL SCIENTIFIC RESOURCES

ADVANCES: The Journal of Mind-Body Health. P.O. Box 3000, Denville, NJ 07834 (1-800-875-2997).

Hafen, Brent Q.; Karren, Keith J.; Frandsen, Kathryn J.; Smith, and N. Lee: *Mind/Body Health: The Health Effects of Attitudes, Emotions, and Relationships.* Boston: Allyn and Bacon, 1996.

Kleinke, Chris L.: *Coping with Life Challenges.* Pacific Grove, CA: Brooks/Cole Publishing Co, 1991. *Introductory college text to the psycho-logical process of coping.*

Ornstein, Robert and Sobel, David: *Healthy Pleasures.* Reading, MA: Addison-Wesley, 1989. *Review of evidence of health benefits from sensuality, optimism, and altruism.*

Ornstein, Robert and Sobel, David: *The Healing Brain.* New York: Simon & Schuster, 1987.

Pelletier, Kenneth R.: *Sound Mind, Sound Body: A New Model for Lifelong Health.* New York: Simon & Schuster, 1994.

Sapolsky, Robert M.: *Why Zebras Don't Get Ulcers: A Guide to Stress, Stress-Related Diseases, and Coping.* New York: W.H. Freeman, 1994.

Sobel, David: "ReThinking Medicine: Improving health outcomes with cost-effective psychosocial interventions." *Psychosomatic Medicine.* 1995: 57:234-244.

1. The Power to Change

Kemper, Donald; Giuffre, Jim; and Drabinski, Gene: *Pathways: A Success Guide for Healthy Living.* Boise, Idaho: Healthwise, Inc., 1985. *Workbook for making changes in stress management, fitness, nutrition, self-care, and lifestyle.*

Prochaska, James O.; Norcross, John C.; and DiClemente, Carlo C: *Changing for Good.* New York: William Morrow and Company, Inc., 1994. *Discussion of the stages of change and the most effective stage-based strategies.*

Seligman, Martin E.P.: *What You Can Change & What You Can't: The Complete Guide to Successful Self-Improvement.* New York: Alfred A. Knopf, 1994.

Mind/Body Health Newsletter (formerly *Mental Medicine Update*), David Sobel , M.D., and Robert Ornstein, Ph.D. (editors)
Center for Health Sciences
c/o ISHK Book Service
P.O. Box 381069
Cambridge, MA 02238-1069
(1-800-222-4745).

A newsletter that includes self-help advice, summaries of recent research, and reviews of books and other resources in the area of mind/body health.

2. Healthy Thinking

Benson, Herbert: *Timeless Healing: The Power and Biology of Belief.* New York: Scribners, 1996.

Burns, David: *The Feeling Good Handbook.* New York: Plume, 1989. *Cognitive therapy techniques to manage depression, anxiety, and communication problems.*

Ellis, Albert and Harper, Robert A.: *A New Guide to Rational Living.* N. Hollywood, CA: Wiltshire Book Co., 1975. *Solve emotional problems by correcting irrational thinking.*

Freeman, Arthur and DeWolf, Rose: *The 10 Dumbest Mistakes Smart People Make and How to Avoid Them.* New York: HarperCollins, 1992.

Greenberger, Dennis and Padesky, Christine A.: *Mind Over Mood: A Cognitive Therapy Treatment Manual for Clients.* New York: The Guilford Press, 1995.

McKay, Matthew; Davis, Martha; Fanning, Patrick: *Thoughts and Feelings: The Art of Cognitive Stress Intervention.* Oakland, CA : New Harbinger, 1981.

Myers, David G.: *The Pursuit of Happiness.* New York: William Morrow, 1992.

Peterson, Christopher and Bossio, Lisa M.: *Health and Optimism.* New York: Free Press, 1991.

Seligman, Martin E.P.: *Learned Optimism.* New York: Knopf, 1990.

3. Humor

American Association of Therapeutic Humor, 222 S. Merrimac, Suite 303, St. Louis, MO 63105 (314-863-6232).

Baim, Margaret and La Roche, Loretta: "Jest 'n' Joy" in Herbert Benson and Eileen Stuart, *The Wellness Book.* New York: Carol Publishing, 1992.

Blumenfeld, Esther and Alpern, Lynne: *The Smile Connection: How to Use Humor in Dealing with People.* Englewood Cliffs, NJ: Prentice-Hall, 1986.

Hageseth, Christian: *A Laughing Place: The Art and Psychology of Positive Humor in Love and Adversity.* Fort Collins, CO: Berwick Publishing Co., 1988.

The Humor Project. 110 Spring Street, Saratoga Springs, NY 12866 (518-587-8770). *Publishes Laughing Matters Magazine, Humor Resources Catalog, and a clearinghouse for theory, research, and practical ideas related to humor.*

Klein, Alan: *The Healing Power of Humor.* Los Angeles: Jeremey P. Tarcher, Inc., 1989.

Metcalf, C.W. and Felible, Roma: *Lighten Up: Survival Skills for People Under Pressure.* Reading, MA: Addison-Wesley, 1992.

4. Enjoy Your Senses

Ackerman, Diane: *A Natural History of the Senses.* New York: Random House, 1990.

American Association for Music Therapy, P.O. Box 80012, Valley Forge, PA 19484 (914-944-9260).

The Bonny Foundation: Institute for Music-Centered Therapies, 2020 Simmons Street, Salina, Kansas 67401 Tel. (913-827-1497), Fax (913-827-5706). *Guided Imagery and Music (GIM)*

Katsh, Shelley and Merle-Fishman, Carol: *The Music Within You*. New York: Fireside/Simon & Schuster, 1985.

Maxwell-Hudson, Claire: *The Complete Book of Massage*. New York: Random House, 1988.

National Association for Music Therapy, 8455 Colesville Rd., Suite 930, Silver Spring, MD 20910 (301-589-3300).

Ornstein, Robert and Sobel, David: *Healthy Pleasures*. Reading, MA: Addison-Wesley, 1989. *Includes fifty pages of annotated notes and references to the health benefits of pleasure and sensuality.*

Tiger, Lionel: *The Pursuit of Pleasure*. Boston: Little, Brown, 1992.

5. Healthy Sex

Barbach, Lonnie and Levine, Linda: *Shared Intimacies: Women's Sexual Experiences*. New York: Bantam, 1981.

Barbach, Lonnie: *For Each Other: Sharing Sexual Intimacy*. New York: Doubleday, 1982.

Barbach, Lonnie: *For Yourself: The Fulfillment of Female Sexuality*. New York: New American Library, 1975.

Castleman, Michael: *Sexual Solutions: A Guide for Men and the Women Who Love Them*. New York: Simon & Schuster, 1989.

Godeck, Gregory. *1001 Ways to Be Romantic*. Weymouth, MA: Casablanca Press, 1993.

Knopf, Jennifer and Seiler, Michael: *Inhibited Sexual Desire*. New York: Warner Books, 1990.

Renshaw, Domeena: *Seven Weeks to Better Sex*. New York: Random House, 1995.

Stoppard, Miriam: *The Magic of Sex*. New York: Dorling-Kindersley, Inc., 1991.

Williams, Warwick: *Rekindling Desire: Bringing Your Sexual Relationship Back to Life*. Oakland, CA: New Harbinger Publications, Inc., 1988.

HEALTH ONLINE

Ferguson, Tom: *Health Online*. Reading, MA: Addison-Wesley, 1996. *A book on how to access online computer health information and support.*

If you have Internet access, check out:

Self-Help Clearinghouse
(http://www.cmhc.com/selfhelp)

Psych Central—
Grohol's Mental Health Page
(http://www.coil.com/~grohol)

Zilbergeld, Bernie: *The New Male Sexuality: The Truth about Men, Sex, and Pleasure*. New York: Bantam Books, 1993.

6. Relaxation

Benson, Herbert and Klipper, Miriam: *The Relaxation Response*. New York: Avon, 1976.

Benson, Herbert and Stuart, Eileen: *The Wellness Book*, New York: Birch Lane Press, 1992.

Davis, Martha; Eshelman, Elizabeth; and McKay, Matthew: *The Relaxation & Stress Reduction Workbook*. Oakland, CA: New Harbinger Publications, 1995.

Goleman, Daniel and Gurin, Joel (Editors): *Mind/Body Medicine: How To Use Your Mind for Better Health*. New York: Consumer Reports Books, 1993.

Kabat-Zinn, Jon: *Full Castatrophe Living: Using the Wisdom of Your Body and Mind to Face Stress, Pain, and Illness*. New York: Delacorte Press, 1990.

Kabat-Zinn, Jon: *Wherever You Go There You Are: Mindfulness Meditation in Everyday Life*. New York: Hyperion, 1994.

Stress Reduction Tapes, P.O. Box 547, Lexington, MA 02173 (508-856-1616) *Mindfulness meditation tapes from Jon Kabat-Zinn.*

Stroebel, Charles: *The Quieting Reflex.* New York: Berkeley Books, 1983.

7. Imagery

Academy for Guided Imagery, P.O. Box 2070, Mill Valley, CA 94942: *Relaxation and imagery tapes, books, and courses.*

Alman, Brian M. and Lambrou, Peter: *Self-Hypnosis: The Complete Manual for Health and Self-Change.* New York: Bruner/Mazel, Inc., 1992.

The American Society of Clinical Hypnosis, 2200 East Devon Avenue, Suite 291, Des Plaines, IL 60018.

Davis, Martha; Eshelman, Elizabeth; and McKay, Matthew: *The Relaxation & Stress Reduction Workbook.* Oakland, CA: New Harbinger Publications, 1995.

Fanning, Patrick: *Visualization for Change.* Oakland, CA: New Harbinger Publications, 1994.

Hadley, Josie and Stuadacher, Carol: *Hypnosis for Change.* Oakland, CA: New Harbinger Publications, 1989.

"Health Journeys" by Belleruth Naparstek, Image Paths, Inc., Box 5714, Cleveland, OH 44101-0714 (1-800-800-8661): *Relaxation and imagery tapes and books.*

Keely, Sean F. and Kelly, Reid J.: *Imagine Yourself Well: Better Health through Self-Hypnosis.* New York: Insight, 1995.

Lusk, Julie T.: *30 Scripts for Relaxation Imagery and Inner Healing.* Volumes 1 and 2. Duluth, MN: Whole Person Associates, 1992-1993.

The Mind/Body Medical Institute, Deaconess Hospital, Division of Behavioral Medicine, One Deaconess Rd., Boston, MA 02215 (617-632-9530)

Naparstek, Belleruth: *Staying Well with Guided Imagery.* New York: Warner Books, 1994.

New Harbinger Publications, 5674 Shattuck Avenue, Oakland, CA 94609 (1-800-748-6273): *Relaxation and imagery tapes and books.*

Rossman, Martin: *Healing Yourself: A Step-by-Step Program for Better Health Through Imagery.* New York: Pocket Books, 1987.

The Society for Clinical and Experimental Hypnosis, 3905 Vincennes Rd., Suite 304, Indianapolis, IN 46268.

Whole Person Associates, Inc., 210 West Michigan, Duluth, MN 55802-1908 (218-727-0500): *Relaxation and imagery tapes and books.*

Zilbergeld, Bernie and Lazarus, Arnold: *Mind Power: Getting What You Want Through Mental Training.* New York: Ivy Books, 1988.

8. Enjoy Physical Activity

Blair, Steven: *Living with Exercise.* Dallas, TX: American Health Publishing Co., 1991.

Lyons, Pat and Burgard, Debby: *Great Shape: The First Fitness Guide for Large Women.* Palo Alto, CA: Bull Publishing, 1990. *Encourages larger women to enjoy movement, improve fitness, and feel good about themselves.*

Stamford, Bryant A. and Shimer, Porter: *Fitness Without Exercise.* New York: Warner, 1990.

Swencionis, Charles and Ryan, E. Davis: *The Lazy Person's Guide to Fitness.* New York: Barricade Books, 1994. *Based on understanding the stages of readiness to change.*

9. Communicate Well

Alberti, Robert E. and Emmons, Michael: *Your Perfect Right.* San Luis Obispo, CA: Impact Press, 1990.

Beck, Aaron T.: *Love Is Never Enough.* New York: Harper and Row, 1988.

Bower, Sharon Anthony and Bower, Gordon H.: *Asserting Yourself.* Reading, MA: Addison-Wesley Publishing, 1991.

McKay, Matthew; Davis, Martha; and Fanning, Patrick: *Messages: The Communication Book*. Oakland, CA: New Harbinger, 1995.

Zimbardo, Philip G.: *Shyness*. Reading, MA: Addison-Wesley, 1990.

10. Healthy Helping

The Clean Yield Group, Box 1880, Greensboro Bend, VT 05842 (802-533-7178): *Publishes* The Clean Yield, *a newsletter on socially responsible investing*.

Council on Economic Priorities, 30 Irving Place, New York, NY 10003 (1-800-729-4237): *Publishes newsletter and materials on socially responsible investing*.

Dass, Ram and Gorman, Paul: *How Can I Help?: Stories and Reflections on Service*. New York: Knopf, 1991.

Domini, Amy L. and Kinder, Peter D.: *Ethical Investing: How to Make Profitable Investments Without Sacrificing Your Principles*. Reading, MA: Addison-Wesley, 1986.

Editors of Conari Press: *Random Acts of Kindness*. Berkeley, CA: Conari Press, 1993.

Franklin Research and Development, 711 Atlantic Avenue, Boston, MA 02111 (617 423-6655): *Publishes* Insight, *a newsletter on socially responsible investing*.

Luks, Allan with Peggy Payne: *The Healing Power of Doing Good: The Health and Spiritual Benefits of Helping Others*. New York: Fawcett Columbine, 1991.

Riessman, Frank and Carroll, David: *Redefining Self-Help*. San Francisco: Jossey-Bass, 1995.

Volunteer Referral Service, 736 Jackson Place, Washington, DC (1-800-879-5400).Volunteers of America, 3939 North Causeway Blvd., Suite 400, Metairie, LA 70002-1777 (1-800-899-0089) or Volunteer's The National Center, 1111 North 19th Street, Arlington, VA 22209;,(703-276-0542). *Also, check with voluntary organizations, houses of worship, hospitals, schools, nursing/eldercare homes, and YMCA's or look in the white or yellow pages under your area of interest or under "volunteer."*

White, Barbara and Madara, Edward: *The Self-Help Sourcebook: The Comprehensive Reference of Self-Help Group Resources* (5th Edition). Denville, NJ: Northwest Covenant Medical Center, 1995. *Description of self-help groups in dozens of categories and information on how to develop your own group*.

Whitsett, Gavin: *Guerrilla Kindness: A Manual of Good Works, Kind Acts, and Thoughtful Deeds*. San Luis Obispo, California: Impact Publishers, 1993.

11. Anxiety

Anxiety Disorders Association of America, 6000 Executive Blvd., Suite 513, Rockville, MD 20852 (301-231-9350).

Barlow, David H. and Craske, Michelle: *Mastery of Your Anxiety and Panic*. Albany, New York: Graywind Publications, 1994.

Bourne, Edumund J.: *The Anxiety and Phobia Workbook*. Oakland: New Harbinger Publications, 1995.

Burns, David: *The Feeling Good Handbook*. New York: Plume, 1989.

National Institute of Mental Health (NIMH), Information Resources and Inquiry Branch, Room 15C-05, 5600 Fishers Lane, Rockville, MD 20892 (1-800-64-PANIC or 301-443-4513).

National Mental Health Association, 1021 Prince St., Alexandria, VA 22314-2971 (1-800-969-6642).

Peurifoy, Reneau Z.: *Anxiety, Phobias and Panic: A Step-by-Step Program for Regaining Control of Your Life*. Life Skills, 1992.

Schiraldi, Glenn R.: *Conquer Anxiety, Worry and Nervous Fatigue: A Guide to Greater Peace*. Ellicott City, MD: Chevron Publishing, 1997.

Zuercher-White, Elke: *An End to Panic: Breathrough Techniques for Overcoming Panic Disorder.* Oakland, CA: New Harbinger, 1995.

12. Depression

Burns, David: *Feeling Good: The New Mood Therapy.* New York: Avon, 1980.

Burns, David: *The Feeling Good Handbook.* New York: Plume, 1989.

Copeland, Mary Ellen: *The Depression Workbook.* Oakland, CA: New Harbinger, 1992.

Copeland, Mary Ellen: *Living Without Depression & Manic Depression: A Workbook for Maintaining Mood Stability.* Oakland, CA: New Harbinger, 1994.

Depression Awareness, Recognition, and Treatment (D/ART) Program, National Institute of Mental Health, Room 10-85, 5600 Fishers Lane, Rockville, MD 20857 (1-800-421-4211).

Lewinsohn, Peter; Munoz, Ricardo; Youngren, Mary; and Zeiss, Antoinette: *Control Your Depression.* New York: Simon & Schuster, 1992.

National Depressive and Manic-Depressive Association, 730 N. Franklin, Suite 501, Chicago, IL 60610 (1-800-826-3632 or 312-642-0049).

National Mental Health Association, 1021 Prince St., Alexandria, VA 22314-2971 (1-800-969-6642).

Rosenthal, Norman E.: *Winter Blues: Seasonal Affective Disorder: What It Is and How to Overcome It.* New York: Guilford Press, 1993. *Includes discussion of phototherapy.*

13. Anger

Casarjian, Robin: *Forgiveness: A Bold Choice for a Peaceful Heart.* New York: Bantam Books, 1993.

Daldrup, Roger J. and Gust, Dodie: *Freedom From Anger.* New York: Pocket Books, 1990.

Eliot, Robert S. and Breo, Dennis: *Is It Worth Dying For?* New York: Bantam Books, 1980. *A self-help stress management program for "hot reactors."*

Hankins, Gary and Hankins, Carol: *Prescription for Anger: Coping with Angry Feelings and Angry People.* New York: Warner Books, 1993.

McKay, Matthew; Rogers, Peter D., and McKay, Judith: *When Anger Hurts.* Oakland, CA: New Harbinger Publications, 1989.

Statman, Jan Berliner: *The Battered Woman's Survival Guide: Breaking the Cycle.* Bellingham, WA: Taylor Publishing, 1990.

Williams, Redford and Williams, Virginia: *Anger Kills: Seventeen Strategies for Controlling the Hostility that Can Harm Your Health.* New York: Random House, 1993.

14. Time Pressure

Burka, Jane and Yuen, Lenora: *Procrastination: Why You Do It, What to Do About It.* Reading, MA: Addison-Wesley, 1983.

Culp, Stephanie: *Streamlining Your Life: A 5-Point Plan for Uncomplicated Living.* Cincinnati: Writer's Digest Books, 1991.

Elgin, Duane: *Voluntary Simplicity.* New York: William Morrow, 1993.

Fanning, Tony and Fanning, Robbie: *Get It All Done and Still Be Human: A Personal Time-Management Workshop.* Menlo Park, CA: Kali House, 1990.

Fiore, Neil: *The Now Habit: A Strategic Program for Overcoming Procrastination and Enjoying Guilt-Free Play.* Los Angeles: Jeremy Tarcher, 1989.

Hunt, Diana and Hait, Pam: *The Tao of Time.* New York: Fireside, 1990.

Josephs, Ray: *How to Gain an Extra Hour Every Day: New Time Strategies That Work.* New York: Penguin, 1992.

Keyes, Ralph: *Timelock: How Life Got So Hectic and What You Can Do About It.* New York: HarperCollins, 1991.

Winston, Stephanie: *Getting Organized: The Easy Way to Put Your Life in Order.* New York: Warner Books, 1978.

15. Sleep Better

National Sleep Foundation, 1367 Connecticut Ave. NW, Suite 200, Washington, DC 20036.

Catalano, Ellen Mohr: *Getting to Sleep.* Oakland, CA : New Harbinger, 1990.

Hauri, Peter and Linde, Shirley: *No More Sleepless Nights.* New York: John Wiley & Sons, 1990.

Jacobs, Gregg D.: *Improving Your Sleep.* In *The Wellness Book* by Herbert Benson and Eileen Stuart, New York: Birch Lane Press, 1992.

Perl, James: *Sleep Right in Five Nights: A Clear and Effective Guide for Conquering Insomnia.* New York: William Morrow & Co., 1993.

16. Surviving Trauma

Colgrove, Melba; Bloomfield, Harold; and McWilliams, Peter: *How to Survive the Loss of a Love.* New York: Bantam, 1991.

Matsakis, Aphrodite: *I Can't Get Over It: A Handbook for Trauma Survivors.* Oakland, CA: New Harbinger 1993.

Pennebaker, James W.: *Opening Up: The Healing Power of Confiding in Others.* New York: Avon Books, 1990.

Staudacher, Carol: *Beyond Grief: A Guide for Recovering from the Death of a Loved One.* Oakland, CA: New Harbinger, 1987.

White, Barbara and Madara, Edward: *The Self-Help Sourcebook: the Comprehensive Reference of Self-Help Group Resources* (5th Edition). Denville, NJ: Northwest Covenant Medical Center, 1995. *Description of self-help groups in dozens of categories and information on how to develop your own group.*

17. Addiction

Birkedahl, Nonie: *The Habit Control Workbook.* Oakland, CA: New Harbinger, 1990.

Ferguson, Tom: *The No-Nag, No-Guilt, Do-It-Your-Own Way Guide to Quitting Smoking.* New York: Ballantine, 1987.

Hotlines and Support Groups: National Council on Alcoholism and Drug Dependence (1-800-662-2255), National Drug and Alcohol Treatment Referral Hotline of the Center for Substance Abuse Treatment (1-800-662-4357), Cocaine Anonymous National Hotline (1-800-347-8998) or check the Yellow Pages for listing of local programs such as AA, Al-Anon, Narcotics Anonymous, etc.

Kishline, Audrey: *Moderate Drinking.* New York: Crown, 1995.

Marlatt, G. A. and Gordon, J. R. (Eds.): *Relapse Prevention.* New York: Guilford Press, 1985.

Peele, Stanton: *The Truth About Addiction and Recovery.* Fireside/Simon & Schuster, 1992.

Prochaska, James O.; Norcross, John C; and DiClemente, Carlo C.: *Changing for Good.* New York: William Morrow, 1994.

18. Chronic Pain

American Chronic Pain Association, PO Box 850, Rocklin, CA 95677, Tel. (916-632-0922), Fax (916-632-3208).

Catalano, Ellen Mohr: *The Chronic Pain Control Workbook.* Oakland, CA: New Harbinger Publications, 1987.

Caudill, Margaret: *Managing Pain Before It Manages You.* New York: Guilford Press, 1995.

Kabat-Zinn, Jon: *Full Catastrophe Living: Using the Wisdom of Your Body and Mind to Face Stress, Pain, and Illness.* New York: Delacorte Press, 1990. *A clinically tested program using "mindfulness" meditation practices.*

National Chronic Pain Outreach Association, 7979 Old Georgetown Rd., Suite 100, Bethesda, MD 20814 (301-652-4948).

Sternbach, Richard A.: *Mastering Pain.* New York: Ballantine Books, 1987.

Turk, Dennis and Nash, Justin: "Chronic Pain: New Ways to Cope" in *Mind/Body Medicine,* edited by Daniel Goleman and Joel Gurin. New York: Consumer Reports Books, 1993.

19. Chronic Illness

Choices in Dying, 200 Varick Street, New York, NY 10014: *Specific information about Durable Power of Attorney for Health Care and state laws for managing the legal aspects of death.*

Dollinger, Malin; Rosenbaum, Ernest H.; and Cable, Greg: *Everyone's Guide to Cancer Therapy: How Cancer is Diagnosed, Treated, and Managed Day to Day.* Kansas City, MO: Andrews and McMeel, 1991.

Franz, Marion; Etzwiler, Donnell; Ostron-Joynes, Judy; and Hollander, Priscilla: *Learning to Live Well with Diabetes.* Minneapolis, MN: DCI/ChroniMed Publishing, 1991.

Jevne, Ronna Fay and Levitan, Alexander: *No Time for Nonsense: Getting Well Against the Odds.* San Diego, CA: LuraMedia, 1989. *A guide to coping with serious chronic illness.*

Kane, Jeff: *Be Sick Well: A Healthy Approach to Chronic Illness.* Oakland, CA: New Harbinger, 1991.

Klein, Robert A. and Landau, Marcia Goodman: *Healing the Body Betrayed: A Self-Paced Self-Help Guide to Regaining Psychological Control of Your Chronic Illness.* Minneapolis, MN: DCI/ChroniMed Publishing, 1992.

Lerner, Michael: *Choices in Healing: Integrating the Best of Conventional and Complementary Approaches to Cancer.* Cambridge, MA: MIT Press, 1994. *Includes level-headed discussion of unconventional and alternative cancer therapies.*

Lorig, Kate and Fries, James: *The Arthritis Helpbook.* Reading, MA: Addison Wesley, 1990.

Lorig, Kate; Holman, Halsted; Sobel, David; Laurent, Diana; Gonzalez, Virginia; and Minor, Marian: *Living a Healthy Life with Chronic Conditions: Self-Management of Heart Disease, Arthritis, Stroke, Diabetes, Asthma, Bronchitis, Emphysema & Others.* Palo Alto, CA: Bull Publishing Co., 1994.

Maurer, Janet R. and Strasberg, Patricia D.: *Building a New Dream: A Family Guide to Coping with Chronic Illness and Disability.* Reading, MA: Addison-Wesley, 1989.

McKay, Judith and Hirano, Nancee: *The Chemotherapy Survival Guide.* Oakland, CA: New Harbinger, 1993.

Pitzele, Sefra Kobrin: *We Are Not Alone: Learning to Live with Chronic Illness.* New York: Workman Publishing, 1986. *Practical, firsthand advice on how to cope with chronic conditions.*

Spiegel, David: *Living Beyond Limits: New Hope and Help for Facing Life-Threatening Illness.* New York: Ballentine/Fawcett, 1994.. *Guide to confronting the emotional challenges of cancer and other life-threatening conditions.*

20. Doctor-Patient Partnership

Barksy, A.J.: *Worried Sick: Our Troubled Quest for Wellness.* Boston: Little Brown, 1988. *Describes the personal and cultural pressures towards expressing psychological distress in physical symptoms (somatization).*

Clayman, Charles B. (Editor): *The American Medical Association Family Medical Guide.* New York: Random House, 1994.

Ferguson, Tom: "Working with Your Doctor" in Goleman, D. and Gurin, J. (editors): *Mind/Body Medicine*. New York: Consumer Union Report Books, 1993.

Freed, Melvyn N. and Graves, Karen J.: *The Patient's Desk Reference: Where to Find Answers to Medical Questions*. New York: Macmillian, 1994. *Listing of print, computer database, health organizations, and government offices.*

Fries, James F.: *Aging Well: The Life Plan for Health and Vitality in Your Later Years*. Reading, MA: Addison-Wesley, 1989.

Griffith, H. Winter: *Complete Guide to Symptoms, Illness, and Surgery*. New York: Putnam, 1989.

Home Medical Advisor Pro, Version 4.0. Merrit Island, Florida: Pixel Perfect, 1994. *CD-ROM health encyclopedia.*

Health Publishing Group: *Dr. Koop's Self-Care Advisor: The Essential Home Health Guide for You and Your Family*. New York: Patient Education Media, Inc., 1996.

Inlander, Charles: *150 Ways to Be a Savvy Medical Consumer*. Allentown, PA: The People's Medical Society, 1992.

Kemper, Donald W.; McIntosh, Kathleen E.; and Roberts, Toni M.: *Healthwise Handbook: A Self-Care Manual for You*. Boise, Idaho: Healthwise (P.O. Box 1989, Boise, ID 83701), 1994.

Kemper, Donald W.; Mettler, Molly; and Alves, Frances: *It's About Time: Better Health Care in a Minute (or Two)*. Boise, Idaho: Healthwise, Inc., 1993.

Larson, David E. (Editor): *Mayo Clinic Family Health Book*. New York: William Morrow, 1990.

Medical HouseCall, Salt Lake City, UT: Applied Medical Infomatics, 1995. *CD-ROM interactive home medical guide and symptom analysis.*

Mettler, Molly and Kemper, Donald: *Healthwise for Life: Medical Self-Care for Healthy Aging*. Boise, ID: Healthwise, Inc., 1992.

Stutz, David R. and Feder, Bernard: *The Savvy Patient: How To Be An Active Participant in Your Medical Care*. Yonkers, NY: Consumer Reports Books, 1990.

Vickery, Donald and Fries, James: *Take Care of Yourself: The Complete Guide to Medical Self-Care*. Reading, MA: Addison-Wesley, 1996.

21. Medical Tests

Guide to Clinical Preventive Services: Report of the US Preventive Services Task Force. Second Edition. Baltimore: Williams and Wilkins, 1996.

Illustrated Guide to Medical Tests. Springhouse, PA: Springhouse Corp., 1993.

Pickney, Cathey and Pickney, Edward R.: *The Patient's Guide to Medical Tests*. New York: Facts on File, 1986.

Sobel, David S. and Ferguson, Tom: *The People's Book of Medical Tests*. New York: Summit Books, 1985.

22. Medications

Consumer Reports Books. *The Complete Drug Reference*. Yonkers, NY: Consumers Union, 1995.

Griffth, H. Winter: *Complete Guide to Prescription & Nonprescription Drugs*. New York: The Body Press/Perigee Books, 1995.

Long, James W. and Rybacki, J.J.: *The Essential Guide to Prescription Drugs*. New York: HarperCollins, 1995.

PDR Family Guide to Prescription Drugs. Montvale, NJ: Medical Economics Data, 1994.

Silverman, Harold M.: *The Pill Book*. New York: Bantam, 1994.

23. Surgery

Acute Pain Management Guideline Panel: *Pain Control After Surgery: A Patient's Guide*. Rockville, MD: Agency for Health Care Policy and Research. Public Health Service, U.S. Department of Health and Human Services, Feb. 1992 (Publication No. AHCPR 92-0021) 1-800-358-9295, AHCPR Publications Clearinghouse, P.O. Box 8547, Silver Spring, MD 20907.

Bennett, Henry L. and Disbrow, Elizabeth A.: "Preparing For Surgery And Other Medical Procedures," in *Mind/Body Medicine*, edited by Daniel Goleman and Joel Gurin, New York: Consumer Reports Books, 1993.

Bradley, Edward L.: *A Patient's Guide to Surgery*. New York: Consumer Reports Books, 1994.

Deardorf, William W. and Reeves, John L.: *Preparing for Surgery: A Mind-Body Approach to Enhance Healing and Recovery*. Oakland, CA: New Harbinger, 1997.

Huddleston, Peggy: *Prepare for Surgery, Heal Faster: A Guide of Mind-Body Techniques*. Cambridge, MA: Angel River Press, 1996.

Huddleston, Peggy: *Prepare for Surgery, Heal Faster: Relaxation/Healing Audio Tape*. Angel River Press, Box 1038, Cambridge, MA 02140-0009 (617-497-9431).

Inlander, Charles B.: *Good Operations, Bad Operations*. New York: Penguin Books, 1993.

Lewis, John: *So Your Doctor Recommended Surgery*. New York: Henry Holt, 1990.

Macho, James and Cable, Greg: *Everyone's Guide to Outpatient Surgery*. Kansas City, Missouri: Somerville House Books, 1994.

Naparstek, Belleruth. *Health Journeys: Surgery Audio Cassette*. Image Paths, Inc., Box 5714, Cleveland, OH 44114-0714 (1-800-800-8661).

Patient Comfort, Inc., 141618 Tyler Foote Rd., Nevada City, CA 95959 (1-800-213-3223). *Provides a selection of audiotapes and materials for surgical preparation including tapes by Henry Bennett, Ph.D.*

Rodgers, Linda. *P.I.P.: Surgical Audiotape Series*, 70 Maple Avenue, Katonah, NY 10536 (914-232-6405).

Youngson, Robert M.: *The Surgery Book: An Illustrated Guide to 73 of the Most Common Operations*. New York: St. Martin's Press, 1993.

Index

Numbers in **boldface** indicate the pages where you can find the most information on the subject.

A

Abstinence 30
Addiction 21-31, **209-214**
Affirmations 26, 47, 89, 97, 103
Aggression 127, 137, 168
AIDS 71, 87, 107, 269
Alcohol 146, 157, 195
Alcoholism 24, 27, **209-214**
Altruism *See Helping*
Anesthesia 269
Anger 11, 16, 25, 46, 54-55, 135, **167-178,**
    203, 219, 226, 229
    Anger Log 172-173
    deflecting others' anger 176
    in a relationship 174
    Test Your Hostility 170
Antibodies *See Immune system*
Antidepressants 158
Anxiety 14, 24, 46, 58, 84, 98, 101, **143-154,**
    226, 264
    and exercise 112, 147
    and helping others 135, 154
    and humor 55
    and medications 146
    and mood 112
    and social skills 153
    and use of imagery 98
    relaxation-induced 85
    See also Stress, Panic, and Fear
Apology 132 *See also Communication*
Aromatherapy 68-70
Arthritis 11, 14, 135-137, 225, 227
Assertiveness **126-128**, 165, 174
Asthma 87, 98, 106-107, 137, 144
Autogenic Training 97, **102**

B

Bibliotherapy 13
Bleeding 98, 263
Blood pressure *See Hypertension*
Boredom 29, 62, 157
Breathing **89-91**, 153, 174, 193, 220
    belly breathing 90
    with imagery 91
    to calm panic 153
    to defuse anger 174
    See also Sleep Apnea
Burnout 140

C

Cancer 11, 15, 40, 87, 106, 111, 135-136,
    193, 227, 239
Change **17-34**
    and imagery 107
    barriers to 25
    breakthrough 18
    excuses 22
    options 23
    pleasurable 18
    readiness for 19, 21
    step-by-step 19
Chemotherapy 87
Childbirth 15, 84, 98
Cholesterol 14, 66, 111, 124, 156, 226
Chronic illness 16, 20, 84, 137, **225-234,**
    247
    and helping 135
    and music 64
Commitment 26-27
Communication **121-132**, **164-165**, 174,
    239, 243
    and doctor-patient communication
        238-244, 254-256

Communication continued
    and hypnosis 101
    and sex 76
    body language 125
    listening 122-125
    See also Assertiveness, Passiveness,
    Aggression, and Criticism
Conflict 130
Contract with yourself 26
Control 20, 30, 40-41, 48, 202, 217
Costs, medical 11, 15, 232
Coping 16, 31-34, 46, 131, 160, 260
Coronary artery disease *See Heart disease*
Cravings 29
Crisis 18, 27 *See also Trauma*
Criticism 131, 132
Crying 56

D

Denial 204-205
Decisions, medical 242-243
Depression 11, 14, 135, 136, **155-165**, 192,
    204, 229
    and bad moods 155, 158
    and imagery 107
    and touch 60
    causes 157
    manic depression 157
    treatment options 158-159
Desensitization 151
Diabetes 11, 14, 85, 106, 111, 238
Digestion 81, 262
    and relaxation 87
    and communication 124
    and sleep 192
Distraction techniques 148-150, 162, 175,
    221
Disease
    See AIDS, Arthritis, Asthma, Heart
    Disease, Cancer, Diabetes, Hypertension,
    Lung Disease, and Chronic Illness
Doctor-patient partnership 235-244
Drug abuse *See Addiction*
Durable power of attorney 234

E

Empathy 177
Endorphins 66, 218
Exercise 24-27, **109-120**
    and anger 174
    and anxiety 112, 147
    and depression 161-162
    and mood 113
    and pain 222-223
    and sex 79
    and sleep 195
    benefits 111
    excuses 115-116
    motivation 118

F

Faith 39 *See also Religion*
Fear *See Anxiety*
Fight or flight response *See Stress*
Food 65-68, 195
Forgiveness 177

G

Grief 46, 201-208
    The Grieving Process 204
    Myths about loss and grief 204-5
Guided imagery *See Imagery*

H

Healing injuries 106
Heart disease 11, 15, 74, 82, 84, 86, 98, 106,
    111, 123, 137, 144, 156, 168, 193, 202
    and anxiety 144
    and bereavement 202
    and depression 156
    and helping 137
    and hostility 168
    and physical activity 111
Helping **133-142**, 165, 177
Hostility *See Anger*
Humor 16, **49-56**
    and anxiety 55
    and anger 174-5
    and immunity 50
    and pain 50

Humor continued
  and stress 50
  benefits 51
  unhealthy 55
Hypertension 62, 66, 111, 123, 144
  and anxiety 144
  and communication 123, 238
  and exercise 111
  and relaxation 84, 86
Hypnosis 87, 100-101

I

Imagery 26, 84, 87, 91, **97-108,** 190, 253
  See also Affirmations, Autogenic Training,
  Hypnosis, and Visualization
Immune system 11, 14, 16, 82, 84, 87, 107,
  263
  and communication 123-124
  and depression 156
  and imagery 98, 107
  and laughter 50, 58
  and music 64
  and optimism 36, 40
  and relaxation 82, 84, 87
  and sleep 193
  and touch 60
  and trauma 202
Infection 107, 135
Infertility 86-87
Insomnia 11, 86, 191, 202 *See also Sleep*

J, K, L

Laughter *See Humor*
Listening **122-125,** 176
Loneliness 29, 157
Longevity 36, 40
Lung disease 87, 98, 106 *See also Asthma*

M

Mania *See Depression*
Massage 14, 59, 60, 220
Medical decisions 242-243, 246-247
Medical jargon 238-239
Medical tests 245-250
  normal values 250

false negatives 250
preventive screening 246-248
risks 248-249
Medication 12, 85, 146, 158, 194, 218-219,
  247, **251-258,** 267
  Medication Calendar 255
Meditation 84, 87, 96 *See also Mindfulness*
Mindfulness 48, 82, 87, **94-95,** 184-185,
  222
Money 140-141
Mood 11, 16, 155, 158-159, 161-162
  and exercise 113
  and helping 135
  and music 65
  and sex 72
Muscle tension 82, 92-93, 106
Music 15, 63-65, 264

N

Narcotics 219
Negative feelings 46, 218-219, 229-230, 264
Negative thinking 35-38, 42-46, 163, 189, 219
Nervous system 59
  autonomic 261
  sympathetic 81, 168
Nursing home 15, 64, 138

O

Optimism 16, **35-48**, 138, 226 *See also*
Pessimism
Osteoporosis 111, 115, 156, 227
Overeating 31 *See also Food*

P

Pain 11, 36, **215-223**
  and distraction 221
  and exercise 222
  and imagery 107
  and laughter 50
  and music 64
  and relaxation 84, 86, 220
  and sex 74
  and surgery 265-266
  Pain Diary 216
Panic 98, 145, **152-153**
Passiveness 127

Pessimism 16, **35-48**, 157, 163-165, 226
  See also Optimism
Pets 141
Phobias 145, 151
Phototherapy 162-163, 198
Physical activity **109-120** *See Exercise*
Placebo effect 251-252
Pleasure 18, **57-70**, 161, 221
Positive thinking 164-165, 264-265 *See also Optimism*
Post Traumatic Stress Disorder 203
Prescriptions 12 *See Medications*
Problem solving 31-34
Procrastination 188-190
Professional help 3, 13, 158, 178, 199, 233
  Working with Health Professionals See Doctor-Patient Partnership

Q-R

Relaxation 16, 58, 61-62, **81-96**, 99-102, 104-105, 108, 147, 220
Relapses 29-30
Religion 14, 39, 208 *See also Spiritual Beliefs*

S

Saunas 60, 195
Seasonal affective disorder 162-163
Second opinion 243, 268
Self-talk 17, 42-45, 89, 100-108, 118, 131, 149, 151, 189-190, 230, 262-3
Sensate focusing 78
Senses **57-70**
  sight 61-62
  smell 69-70
  sound 63-65
  taste 65-68
  touch 59-60
Sex **71-79**
  and physical health 72, 74
  and mental health 72, 75
  monotony 75-76
  misconceptions 72, 73
  shyness 153-154
Side effects 12, 56, 258

Simplicity 184
Skin conditions 84, 87, 98
Sleep 14, 64, 84, 98, **191-200**
  and exercise 195
  sleep apnea 193
Smoking 14, 20, 23-24, 27, 29-30, 101, 136, 195, 209-214, 267
Social support 27, 117, 136, 142, 206, 208, 231
  See also Helping
Somatization 232-233
Spiritual beliefs 14, 39, 208
Stages of change *See Change*
Stress 11, 14, 16, 31-34, 50, 58, 62, 81-83, 106, 112-113, 144, 168, 180-182
Surgery 11, 15, 36, 41, 64, 84, 87, 98, **259-270**

T

Taste 65-68, 95
Tension 91, 98, 106, 181 *See also Stress*
Thinking **35-48**, 163-164, 171-174, 189, 219-220
Time
  pressure 16, **179-190**
  priorities 184
  management 16, 179-190
  Time Log 185-6
Touch 59-60, 124
Trauma 16, **201-208**

U

Unexplained symptoms 15, 233

V

Visualization 84, 104-105
Volunteering *See Helping*

W

Weight 111
Worry 44, 84, **150**, 196 *See also Anxiety*
Writing 178, 207, 230

X Y Z

Yoga 120